SUPPORTING CHILDREN'S SPEECH, LANGUAGE AND COMMUNICATION NEEDS

This book is the definitive text on understanding and supporting children's speech, language and communication needs (SLCN). Written by experts, it presents evidence-based approaches in a highly accessible format. Wide-ranging in scope, *Supporting Children's Speech, Language and Communication Needs*

- covers best practice for many groups of children, including those with speech sound disorders, Developmental Language Disorder (DLD) and neurodevelopmental differences
- discusses specialist populations, including acquired brain injury and cleft lip and palate, as well as childhood onset eating, drinking and swallowing difficulties
- features chapters on inclusive communication environments, Alternative and Augmentative Communication (AAC), communication partners, the whole systems approach and evidencing impact, exploring cross-cutting themes.

Case studies are included throughout to bring learning to life, and recommended online sources of further information are included. Comprehensive, authoritative and up to date, this book will prove indispensable for students and practitioners in speech and language therapy.

Susan McCool is a Principal Teaching Fellow in speech and language therapy at the University of Strathclyde, Glasgow, UK. She is the author of *Working with Child and Adolescent Mental Health: The Central Role of Language and Communication*.

SUPPORTING CHILDREN'S SPEECH, LANGUAGE AND COMMUNICATION NEEDS

Edited by Susan McCool

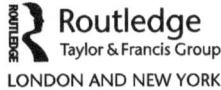

Designed cover image: Getty Images

First published 2026
by Routledge
4 Park Square, Milton Park, Abingdon, Oxon OX14 4RN

and by Routledge
605 Third Avenue, New York, NY 10158

Routledge is an imprint of the Taylor & Francis Group, an informa business

© 2026 selection and editorial matter, Susan McCool; individual chapters, the contributors

The right of Susan McCool to be identified as the author of the editorial material, and of the authors for their individual chapters, has been asserted in accordance with sections 77 and 78 of the Copyright, Designs and Patents Act 1988.

All rights reserved. No part of this book may be reprinted or reproduced or utilised in any form or by any electronic, mechanical, or other means, now known or hereafter invented, including photocopying and recording, or in any information storage or retrieval system, without permission in writing from the publishers.

Trademark notice: Product or corporate names may be trademarks or registered trademarks, and are used only for identification and explanation without intent to infringe.

British Library Cataloguing-in-Publication Data
A catalogue record for this book is available from the British Library

ISBN: 978-1-041-13816-7 (hbk)
ISBN: 978-1-041-13810-5 (pbk)
ISBN: 978-1-003-67162-6 (ebk)

DOI: 10.4324/9781003671626

Typeset in Interstate
by Apex CoVantage, LLC

In memory of Judy Halden, whose significant contribution to speech and language therapy will long be remembered and valued.

CONTENTS

List of contributors — ix

Introduction — 1
Susan McCool

Part I   Understanding and supporting children's speech, language and communication needs — 3

1   **Understanding and supporting children's speech, language and communication needs** — 5
    Susan McCool

2   **A 'whole system' approach to meeting speech, language and communication needs** — 18
    Marie Gascoigne

3   **Inclusive communication** — 35
    Kim Hartley Kean

4   **Augmentative and Alternative Communication (AAC)** — 53
    Janice Murray

5   **Communication partners** — 62
    Hayley Moroke

6   **So what? And prove it!: Evidencing impact** — 74
    Marie Gascoigne

Part II   Speech — 87

7   **Speech Sound Disorders (SSDs)** — 89
    Joanne Cleland and Helen Stringer

8   **Voice** — 101
    Wendy Cohen

Part III Language   115

9 Promoting early language development   117
Sheena Reilly and Cristina McKean

10 Developmental Language Disorder (DLD)   136
Courtenay Norbury and Susan Ebbels

Part IV Communication   151

11 Severe and profound learning disabilities: a school-based approach   153
Rachel Sawford and Ann Miles

12 Stammering   169
Ben Bolton-Grant

13 Neurodivergent children: a neuro-affirming lens on autism, ADHD and beyond   186
Lynne Bremner and Marion Rutherford

14 Social, emotional and mental health needs: trauma-informed and anxiety-aware care   208
Susan McCool

Part V Selected populations with specialist needs   223

15 Deaf children   225
Sarah Beazley and Judy Halden

16 Cleft lip and palate   241
Stephanie van Eeden and Julie Davies

17 Acquired Brain Injury (ABI)   257
Katherine Buckeridge, Helen Cullimore, Lucy Cuthbertson and Rhiannon Halfpenny

18 Childhood onset eating, drinking and swallowing difficulties   277
Diane Sellers, Ailish Harrison, Sally Morgan and Mari Viviers

Index   303

CONTRIBUTORS

Sarah Beazley is a specialist speech and language therapist who has worked with deaf people since 1983 and as a lecturer on a range of university courses. Sarah has worked professionally in West Asia and is an Executive Editor for the international journal *Disability & Society*. She continues to train practitioners in their work with deaf children. Her publications include *Working with Deaf Children and Young People: A Guide for Practitioners* (with J. Halden, Routledge, 2025).

Ben Bolton-Grant is a speech and language therapist, lecturer and Course Director at Leeds Beckett University, where he trains speech and language therapy students with a particular focus on stammering and professional practice. Ben's clinical experience spans both the NHS and independent practice. Currently, he is a Director of Talking Out Ltd, supporting teenagers who stammer and their families through online and residential group therapy. Ben is committed to fostering acceptance and empowerment for those who stammer. His work bridges clinical expertise and academia, ensuring the next generation of therapists is equipped to deliver inclusive, client-centred care.

Lynne Bremner is a speech and language therapist with over 20 years of experience working with neurodivergent children and young people, with a focus on the diagnostic process. As an educator, she leads the undergraduate speech and language therapy programmes at Queen Margaret University, Musselburgh, where her teaching and research focus on neurodivergence. Lynne is committed to creating an inclusive learning environment, to foster belonging for neurodivergent students. In her role with the National Autism Implementation Team, she contributes to advancing understanding and driving systemic changes in health, education, and employment to ensure neurodivergent individuals can participate fully and thrive.

Katherine Buckeridge worked in the NHS for 20 years, specialising in helping children and young people with neurodisability. She became fascinated by acquired brain injury during her time working on a paediatric rehabilitation unit and supporting children with their return to school. In 2016, Katherine completed a Clinical Research Masters. Her research explored adolescents' experiences of communication following acquired brain injury. Her PhD study aims to develop an instrument to measure communication outcomes for non-speaking children with neurodisability. Katherine now works as an independent SLT in the Southeast of England and provides supervision to other specialist therapists.

Joanne Cleland is Professor of Speech and Language Therapy at the University of Strathclyde, Glasgow, UK. Her research and teaching focus on assessment and diagnosis of childhood speech sound disorders and innovative approaches to intervention for articulatory and motor speech sound disorders. She has expertise in articulatory instrumentation, such as ultrasound tongue imaging, for both theoretical research and for biofeedback interventions.

Wendy Cohen qualified as a speech and language therapist in 1993. After working in a variety of NHS settings and academic settings with adults and children with a range of speech, language and communication needs, Wendy joined the University of Strathclyde in 2005. Since 2009, Wendy has worked closely with colleagues from the Ear Nose and Throat department at the Royal Hospital for Children, Glasgow, helping set up their dedicated paediatric voice clinic. Wendy's research focuses on assessment and interventions for children with voice disorder alongside teaching undergraduate SLT students at the University of Strathclyde.

Helen Cullimore qualified with a Joint Honours BSC in Speech and Psychology at the University of Newcastle-upon-Tyne in 1996. Helen's first SLT roles were in community paediatrics and Special Schools. Helen found her passion for acquired brain injury in 1999 when she started working at Frenchay Hospital, with adults and children. Following the centralisation of children's services and closure of Frenchay Hospital in 2004, Helen transferred to Bristol Children's Hospital, where she is the Lead SLT for neurorehabilitation and works with children and young people with acquired brain injury from admission to outpatient care.

Lucy Cuthbertson has had a rewarding career as a speech and language therapist. Through her work in acute paediatric and neonatal services, for over 30 years, she has gained extensive experience of neurology. Lucy has supported brain-injured children from their hospital admission, following neurosurgery, during neurorehabilitation and reintegration into school. She was a founder member of the speech and language therapists' interest group in paediatric acquired brain injury (RCSLT's ABICA CEN) and is contributing to the development of the next generation of therapists through her roles in higher education. Lucy works independently and in the NHS across the South of England.

Julie Davies is a highly experienced speech and language therapist, specialising in cleft care since 1997 within the Northwest, North Wales, and Isle of Man Cleft Network, based at the Royal Manchester Children's Hospital. Julie has presented and published work nationally and internationally, showcasing her expertise. She is currently pursuing a Professional Doctorate in Health Psychology, with a focus on qualitative research – including photovoice and participatory action research – behaviour change, and empowering young people with cleft to feel more confident about their appearance. Julie is dedicated to advancing her field and supporting her patients with a compassionate, evidence-based approach.

Susan Ebbels is a speech and language therapist and Director of Moor House Research and Training Institute at Moor House School & College, Surrey, UK, a special school for children with Developmental Language Disorder (DLD) aged 7-19. She is on the editorial boards of *International Journal of Language and Communication Disorders* and *Child Language Teaching and Therapy*. She has an honorary lectureship at UCL and is also a specialist advisor for Royal College of Speech and Language Therapists. She has carried out and coordinated many intervention studies, with a particular focus on improving the comprehension and production of grammar in children with language disorders using her SHAPE CODING™ system. She delivers regular courses both on the SHAPE CODING™ system and on the current evidence base for school-aged children with DLD.

Marie Gascoigne is a speech and language therapist who has worked as a practitioner in mainstream schools as a specialist in DLD, an academic and researcher, a lead for AHPs in a London Trust and, for the past 18 years, as an advisor and consultant. Marie's interest in systems to support children and young people began after completing an MBA which led to the creation of the Balanced System® as a whole system outcome-based approach for meeting needs within integrated services. Marie has a longstanding interest in influencing policy and served as a Trustee of the Royal College of Speech and Language Therapists, chairing the then Policy and Partnership Board. Marie is currently Director of Better Communication CIC, the not-for-profit organisation she founded in 2011.

Judy Halden was dual qualified as an SLT and a teacher for deaf children. She worked with deaf people from 1978, setting up and running specialist speech and language services for deaf children and for both deaf and deafened adults. She was an adviser, lecturer, and supervisor on the Hertfordshire University course for teachers of deaf children, as well as an honorary research associate and lecturer at University College London's Department of Psychology and Language Sciences. Judy's publications in the field of deafness include *Working with Deaf Children and Young People: A Guide for Practitioners* (with S. Beazley, Routledge, 2025).

Rhiannon Halfpenny is a speech and language therapist who specialises in supporting children with acquired brain injuries in acute and early rehabilitation settings. She completed an NIHR-funded Pre-Doctoral Clinical Academic Fellowship focused on dysphagia rehabilitation in children after brain injury, an endeavour sparked by her frustration at the lack of child-specific research in this area. She has worked in both community and acute settings, including Northwick Park and Great Ormond Street Hospital. Currently, Rhiannon is a Clinical Specialist for Acute Paediatrics at Nottingham Children's Hospital.

Ailish Harrison has special interests in neonatal feeding difficulties and children and young people with feeding aversion and restricted diets. Ailish is an active member of the research community with past projects focusing on service provision for children with ARFID in the UK, and her current projects include therapeutic interventions for premature babies with feeding aversion. She is currently a Senior Specialist speech and language therapist in the Feeding Team at Sheffield Children's Hospital

Kim Hartley Kean is a speech and language therapist. She has dedicated much of her career to a vision of communication equity through universal implementation of inclusive communication good practice. She has worked as a clinician with children and adults; designed and led many inclusive communication national and local projects; acted as an inclusive communication expert adviser to national and local government and played a key role in securing investment, policy and the first UK law to mention inclusive communication. She is currently a founding Director of Communication Inclusion People CIC.

Susan McCool is a speech and language therapist whose career has combined clinical practice, university education, supervision and mentoring, consulting and advising, research and writing. Susan has extensive experience supporting children who have complex profiles, taking account of relational and contextual considerations. Her teaching and writing focus on communication support in contexts involving neurodevelopmental differences and social, emotional and mental health. She has a special interest in resilience. She is currently a Principal Teaching Fellow at the University of Strathclyde, Glasgow.

Cristina McKean is Professor of Child Language Development & Disorders at the University of Oxford's Department of Education. A former speech and language therapist, she previously held academic positions at Newcastle University, UK, and the Murdoch Children's Research Institute in Australia, where she retains honorary positions. A Fellow of the Royal College of Speech and Language Therapists and former Editor-in-Chief of the *International Journal of Language and Communication Disorders*, she leads interdisciplinary and international research on child language development. Her work informs theory, policy, and practice, focusing on language trajectories, early risk identification, intervention development, and equitable service provision.

Ann Miles is a special education teacher who spent her career working in schools for children with learning disabilities. Drawing upon her classroom experience and extensive knowledge of early communication, she has packaged up all the elements of Communication at the Heart of the School (CATHS) to share with other professionals. Ann is a firm believer that, for communication to be successful, it needs to be both natural and meaningful. The development of communication skills should be embedded within all aspects of teaching and the curriculum.

Sally Morgan is a speech and language therapist with expertise in working with children and young people with complex learning and healthcare needs across various London boroughs. She is a Senior Lecturer and Clinical Research Fellow at City St George's, University of London, through a Barts Charity Allied Health Professionals Clinical Doctoral Fellowship.

Her research project is exploring how speech and language therapists and family carers can work together to improve the Safety, Efficiency and Enjoyment of Mealtimes for children with neurodisability and dysphagia (not as simple as it may SEEM).

Hayley Moroke is a speech and language therapist currently working within an NHS service in Scotland, where she has experience supporting and implementing Inclusive communication environments in educational establishments. She also works closely with families to help support their child or young person's SLCN. Hayley also has her own consultancy where she supports implementation of accessible information and delivers training on SLCN, usually with a focus on neurodevelopmental differences. She comes with a unique understanding of SLCN, bringing her professional and parental experience of communication differences together to best support families and young people.

Janice Murray is Professor Emeritus at Manchester Metropolitan University, and a Fellow of Royal College of Speech & Language Therapists (RCSLT). She was the lead author for the RCSLT guidance on augmentative and alternative communication (AAC) (2024). Janice has previously managed speech and language therapy undergraduate and postgraduate education programmes. She has chaired Communication Matters, the AAC Committee for the International Association of Communication Sciences and Disorders (IALP), and the Council for the International Society for Augmentative and Alternative Communication (ISAAC). She has been awarded over 40 grants and published widely on clinical decision-making and aided language acquisition.

Courtenay Norbury is Professor of Developmental Disorders of Language and Communication at Psychology and Language Sciences, University College London and the Vice Dean Research for the Faculty of Brain Sciences. She is the co-director of the Well-being and Language Lab at UCL and is a Fellow of the Royal College of Speech and Language Therapists. She obtained her PhD in Experimental Psychology at the University of Oxford, working with Professor Dorothy Bishop on the overlapping language profiles that characterise autism and developmental language disorder. Professor Norbury's current research focuses on language disorders and how language interacts with other aspects of social and cognitive development. She leads SCALES, a population study of language development and disorder from school entry. She is also a founding member of the RADLD campaign (https://radld.org/).

Sheena Reilly is Professor Emeritus at Griffith University, Australia. Over the course of her career, she has led multidisciplinary research teams responsible for a series of landmark studies that have transformed our current day understanding of the epidemiological and natural history of common and debilitating childhood speech and language problems. In 2020, Sheena was made a Member of the Order of Australia in the Queen's Birthday Honours, for significant service to tertiary education, medical research, and paediatric speech pathology. She is an inaugural Fellow of the Australian Academy of Health and Medical Sciences and a Fellow of the Academy of Social Sciences Australia.

Marion Rutherford currently co-leads the National Autism Implementation Team (NAIT) and the Neuro-affirming Community of Practice in Scotland, based at Queen Margaret University, Musselburgh. She graduated in 1992 and has worked as a practitioner and research speech and language therapist since then. Her work has developed from a focus on understanding and supporting autistic children and their families to a broader focus on cross-sector support for neurodivergent people of all ages. Recent publications have focused on neurodevelopmental pathways for assessment and diagnosis, professional learning and practice change aligned to the neurodiversity paradigm.

Rachel Sawford is a speech and language therapist who works with schools to help children with a learning disability develop their communication skills. Rachel believes that speech and language therapists have the biggest impact when they give time to developing good quality environments where all children can benefit. She recognises that all those around the child have a role to play in supporting their communication. Rachel is currently working at the Chiltern School to implement the Communication at the Heart of the School approach (CATHS). She continues to support other therapists working with CATHS in a variety of other settings, including in mainstream and adults with learning disabilities.

Diane Sellers is a Senior Clinical Research Fellow and Advanced Clinical Practitioner speech and language therapist with more than 30 years' experience working with children and young people with neuro-disability. She has worked in specialist integrated multi-disciplinary teams at Chailey Clinical Services, to treat and manage children's difficulties in eating, drinking and swallowing and saliva control, as well as sensori-motor speech disturbances. Dr Sellers is the lead author of the Eating and Drinking Ability Classification System for people with cerebral palsy; work has been completed or is ongoing to translate EDACS into more than 36 languages. With over £1.7 million in research funding, she has led four original research projects and acted as co-investigator for five other research projects all with international impact.

Helen Stringer is a Professor of Childhood Speech Sound Disorders and Behaviour Change at Newcastle University, UK. She was lead author on the Royal College of Speech and Language Therapists' 2024 guidance for speech sound disorder and the position paper on childhood apraxia of speech. Behaviour change theory underpins her research into the effectiveness and implementation of speech and language therapy interventions.

Stephanie van Eeden is a speech and language therapist and lecturer in the School of Education, Communication, and Language Sciences at Newcastle University. Dr van Eeden's expertise lies in speech and language sciences, particularly related to cleft lip and palate. Working with the cleft lip and palate team in Newcastle-upon-Tyne, UK, since 2004, she has been a key contributor to improving communication outcomes for individuals with cleft lip and palate. Dr van Eeden completed her PhD in the language and listening skills of children with cleft lip and palate. She has published and presented widely on speech and language outcomes in cleft lip and palate and factors which impact development in this population.

Mari Viviers qualified as a speech and language therapist in 2003 (University of Pretoria, South Africa). She completed her doctorate in 2017 on infant feeding with a specific focus on neonatal dysphagia in premature and high-risk infants. She has worked in NICU and PICU for the past 22 years. Currently she is the Service Lead for Paediatric Speech and Language Therapy, St Mary's Hospital, Imperial College NHS Foundation Trust. London. She has presented nationally and internationally at various conferences and has published numerous peer-reviewed journal articles and book chapters.

Introduction

Susan McCool

Speech and language therapy (SLT) has the power to transform children's lives and futures. Since the developmental phase of life holds so much flexibility and promise for children, the right SLT support at the right time can have an extraordinary impact on children's current and future participation in living, learning and loving. It is no surprise, then, that many new avenues are opening up into this rewarding and fulfilling profession, attracting more learners and practitioners than ever before.

SLT practice is enormously varied, continually expanding across sectors and settings, populations and practices. Correspondingly, SLT students and practitioners face the challenge of extending their learning across an ever-wider range of topics. At the same time, while online information proliferates, it is harder than ever to access reliable learning material and evaluate its credibility. This book gathers the essential information for ethical and evidence-based practice in supporting children's speech, language and communication needs (SLCN). It offers short, clear chapters that are accessible for busy students and practitioners.

Many contributors to this book are highly esteemed international experts who publish widely in their topic. Many are experienced university educators who understand curriculum requirements and Standards of Proficiency in SLT. Others are skilled professionals, bringing valuable expertise and application. As Editor, I am truly indebted to them all. The book is so much richer for the blend of perspectives it has woven together.

Difficult decisions had to be made in determining the content and structure of this book. For instance, it was not possible to include every conceivable group that benefits from SLT involvement. Instead, Part I offers principles that readers can apply widely, and later chapters signpost additional resources where relevant.

Equally, terminology was carefully considered. With the emergence of the social justice movement and neurodiversity paradigm, seismic shifts are affecting how professionals think about and speak of the people they serve. This (r)evolution is more apparent in some branches of SLT practice than in others, and for good reason. Children are human beings first and foremost, with unique and developing personalities and potential. Nonetheless, many children's SLCN are associated with medical needs, or may become so in the future, so children rightly depend on practitioners being alert to that reality. The chapters in this book, therefore, reflect both linguistic and conceptual flux and growth.

The structure of the book

This book is divided into five Parts:

Part I introduces children's SLCN and covers cross-cutting themes, such as inclusive communication (and Augmentative and Alternative Communication) and SLT roles with communication partners. This first Part is bookended by chapters focusing on effective and efficient delivery of services and evidencing meaningful impact.

Part II focuses on speech, with chapters on speech sound disorders and voice.

Part III turns to language needs. It opens with a chapter on promoting early language development through a public health approach. This is followed by a chapter on Developmental Language Disorder.

Part IV's topic is communication needs, and chapters in this Part all highlight the crucial importance of children's communication environments. Varied topics include children with severe and profound learning disabilities and those described as having social, emotional and mental health needs. Chapters on stammering and neurodivergent children fully embrace the neurodiversity paradigm as applied to SLT practice.

Part V considers selected populations with special needs, including deaf children, those with cleft conditions and those who have acquired a brain injury during their development. This Part ends with a chapter on support needs in eating, drinking and swallowing. Many of the children covered in the preceding chapters will also have needs in this important and growing area of SLT practice, and its inclusion here allows appropriate consideration of complexity.

For ease of access, chapters follow a simple, common structure. Each opens with a list of key learning points readers can expect to gain, then goes on to outline key information in each topic and highlight important points about SLT practice in that area. Chapters then proceed with separate sections on understanding and supporting relevant aspects of children's SLCN. All chapters contain a case study or similar illustration of application, and all conclude with a useful summary to consolidate readers' learning.

This book is authoritative, comprehensive and up-to-date. Time-pressed SLT students and busy practitioners will appreciate the way it offers a wealth of evidence-based information in an accessible format. It is the definitive guide to understanding and supporting children's SLCN.

PART I

Understanding and supporting children's speech, language and communication needs

1 Understanding and supporting children's speech, language and communication needs

Susan McCool

What you'll learn in this chapter

- Key principles of child development: that it is holistic, cumulative and considered to be influenced by multiple determinants, both biological and social
- Needs-based and rights-based approaches rightly draw attention to the nature and intensity of supports that children need to thrive, moving away from outdated 'deficits-based' views
- Speech and language therapy typically resists the false dichotomy of medical versus social models; preferring instead biopsychosocial models as illustrated by the International Classification of Function, Disability and Health: Children and Youth version (ICF:CY)
- The meaning of key concepts: speech, language and communication; and models of communication, including Content/Form/Use and Means, Reasons & Opportunities
- Key tenets of supporting children's speech, language and communication needs (SLCN): public health, anti-discrimination, cultural inquisitiveness, strengths-based, collaboration and evidence-based practice
- The people and places around children with speech, language and communication needs (SLCN) can do most to support them
- Understanding and supporting children's SLCN are continual, inter-related processes.
- The AWEsome and EPIC approaches outline the steps in understanding and supporting children's SLCN.

Let's think about children and childhood

This book is about supporting children, so it is worth taking a moment to first understand what we mean when we talk about children. This book adopts the simple and effective definition that a child is any person under the age of 18 (UNICEF UK, 1989).

Being in the childhood period of life carries with it important developmental accomplishments, experiences, needs and rights. It is worthwhile, therefore, to understand essential features of this life stage. In this, we are guided by core principles of child development: that it is holistic and cumulative; that it is influenced by multiple determinants; that it typically occurs in a broadly predictable sequence and direction, yet there is tremendous individual variation (see Table 1.1).

- Children's development is *holistic*. Development in one area impacts, and is in turn affected by, change in other areas.
- Development is *cumulative*. Early development forms the basis of later change.
- Development has *multiple determinants*, both biological and social.
- Development (typically) occurs in a *predictable sequence and direction*.
- Development shows tremendous *individual variation*, reflecting the complex interplay of multiple determinants with unique child factors. The child is both shaped by, and in turn impacts upon, their context.

Table 1.1 Principles of child development
Source: adapted from Neaum (2022).

Childhood is a time of remarkable change. Development occurs simultaneously across an array of areas: physiological, neurological, motoric, sensorial, emotional, relational, social, linguistic, cognitive and moral. Importantly, these strands of development are highly interdependent; change in one area triggers change in related areas, in a process of developmental cascades. Therefore, it can be helpful to view these dimensions as forming a network or a web formation, rather than a linear model.

Later developing skills are built on the foundations of earlier acquired skills. This underscores the importance of ensuring time and support for consolidation of newly acquired skills. Typical development follows broadly predictable patterns in the order in which new skills are developed, although each child's unique biopsychosocial circumstances can impact the pace and/or pattern of development. Increasingly, it is noted that neurodevelopmental differences involve alternative developmental pathways.

Contemporary views consider that child development reflects a multi-faceted mix of both biological maturation and experiences shaped by each child's unique relational and social context. The milieu around the child operates at different levels, from relationships with close caregivers in the family, through community settings, to wider societal influences shaped by historical, cultural, political and economic influences.

Crucially, children are seen as active agents in their own lives, participating in reciprocal exchanges within their relational and social contexts. This means that their specific environment will both shape, and be influenced by, their own unfolding uniqueness. This dynamic process will continue throughout childhood and beyond.

A lifespan approach is increasingly advocated, noting that childhood experiences shape the developing human in fundamental ways, both physiological and psychological. Childhood influences are now known to exert powerful influences on the individual throughout life.

Support needs: what does this mean?

This book focuses on supporting children's needs, so we start this section by considering what support needs means in this context. Importantly, we contrast the contemporary concept of having support needs with now-outdated deficit-based notions. This leads us to critically examine models frequently used to guide thinking in this context. This chapter advocates for holistic and multidimensional conceptions of children's support needs, citing as an example the International Classification of Functioning, Disability and Health: Children and Youth version (ICF:CY, WHO, 2007).

Support needs versus 'having deficits'

All children need support to progress in their development, because childhood intrinsically involves dependence on others, to varying degrees. Some children need different or additional support so they can make the most of their lives and participate in ways that are meaningful and fulfilling.

Importantly, the concept of additional support needs places the onus on people and places around children to provide support; by reducing or removing barriers to children's participation. Within this framing, needs may arise from multiple sources, including differences in the child's biology, psychology or a myriad of social determinants.

In this view, entitlement to support is emphatically *not* reliant on the child surpassing arbitrary diagnostic thresholds or fulfilling a predetermined level of deficiencies (Moscardini, 2018). Instead, we consider the nature and intensity of support children need to enable them to thrive, based on all their unique circumstances at any given time. Rather than bowing down to the rigid requirements of bureaucracies within services, this approach is geared towards children, focused on families, and orientated around communities.

The profession of speech and language therapy (SLT) must participate in these conceptual debates and reflections, situated as it is at the nexus of both medically and socially focused milieu. For a discipline highly focused on language and communication, it is perhaps inevitable that its nomenclature comes under particularly sharp scrutiny. In that respect, the terms used within the profession are subject to ongoing critique, review and change. Differences of opinion exist while that process plays out, as can be seen in the linguistic variation across chapters in this book. Branches of children's SLT services traditionally aligned with medical services are more inclined towards terms such as 'disorders' whereas those more aligned with social and community perspectives are more likely to consciously adopt language such as 'differences' and 'support needs'.

When we focus on support requirements, attention shifts to how environments must change. We ask how the right support can empower the child and those around them to access experiences and resources, to harness strengths, and to move towards their own goals and priorities. When it is accepted that children are entitled to support, we see that they have every right to expect it. This is consistent with human rights-based approaches, as enshrined in the United Nations Convention on the Rights of the Child (UNICEF UK, 1989). This internationally sanctioned agreement sets out the fundamental rights of any child, irrespective of their needs, abilities or life situation. Here are the Articles that are most immediately impactful in the context of SLCN:

- Right to develop to their full potential
- Right to live a full life with dignity and, as far as possible, independence and to play an active part in the community

- Right to a standard of living that is good enough to meet their physical and social needs and support their development
- Right to relax, play and take part in a wide range of cultural and artistic activities
- Right to meet with other children and join groups
- Right to an education that develops their personality, talents and abilities to the full
- Right to express their views, feelings and wishes in all matters affecting them, and to have their views considered and taken seriously
- Right to express their thoughts and opinions and to access all kinds of information
- Right for respect for the child's evolving capacity to make their own choices.

Medical, social and multi-dimensional models

The medical model was dominant within service provision for decades, and it formed the ground in which the roots of the speech and language therapy profession grew. This approach involves identifying, within an individual, patterns of difference or disruption that are associated with processes of disease or disorder.

The medical model has faced strong criticism for veering towards a deficit-based approach, which pejoratively locates 'difficulties' within individuals (Knight et al., 2023). Such deficit-based framing is increasingly acknowledged to problematise children, while simultaneously absolving systems and society of their responsibilities. Indeed, deficit-based narratives are increasingly considered ableist, in that they perpetuate a focus on fixing presumed wrongs and aiming at supposedly normal function. Such positions are therefore rightly subject to increasing challenge within speech and language therapy (DeThorne and Gerlach-Houck, 2022). Much current thinking would have us embrace the social model instead. This places responsibility for disablement squarely on society. It helpfully focuses attention on dismantling societal barriers to access, activity and inclusion.

It can be argued, however, that people's lives are so unique and multifactorial that a rounded understanding is not well served by any one-sided view. Medical aspects are a formative component in many children's lives, and to exclude them from consideration limits our understanding of their impact. An appreciation of medical consequences, for example, can help us consider possibilities such as trauma arising from essential but invasive medical care; or disruptions to early child-caregiver attachment resulting from required medical interventions (Yehuda, 2016). We can consider the impact on a child's developing sense of self from ongoing exposure to the pain, discomfort, fear and lack of privacy that can accompany many developmental conditions in childhood and beyond. Further, understanding patterns within medical syndromes from a lifespan perspective allows us to proactively anticipate the support needs children may go on to have in adolescence, mid-life or beyond. This chapter therefore resists an artificial binary choice between the medical model and the social model, seeking instead a more multi-dimensional approach.

Speech and language therapy has long advocated for multi-dimensional models that allow us to appreciate the full complexity of people's experience and the dynamic interactivity between people and multiple aspects of their environment (their social ecology) over time. Implicitly, but firmly, this stance resists the forced and, frankly, false dichotomy between the medical and social models. Instead, we seek frameworks that help us understand the true richness and complexity of children's lives.

Most influential within speech and language therapy in the UK has been the International Classification of Functioning, Disability and Health: Children and Youth version (ICF:CY; WHO, 2007). It provides a framework that transcends diagnosis; instead providing a holistic and comprehensive profile. Even within conceptually contested landscapes such as neurodivergence, the ICF:CY is valued for its ability to reconcile seemingly opposing perspectives in an integrated and multi-faceted manner (Bölte et al., 2021). Many of the chapters in this book draw explicitly or implicitly on it.

The ICF:CY outlines a biopsychosocial model, wherein disability (dysfunction) is thought to arise from one or more of the following: impairment in body structures or functioning; limitations in the actions the child can accomplish (activities); and restrictions in the child's participation in expectable life situations. A key concept is the gap between children's capacity (maximum functioning in an optimally facilitative context) and their current level of functioning. Impacting on that gap are two interacting sets of contextual factors: personal and environmental factors. The latter includes a wealth of factors relating to children's physical, social and psychological environments.

Used thoughtfully, the ICF:CY model promotes consideration of all inter-related factors that may restrict a child's meaningful engagement in daily living and learning situations. The framework prompts decisions aimed at reducing or removing constraints. By focusing efforts on what children feel and how they function, it supports them to attain meaningful goals.

Speech, language and communication needs

Understanding the terms

This section briefly outlines what the terms speech, language and communication refer to, before going on to consider what it means for children to have support needs in this aspect of their development and functioning. It is beyond the scope of this book to cover these aspects in the detail required by students on speech and language therapy courses, where whole modules will be devoted to the academic study of these concepts.

Communication is the broadest of the three terms. It encompasses all ways of conveying meaning through the sending and receiving of communicative signals. This process can be intentional or not; and it contains both receptive and expressive elements. Messages can be conveyed by multiple means, including verbal, non-verbal, paralinguistic, written, and symbolic forms. Even hesitations, pauses or silences communicate – often powerfully! Communication is typically complex, with multiple and often contradictory messages being exchanged simultaneously within a fast-flowing, multi-way, relationally and contextually bound social encounter.

Nesting within the scope of communication, and a particular form of it, is language. It involves the rules-based generation of novel utterances using lexical items and grammar in particular combinations or by employing particular constructs. Language can be conveyed in spoken form, but also via sign or other modalities such as writing.

Speech nestles within language. It is a form of language, expressed by the production and sequencing of sounds through the co-ordination of articulatory, phonatory and respiratory systems.

Another helpful way to think about communication is to differentiate between three domains: content, form and use. First introduced by Bloom and Lahey (1978), this simple classification has stood the test of time, proving useful and effective for understanding the aspects on which communication disruption might have an impact (Paul, Norbury and Gosse, 2024).

First, we consider *content*, which relates to the meaning that is being conveyed (and interpreted) and how that happens. Then, through the *form* of communicative messages, participants in a communicative exchange can hone (and decode) signals for optimum clarity and precision. This includes morphology and syntax: the rules by which selected elements (for example, verb endings, plural markers or pronouns) and the chosen order in which grammatical elements are combined, together convey (or help us understand) specific intentions. The domain relating to *use* is critical but can often be overlooked by people who do not have a rounded appreciation of linguistics and social communication. Use refers to the deployment (or interpretation) of combinations of communicative signals as deemed appropriate to a specific social context. Humans have developed complex and often unspoken cultural codes about language and communication use. These codes powerfully denote key signifiers like social status, politeness, formality and familiarity. Competence in social communication requires deft handling of complex, multi-layered, fast-changing, and often subtle (or concealed) signals that relate to both the environment and any interlocutors. In spoken exchanges, for example, simultaneous signals can be verbal (deploying euphemism), non-verbal (such as having a bowed head and looking down) and paralinguistic (uttered in a low tone, with low stress). Decisions such as whether to interrupt, or to correct misinterpretations, will be affected by the participants' understanding of the social conventions of that context. This requires skill in pragmatic functioning.

Another representation of communication that has proven to be of lasting utility is the idea of having means, reasons and opportunities to communicate. Originally devised by speech and language therapists Money and Thurman (1994) as a model to introduce teachers to the concept of functional communication, it has become firmly established as a simple and effective way of highlighting the crucial interaction between individuals and their environments if we are to promote and enable communication. The model elegantly encapsulates key components of inclusive communication. It highlights the impetus to effect change within people's physical, social and psychological environment to ensure that communication is effectively supported.

Means refers to the myriad *ways* in which people communicate. Importantly, this can include alternative and augmentative means of communicating, incorporating the full gamut of conventional and less conventional methods. The *Reasons* domain prompts consideration of *why* people communicate. Reasons run the full spectrum from conveying basic needs and wants, through communicating to establish or develop relationships, to communicating for the sheer pleasure of it. Crucial within this realm is the concept of motivation: do people sense that their communication will have any impact? This idea is closely connected to the notion of communicative agency. Coming third in the trio of interrelated concepts, *Opportunities* denotes people's chances to communicate. It includes important elements, such as the timing, place and participants involved in shaping potential communication events.

What does it mean for children to have SLCN?

Speech, language and communication are used to establish and maintain social bonds, so they are essential to all humans for developing and maintaining a sense of belonging, and to feeling safe, seen and valued. These aspects are therefore central to wellbeing at any age.

For children, who depend on others to learn how to navigate their way in the world, these domains carry even greater magnitude. Attachment relationships are created within and through communicative engagements. These profoundly affect how children come to see themselves, their relationships and their place within the wider world. Language develops through guided exposure and is closely associated with social thinking and feeling. Inner language holds key roles in self-soothing and self-regulation, which have impacts on how children are perceived and, in turn, affect how others interact with them (McCool, 2024). Speech, language and communication together shape the realm within which children engage and learn, both informally and in academic settings. Language concepts, and literacy skills, unlock learning in curricular areas as disparate and as essential as mathematics, history and personal, social, health and economic education (PSHE). Entering late childhood and adolescence, substantially higher-level language competence becomes needed to navigate the intensified social, conceptual and personal challenge that accompanies this phase.

Disruptions within speech, language and communication can therefore lead to functional challenges that ripple across multiple areas of development and multiple settings. The impact of SLCN in the childhood period can be foundational and profound.

What does it mean for children to have needs in speech, language or communication? In short, they need people to ensure that they can access suitable means of communication; that they have suitable chances to take part in communication; and that their experience of communication is motivating, rewarding and fulfilling.

Fundamentally, children need the people around them to flexibly alter their physical, social and psychological environments so that they encounter the 'just right' balance of communication challenge and support. They need people to work with them and their close contacts to ensure that they can together access and enjoy positive and emotionally sustaining communicative connections and engagements. Moreover, children need to be surrounded by people who are willing and able to proactively anticipate and address potential communication barriers, working to reduce or remove them in a timely, effective, appropriate and acceptable manner. On those occasions where it is possible to eliminate an underlying condition or to substantially reduce associated impairment, children and their close contacts need guidance on personally tailored options from the range of evidence-based interventions. Equally, children need access to, and encouragement to use, strategies to work around any remaining communication barriers. They may need support to advocate for their communication support needs. To make this possible, they need support to see themselves as active and engaged participants in communication, with the power to contribute, to influence their surroundings, and to make choices.

Supporting children's speech, language and communication needs

So far in this chapter we have reviewed key principles of child development, including the idea that development has multiple determinants, both biological and social. We have focused on the contemporary concept of children's entitlement to additional support and discussed how this can be viewed through a biopsychosocial lens. We have considered what it means for children to have speech, language and communication needs, highlighting children's reliance on people around them to anticipate and meet their needs through supportive surroundings, connections, interactions and interventions.

Ultimately, this issues a call to action for speech and language therapists that goes far beyond a refresh of the terms or the frameworks we use. It necessitates a fundamental shift of orientation. It prompts a radical rethink of the questions about why SLT might get involved in children's lives and what we might be hoping to influence: who, which, when, where, what, how, and perhaps most critically, for what purpose? Whose interests are being served, and is this the best way to achieve those ends?

This final section of the chapter begins by reviewing some of the principles that help us to rise to this challenge. We begin by considering the shift towards public health approaches in SLT, sitting this alongside the drive for equitable and inclusive services. We then think about some of the key tenets governing SLT practice for children in the UK today: strengths-based, collaborative and evidence-based practice. Next, we explore a model of practice in which parallel processes of understanding and supporting children's needs continually influence and reciprocally reinforce each other: the AWEsome and EPIC approaches to understanding and supporting children's speech, language and communication needs.

Public health, anti-discriminatory practice and cultural inquisitiveness

Support-based and right-based perspectives alter roles and responsibilities, placing more emphasis on prevention, advocacy, and empowerment. Promoting communication-related quality of life becomes a focus for SLTs; regardless of whether our job involves meeting the needs of individuals or populations; and whether we aim to do so directly or by engaging children's close contacts as conduits.

More than ever before, SLT roles and activities are geared towards anticipating and promoting the communication needs of populations who are known to be more vulnerable in their communication development, should appropriate support not be accessible. This includes underserved populations, including those experiencing poverty and social disadvantage, and those from minority or marginalised groups.

This aligns with the imperative that SLTs must 'promote and protect the interests of service users and carers' and the requirement that, as such, they must actively prevent and tackle discrimination in all its forms (HCPC, 2023). Anti-discriminatory practice prompts wider consideration of children's broader ecologies, taking full account of social disadvantage and inequalities (Royal College of Speech and Language Therapists, RCSLT, 2023) and social, cultural and linguistic diversity (Pert, 2022). It requires a searching examination of whether, and to what extent, whole services or individual practitioners, by design or unwittingly, limit opportunities for underserved children to access or optimally benefit from their services. In the words of the RCSLT (2023, p. 7) 'SLTs should be providing fair, culturally and linguistically appropriate and inclusive services to all.'

Strengths-based, collaborative and evidence-based practice

The strengths-based approach exemplifies the paradigm shift away from focusing on what people and systems cannot do, to looking instead at what is currently working well. It is about seeking opportunities to support, complement and boost existing capabilities. Importantly, it should not be used as a cover for minimising concerns, or for presenting an unrealistically positive spin on situations. Instead, it is about working with people and systems to identify current strengths, to clarify their motivations, and to support them in mobilising the resources that will help them succeed in achieving meaningful goals.

Collaboration is therefore key in strengths-based practice. If the impetus is to move towards goals that are meaningful, then it is essential to place the relevant child, family or community at the heart of decision-making. Common parlance now talks about the 'Team Around the Child' (TAC) approach, especially for children with complex needs requiring support from different agencies. It provides a framework to connect and engage all relevant parties, including the parents/caregivers and practitioners from different disciplines and agencies. It aims to provide both co-ordination and clear, consistent communication. Often a lead professional is appointed to bring it all together and ensure the process stays on track. The intention is to identify needs and plan support in an integrated manner that is child- and family-centred. That is a laudable aspiration. Too often, it can be hampered by siloed structures, logistical constraints and inter-professional tensions.

Evidence-based practice (EBP) is a requirement for SLTs. It refers to a process of systematic review and careful evaluation of varied forms of evidence, so that decisions and actions are well informed. Sometimes it is mistakenly assumed to exclusively involve consulting peer-reviewed research, or the guidelines based on it. While critical evaluation of published research forms an important part of EBP, all research has its limitations; notably, that it is usually conducted in conditions that don't represent the messy realities of real-world practice; and it is normally carried out on specially selected populations who may not be comparable to everyday clients. So, evaluations and audits of real-world practice also play an important role, alongside practitioner expertise and the perspectives of people and systems with relevant experience of services. One of the key skills for any practitioner engaging in EBP is the ability to evaluate multiple sources of information, weighing up the extent to which conclusions are valid, reliable, trustworthy and applicable to the given context. That skill takes time and effort to develop and maintain.

Understanding and supporting children's SLCN: A two-way process

If we are to support children's speech, language and communication needs in meaningful ways we must first understand those needs. Once we have a rounded appreciation of

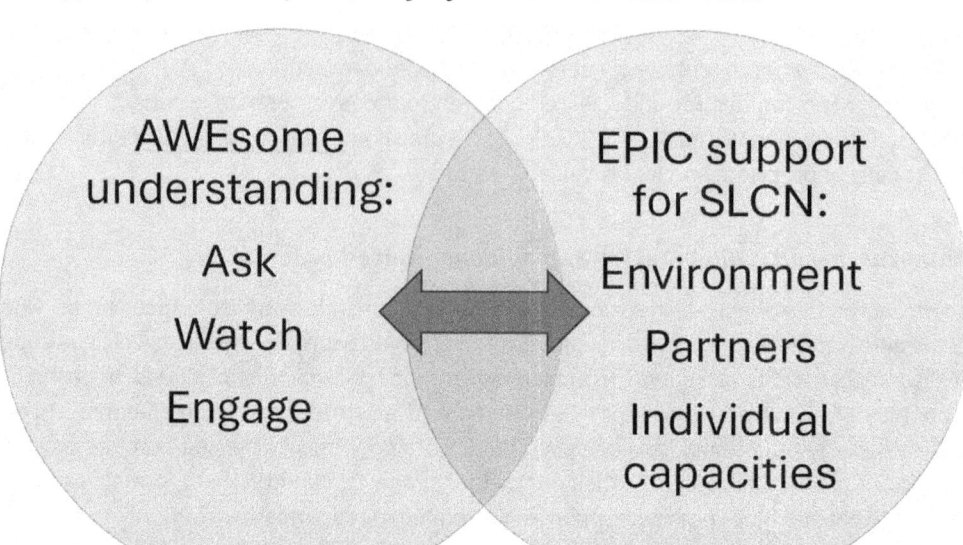

Figure 1.1 The continual two-way process of understanding and supporting children's SLCN: the AWEsome and EPIC approaches

children's needs (whether populations or individuals), we can work together with relevant others to co-create functional goals that meet with the strengths and aspirations of children and their families, and we can jointly plan evidence-based ways to harness resources and move towards achieving goals. As that process unfolds, there should be continual reappraisal of needs: considering whether priorities may be shifting, perspectives may be altering or circumstances changing. Correspondingly, adjustments may be applied to the support plan. And so, the cycle continues, in a two-way process of influence and adaptation between understanding and supporting children's SLCN. This process is depicted in Figure 1.1.

Understanding children's SLCN

The combined approach to understanding children's SLCN is captured with the acronym AWEsome (see Figure 1.1), reminding us of the three main strategies involved: *A*sk, *W*atch and *E*ngage (McCool, 2024). Drawing on information from all three elements allows us to compensate for the limitations inherent in any individual strategy, producing a rounded and authentic appreciation.

- *Asking* involves hearing the views of children, families and key others. Various methods support this important step; including informal and published checklists; as well as conversations, which may or may not be guided by interview protocols. Methods should employ inclusive communication strategies as appropriate.
- *Watching* refers to observation, which is most ecologically valid when capturing events in real-time and in real-world situations. While direct observation can be useful, it is

important that it is as unobtrusive as possible, as the experience of being watched can alter typical patterns of interaction and bring about changes from usual contextual influences. Video-recorded material is increasingly used to enrich observations. Various frameworks are available to guide analysis of observational data, focusing on different aspects of speech, language and communication and representing different levels of detail and structure.

- *Engaging* relates to those activities where a therapist directly interacts with the person or group whose speech, language or communication needs are under consideration, with the intention of understanding more about their needs. Methods span a broad continuum of formality, from static to dynamic. All methods have some advantages and some limitations. The chosen engagement activity will depend on the nature of the information required and its purpose. The trick is choosing the best for the circumstances.

Supporting children's SLCN

A multi-faceted approach to supporting children's SLCN is reflected in the acronym EPIC (see Figure 1.1). This prompts us to consider the main levels towards which support may be offered: the communication environment, communication partners, and children's individual capabilities:

- *Environment* relates to all aspects of children's environments that impact on the communication support available to them. This can include aspects of the physical, social and psychological environment. Increasingly, we acknowledge that adapting environments can generate beneficial impact for many children, and many schools and units work towards accreditation schemes that celebrate their achievements in providing 'communication friendly' spaces. Moreover, we are often concerned with the 'goodness of fit' between children and the environments they spend time in, so efforts may be directed at promoting further adaptations to meet the needs of specific groups or indeed individual children. For all-round benefit, it is important that children encounter consistency in communication approaches across the different environments they experience.
- *Partners* refers to efforts directed at supporting children's communication partners, equipping them with the knowledge, skills and motivation to support children's SLCN. For optimum benefit, approaches should involve a combination of socio-emotional support, relevant information and strategies to enhance interaction. Those strategies should be individually tailored and based on existing strengths. Parents and caregivers are regular participants in these collaborative initiatives with SLTs. Educators, siblings, grandparents and other community members may also participate. Several published parent-mediated intervention schemes and educator-focused training packages exist. Ideally, selection should depend on participant preference. For example, some participants might be drawn to the motivational effects and social support available through group delivery, whereas others may prefer the flexibility afforded via individual approaches.

- *Individual Capabilities* in this context reflect efforts to enhance the effectiveness of children's speech, language or communication. That might involve encouraging more consistent use of previously acquired skills, especially if they are used in some contexts but not in others. It might include supporting the acquisition of new speech, language or communication skills. Collaborative efforts may extend to skills in communication-adjacent areas such as self-regulation and self-esteem. Equally, intervention may focus on boosting communicative function and participation through children learning compensatory strategies, such as saying when they have not understood, or advocating for communication support needs.

Often, a comprehensive approach will involve more than one goal, with a coherent package involving aspects of the environment, partners and individual capabilities.

Summary

This chapter reviewed key principles of child development, including the idea that development has multiple determinants, both biological and social. It examined the contemporary concept of children's entitlement to additional support and discussed how this can be viewed through a biopsychosocial lens. It considered what it means for children to have speech, language and communication needs (SLCN), highlighting children's reliance on people around them to anticipate and meet their needs through supportive surroundings, connections and interventions. The chapter reviewed key principles in supporting children's SLCN, including the shift towards public health approaches in SLT, the drive for equitable and inclusive services, and the need for strengths-based, collaborative and evidence-based practice. It proposed a model of practice in which twin processes continually influence and reciprocally reinforce each other: the AWEsome and EPIC approaches to understanding and supporting children's speech, language and communication needs.

References

Bloom, L. and Lahey, M. (1978) *Language Development and Language Disorders*. New York: John Wiley and Sons.

Bölte, S., Lawson, W., Marschik, P.B., and Girdler, S. (2021) 'Reconciling the seemingly irreconcilable: The WHO's ICF system integrates biological and psychosocial environmental determinants of autism and ADHD. *BioEssays*, 43(9). https://doi.org/10.1002/bies.202000254

DeThorne, L.S. and Gerlach-Houck, H. (2022) 'Resisting ableism in school-based speech-language therapy: an invitation to change', *Language, Speech and Hearing Services in Schools*, 54, 1–7. https://doi.org/10.1080/00131911.2023.2222235.

HCPC (Health and Care Professions Council) (2023) *Standards of Proficiency: Speech and Language Therapists*. London: HCPC. https://www.hcpc-uk.org/globalassets/resources/standards/standards-of-proficiency---speech-and-language-therapists.pdf.

Knight, C., Conn, C., Crick, T. and Brooks, S. (2023) 'Divergences in the framing of inclusive education across the UK: A four nations critical policy', *Educational Review*, pp. 1–18. https://doi.org/10.1080/00131911.2023.2222235.

McCool, S. (2024) *Working with Child and Adolescent Mental Health: The Central Role of Language and Communication*. London: Routledge.

Money, D. and Thurman, S. (1994) 'Talkabout communication', *Bulletin of the College of Speech and Language Therapists*, 12–13.

Moscardini, L. (2018) 'Additional support needs', in Bryce, T.G.K., Humes, W.M., Kennedy, A. and Gillies, D. (eds) *Scottish Education*. Edinburgh: Edinburgh University Press, pp. 707-716.

Neaum, S. (2022) *Child Development for Early Years Students and Practitioners*. 5th edn. Exeter: Learning Matters.

Paul, R., Norbury, C., and Gosse, C. (2024) *Language Disorders from Infancy Through Adolescence: Listening, Speaking, Reading, Writing and Communicating*. 6th edn. St Louis: Elsevier.

Pert, S. (2022) *Working with Children Experiencing Speech and Language Disorders in a Bilingual Context: A Home Language Approach*. London: Routledge.

RCSLT (Royal College of Speech and Language Therapists) (2023) *Addressing Health Inequalities*. London: Royal College of Speech and Language Therapists. Available at: https://www.rcslt.org/learning/diversity-inclusion-and-anti-racism/health-inequalities/addressing-health-inequalities/ (accessed 11 March 2025).

UNICEF UK (1989) *The United Nations Convention on the Rights of the Child*. Available at: https://www.unicef.org/child-rights-convention (accessed 8 March 2025).

WHO (World Health Organization) (2007) *International Classification of Functioning, Disability and Health: Children and Youth Version: ICF:CY*. Geneva: World Health Organization.

Yehuda, N. (2016) *Communicating Trauma: Clinical Presentations and Interventions with Traumatized Children*. Abingdon: Routledge.

2 A 'whole system' approach to meeting speech, language and communication needs

Marie Gascoigne

What you'll learn in this chapter

- The importance of understanding the child or young person's skills, development, needs and outcomes in the context of the system in which they live
- The factors which need to be analysed at the system level to provide that contextual framework
- The implications for funding, service design and delivery of taking a whole system approach in any given population
- The opportunities for the role of the speech and language therapist (SLT) as a practitioner within a whole system approach.

Introduction

The intended outcome of this chapter is to introduce readers to the concepts and key information needed to consider the child, young person and their family at the centre of the 'whole system'. This crucial perspective will then facilitate understanding of more specific speech, language and communication need profiles that will be detailed in later chapters, *in context*. We shall focus on key aspects of understanding a whole system and what it means for service planning, design and delivery to ensure we have the greatest *impact* on the speech, language and communication skills of the children and young people we serve. The important topic of impact will form the basis of Chapter 6.

As you read this chapter, you are invited to consider how your role as a practitioner, operational or strategic leader can, and should, both influence and be influenced by the broader context for the child or young person.

Why a whole system approach?

There are several reasons why it is important to think about supporting speech, language and communication needs (SLCN) for children and young people through a whole system approach.

First, no child or young person exists in isolation. They are at the centre of a system or network consisting of home and family, those who have immediate contact with them in their day-to-day lives beyond the home, and beyond these, local, national and perhaps even global

DOI: 10.4324/9781003671626-4

networks that impact on them directly or indirectly. This bioecological system view as first described by Bronfenbrenner (1979) has been highly influential in providing a framework where a child's development is understood through the influences and interactions of systems around the child. Their individual needs must be understood in context.

The second reason for taking a whole system approach lies with the reality that most children and young people who will face challenges with elements of their speech, language and communication are not readily identifiable from birth and in the first years of life. Services that support speech, language and communication development must be proactive and anticipatory. There is a growing evidence base indicating the need for a public health role within the SLT profession. This chapter highlights the importance of a public health philosophy in underpinning planned outcomes for children and young people, including those who emerge as having more specific and long-term needs. This requires the outcomes to be clearly articulated, based on the contributions of all the elements of the system around the child or young person.

This brings us to the third reason for taking a whole system, population-based approach to understanding need. The structures and systems in public services, from government departments through to education, health and care services, do not naturally lend themselves to a whole system infrastructure. This challenge is not a new one and the aspiration of integrated services has been present in the policies of all the UK administrations at various points over the past 20 years. Thinking more specifically about supporting children and young people with SLCN, the Royal College of Speech and Language Therapists' Position Paper, 'Supporting children with speech, language and communication needs within integrated children's services' (Gascoigne, 2006), set out clear recommendations for integrated working.

What is involved in a whole system approach to speech, language and communication needs?

Gascoigne (2006) first introduced the concept of the SLT supporting the wider system across three levels of potential need. First, there is the *universal need* for all children in a population. Next, there is *targeted need* in those who are 'vulnerable' (or, as we would now describe it, have increased risk factors). Third, we consider those with *more specific and specialist need*. This concept has been widely adopted as the basis for what have become variously described as 'tiered approaches' or 'hierarchical organisations' of interventions. This concept is still considered relevant almost 20 years after its first publication (Law and Charlton, 2022).

Gascoigne (2024) extended the early concepts of needing to provide support across the whole system by building an outcomes-based framework for understanding not only need, but also the design, implementation and outcome measurement of a whole system approach. The addition of the Five Strands outcome areas resulted in a comprehensive set of outcome indicators for a system through which an individual child, young person and their family should be able to have their needs met in the most impactful way. These Five Strands outcome areas encompass:

1. Family and Young Person Support
2. Enhancing Environments

20 *Supporting Children's Speech, Language and Communication Needs*

3. Developing Workforce
4. Early Identification
5. Effective Intervention

This enhanced model is known as the Balanced System® (see Figure 2.1) and has continued to evolve continuously with tools and templates to support needs analysis and system transformation (see recommended resources at the end of this chapter).

It is important to distinguish between the levels of need in a population, the provision offered across levels, and the level of skills and competence in the workforce. The relationship between population, provision and the workforce is not a linear 'one size fits all' but is dependent on the most effective way to achieve functional impact, which could differ from

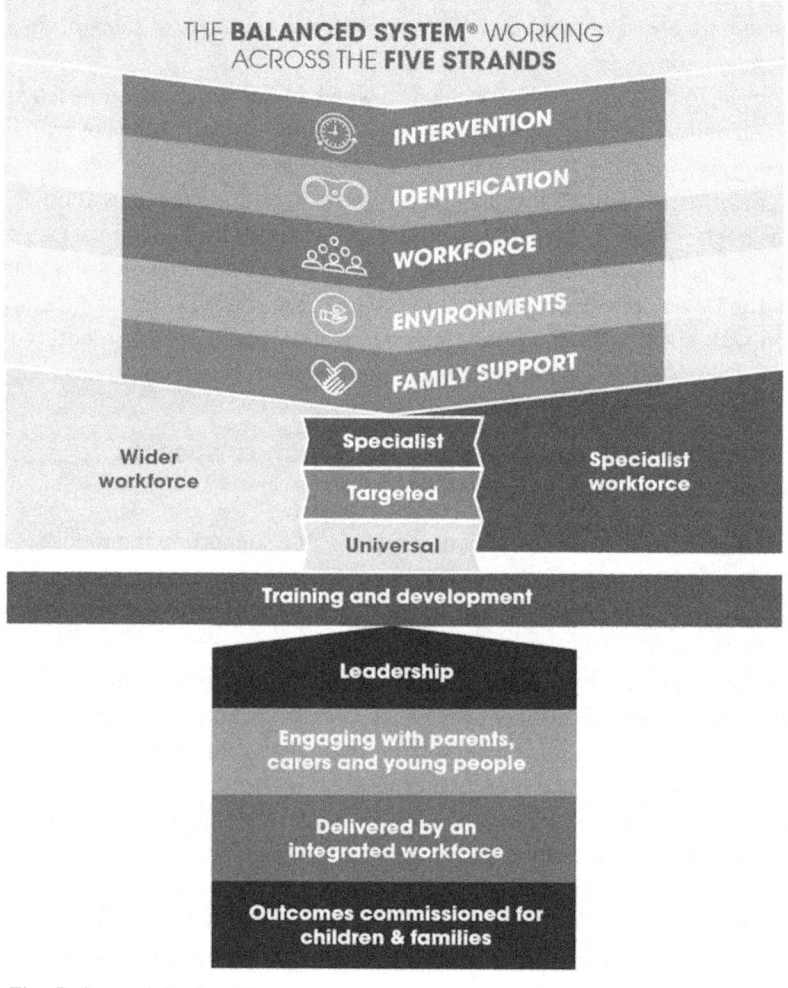

Figure 2.1 The Balanced System®
Source: Marie Gascoigne, 2008-2025.

one child to the next, depending on both within-child factors and their context. The whole system needs to be both comprehensive and flexible to generate the greatest impact for children and young people.

How to go about building a whole system approach?

An effective whole system approach requires the following key steps: (1) understand, (2) plan, (3) do, and (4) review. Much of this process may seem beyond the scope of a speech and language therapy practitioner who regards their primary role as working with individual children, young people and families. However, it is crucial for all practitioners to understand what they do as part of the whole system and to appreciate that the effectiveness and impact of the therapist contribution are dependent on that relationship with the whole system. We are going to begin, then, by looking at a whole system journey through the lens of a commissioner or, ideally, joint commissioning group seeking to fund, commission and secure provision for a population of children and young people.

Understand

Defining the system

To apply a whole system approach, the starting point is to define the system in question. This sounds straightforward but there are a few common challenges in getting past this basic starting point. These typically include geographical, organisational, cultural and professional differences in system definition. For example, taking the interface between geographical and organisational system footprints, in Scotland, Wales and Northern Ireland, a Health Board or Trust will often cover several Local Authorities, and in England the boundaries of Integrated Care Boards, Local Authorities and NHS Provider organisations are frequently different from one another. These geographical challenges are potentially significant in so far as they can create artificial barriers to sensible whole system planning and delivery.

Organisational system differences in definition could be illustrated by a contrasting a school system, with classes, subjects, attainment targets and a workforce made up of teachers, teaching assistants and meal-time supervisors, as opposed to a speech and language therapy department within a health provider where the organisational systems are likely to involve teams of professionals, sometimes organised into multi-professional groups (though not always), and with the language of patients or clients, face-to-face contacts and system requirements that start from a medical basis.

In addition, there can be different views about the role of the SLT in a system and the approach to be taken in considering need and planning service delivery. Some would still take a more traditional medical perspective, often based on a deficit model. These approaches will result in systems made up of diagnostic category-led teams and pathways, in contrast to an ecological, population-based approach, such as the Balanced System®.

Learning points 2.1

- *Strategic*: Identify your population footprint and the commissioners with responsibility for children and young people's health, education and care needs across that footprint.
- *Operational*: Understand the population and ensure it is informing service design and delivery.
- *Practitioner*: Understand the population characteristics, communities, culture and diversity to ensure service delivery is child-, young person- and family-led.

Articulating the vision

To take a whole system approach to the needs of a population, there must be some level of system definition of the desired outcome. This may seem obvious but in practice is potentially complicated by different perspectives of what 'good' looks like at different levels of the system. The Balanced System® identifies outcomes across Five Strands as well as at universal, targeted and specialist levels. This results in a scaffold containing 15 high-level outcomes. That framework is core to the processes that are then required to identify need, plan a response, transform the system offer and review the impact on those outcome areas. The Balanced System® Outcomes Framework (Figure 2.2) is an example of how to take a whole system approach to delivering sustainable change.

The outcomes framework sets out ambitions for the system supporting SLCN in any given area. If the system is working well, it should be possible to identify the contribution of a wide range of system partners, including SLTs, for every one of the 15 outcome areas. This is a key point – the SLTs may be among the specialist workforce in relation to SLCN but they have a contribution to make across the whole outcome framework if the system is to be effective. Equally as important is the recognition of the contribution of other elements of the workforce to achieve the same outcomes: health visitors, teachers, teaching assistants, educational psychologists, paediatricians, early years workers, to name but a few. Most importantly of all, the contribution of families, parents and carers should be identified and recognised as central to the impact of the system.

Learning points 2.2

- *Strategic*: Agree the shared ambitions for the population you serve across the local system, including commissioners from Health and Local Authority perspectives, schools and settings, and, of course children, young people and families.
- *Operational*: Design service delivery with child, young person and family outcomes at the core, as opposed to expecting families to fit in with service design.
- *Practitioner*: Ensure that the support you offer is clearly linked to the functional outcomes for children, young people and families.

A 'whole system' approach to SLCN 23

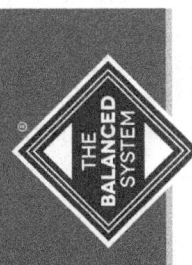

Figure 2.2 The Balanced System® high level outcomes
Public Health England Guidance 2021: www.gov.uk/government/publications/public-health.

Analyse the context of the system

If the vision is to implement a whole system approach in any given area, then the process must begin with an analysis of the needs of the population. As discussed above, 'population' usually will be a geographically defined population, and in terms of how Local Authority and Health structures are organised, that population will typically be based on data that are derived from where people live. However, it is possible to look at a school community as a 'system' and an example of this will be explored later.

Gascoigne (2024) provides a concise, high-level outline of applying the Balanced System® to the population that is the City of Birmingham. This is a relatively 'simple' system in that the City of Birmingham as a Local Authority and the NHS provider organisation that employs the speech and language therapy service are coterminous. However, even in this relatively uncomplicated geography, the Integrated Care Board that is responsible for the 'health' commissioning for children and young people in Birmingham also has responsibility for the neighbouring Local Authority of Solihull. Equally there is a significant contribution to the outcomes for children and young people made by the independent SLT services that are commissioned by some schools across the city.

Regardless of the simplicity or complexity of your system, some key datasets are essential to understand the context of the system. Figure 2.3 summarises these key elements of quantitative and qualitative data.

Understanding need uses publicly available data that can be used to predict the potential need in any given population, which could be a country, a Local Authority, a school or community (Figure 2.3, Box 1). This is contrasted with understanding demand. Demand requires data from the local system that indicate the numbers, and characteristics, of children and young people that are being identified or are seeking support in any given area (Figure 2.3, Box 2). It is important that the distinction is clear. For example, referral patterns across the wards of an area may not match the predicted pattern of need. This could be for several reasons including how accessible the service is for families in certain circumstances, where there may be potential unmet need.

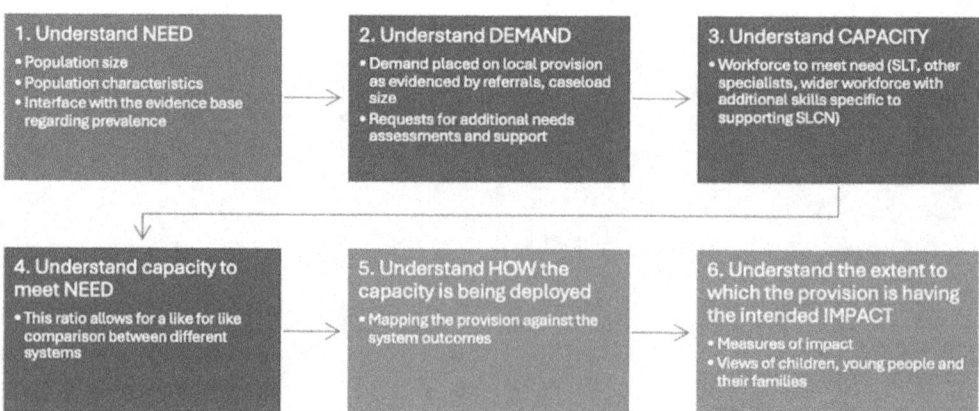

Figure 2.3 Summary of the 'understand' phase of the Balanced System® needs analysis

To understand the capacity in the system to meet the need in a population, the workforce that contributes to outcomes for children and young people and their families must be captured. This workforce includes the speech and language therapy workforce, but also specialist teachers, assistant practitioners, and members of the wider workforce who may have specific roles in their schools or settings for supporting speech, language and communication (Figure 2.3, Box 3). Once there is a clear picture of the workforce within the system, it is possible to calculate the capacity to meet the needs of a specific area (Figure 2.3, Box 4).

This approach is important because it is possible to have two populations that are the same size but whose demographic factors mean that the risk factors associated with speech, language and communication can be anticipated to be greater in one than the other. For instance, the number of children and young people in X and Y are roughly equal. However, the demographic data indicate that the socio-economic challenges in X are significantly greater than in Y. This means that we can anticipate that in addition to the prevalence of SLCN that we can expect in any population (7–10%) the additional contextual need in X means that if we are planning service delivery, we should expect X to have more need at a population level. This is important, as when we look at the workforce available to meet the potential need, the conclusion that can be drawn is that population X may require more therapy capacity to meet the needs than population Y. This disparity may also warrant different qualitative approaches. For example, the Scottish Government commissioned a needs analysis of all the speech and language provision in Scotland using this approach (Gascoigne, 2021). Using this methodology, it was demonstrated that the area with the highest predicted need had the lowest resources available.

So far, the data that have been considered are quantitative. However, to really understand how the needs are being met across the system it is important to capture a qualitative description of how the shared outcomes are being met. What is the available workforce doing in terms of activities to support children and young people and how do they know it is working? The last two boxes in Figure 2.3 refer to mapping the current provision against the high-level outcomes and, alongside that, describing any evidence of impact for the provision.

Learning points 2.3

- *Strategic*: Understanding the context of the whole system requires quantitative and qualitative analysis of the local system data. The model of service delivery and evidence of impact are as important as the quantitative measures in evaluating the whole system.
- *Operational*: Understanding where can be predicted to have greater need will enable more tailored deployment of resources and may require different service delivery based on population need.
- *Practitioner*: Understanding the qualitative information regarding the children and families you are working with is critical to evaluating what support is going to be most impactful for them at a given time.

Planning delivery to meet need in a whole system

Understanding patterns of predicted need in a population is relevant across the age range. Why is this important? Gascoigne and Gross (2017) summarised the risk factors and enabling strategies identified in the evidence base for children's language and communication skills. Drawing on the evidence from longitudinal cohort studies, the implications of having, for instance, poor vocabulary, communication and language skills at age 5, include finding school more challenging to enjoy at age 7 (Moss and Washbrook, 2016), being less able to achieve than peers at English and Maths curriculum at age 11 (Save the Children, 2016) and being twice as likely to have mental health challenges and struggle in employment in their thirties (Law et al., 2009).

There have been significant developments in public health screening for SLCN, however, evidence from long-term studies has found that while early identification is positive, some children who are identified as having a vulnerability for speech, language and communication aged 2 years will go on to be fine at school entry aged 4 years, while others who are not identified at 2 years will go on to demonstrate difficulties (Reilly et al., 2018). Alongside these findings, evidence regarding the prevalence of developmental language disorder (DLD) suggests that 7.58% of children and young people may have a profile for DLD (Norbury et al., 2016), however, these children are not readily identifiable in the pre-school population yet are part of every population-based cohort.

From a service delivery perspective, then, understanding the population risk factors provides two main opportunities. We can direct expertise, advice and provision to those parts of an area where it is predicted that there may be more need; and we can establish strong, enabling and protective practice for those who will go on to be identified as part of the DLD cohort in the area. So, having the potential to increase targeted support in a whole community based on predicted need provides a powerful opportunity to develop the speech, language and communication skills of all the children in that community. That includes all those at risk of SLCN, even those who will go on to be identified for additional, more individualised support and who will benefit from having experienced enhanced support before being identified.

As we look at older cohorts of children and young people, the same principles apply. If we take a whole system approach to understanding the needs in the school-age population, it is possible to identify school communities where data support predictions of need in the school system. Schools report a rich dataset in all parts of the UK. By capturing the size and demographics of the school population, and the levels of identified special educational needs and disabilities (SEND)/additional support needs (ASN), it is possible to predict which schools in an area will have more needs relative to the others. This baseline then facilitates planning. For example, the analysis can be used to indicate where targeted interventions might be prioritised for all children and young people across a school cohort (so effectively being delivered universally in that specific school context), or which schools it should be anticipated will have greater numbers of children on the SLT caseload.

Doing and reviewing within the whole system approach: core delivery principles

Within the Balanced System® approach, five core delivery principles have been identified to ensure that the available resource is being used for the greatest functional impact to deliver the high-level outcomes. Figure 2.4 illustrates how these are inter-related.

The first of these, *Impact* is the subject of a dedicated chapter in this book because ensuring that impact drives the delivery of provision is so fundamental (see Chapter 6). The 'engine of change' in the Balanced System® whole system approach is the combination of *easy access*, *place-based* and ensuring *robust targeted support* between the universal and specialist levels of offer. These three central principles are inter-dependent, however, the following section endeavours to highlight the key elements of each and how they interact across the age range. Finally, *information* that is quality assured and accessible to families and wider system partners is crucial to ensuring consistency of support in an area.

Easy access

Easy access as a principle is exactly what it says! Systems are typically not designed to enable families to access expert advice as simply and quickly as possible. The 'refer – assess – treat' paradigm when applied to a high-frequency, high-volume need such as speech, language and communication is destined to create excessive waiting times for all those referred. In fact, a significant proportion could receive impactful advice or support in their child's functional

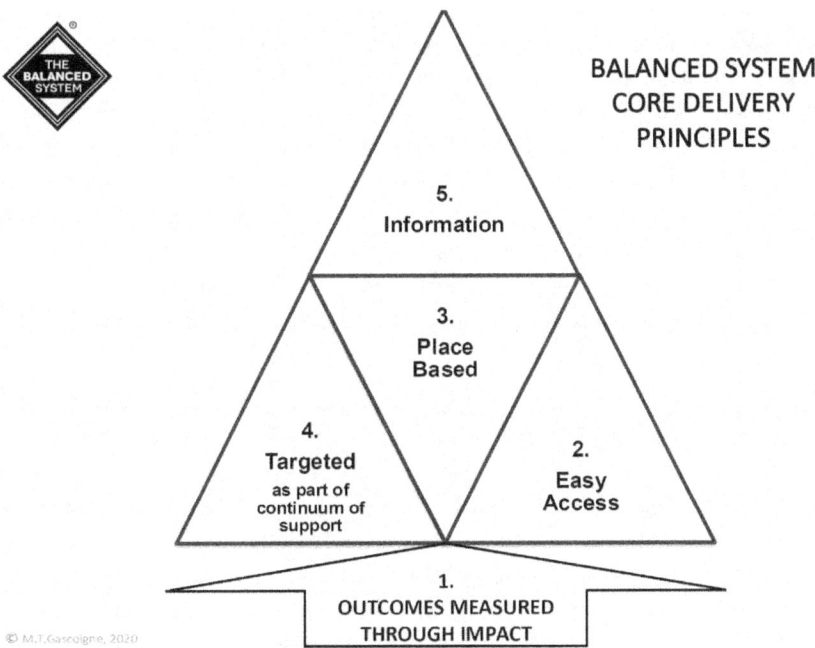

Figure 2.4 The Balanced System® core delivery principles

environment, even if they also require additional support or intervention alongside. The 'easy access' principle of the Balanced System® delivery model challenges the status quo. It suggests that SLTs should be available in community settings that families attend for other purposes, with dedicated sessions available to meet families and discuss their concerns.

However, it is important to avoid a 'cliff edge' where a child requires additional support and the medical model referral processes typically require the family to then attend a health setting and engage with a new team of therapists. The easy access principle applies across the whole continuum of support, including for those who go on to need more individualised specialist intervention. Within a given geography, the expectation would be to provide a regular, advertised opportunity for an open access 'drop-in' session for families at which they can expect to have access to an SLT who can provide not only information and advice but also an initial assessment of a child's needs. This will determine whether further detailed assessment is necessary, whether a community-based targeted offer would be appropriate, or whether signposting to advice and resources is an appropriate first step.

This idea was first developed as part of the redesign of the SLT service in Hackney and the City of London and was given the title 'Talkin Walk-in'. Since then, the concept has been adopted and developed in many services across the UK, with outcome data showing sustained impact, including reduction in waiting times and increased access to support (Gascoigne et al., 2023).

Learning points 2.4

- *Strategic*: Easy access provides a strategic approach to ensuring that children and families are supported appropriately without the need for a lengthy waiting list, alongside enabling access to more in-depth assessment and intervention for those who require this additionally.
- *Operational*: Using understanding of the variations in population need across your area facilitates decision-making as to where to focus the easy access opportunities.
- *Practitioner*: Easy access to support that is proportional and impactful can be achieved by challenging the traditional 'refer – assess – treat' paradigm and enabling families to engage with SLT expertise in functional contexts.

Place-based

Easy access at school age is intrinsically linked with being 'place-based' and can be achieved through the establishment of a link SLT for every school in the local system. This is more than having an identified 'named' therapist linked to each school. Many SLT services visit schools to support children and young people in context, however, the additionality of the link therapist within this approach is that the link therapist builds a working relationship with the school and oversees the needs of any child within the school identified with SLCN. From an easy access perspective, the liaison with the school special educational needs co-ordinator or additional support needs lead means there are regular opportunities to discuss concerns. Working as part of the school extended team means that class-based guidance and strategies can be implemented which will improve support for speech, language and communication of all children, including those who may be emerging as having greater needs. This in turn impacts the easy access to more specialist interventions for those who need that support, typically provided in school.

The link therapist approach not only provides a mechanism for supporting children and young people in context and developing the system around them, but is also efficient, as their time is consolidated and therefore economies of scale are achieved through reduced travel and being able to use time in school flexibly. For example, by allocating time to a school for a day (where the plan is to see a range of children, liaise with school staff, and run some targeted activities alongside school staff, both as intervention and workforce development), there is maximum opportunity to use time effectively. If a child due for some individualised support is away from school, there will be many more activities that can make use of that time profitably, whether working with other known children or as an element of the infrastructure support to the whole school system. The link therapist is also key to collaboration and integrated working with colleagues across the education context, including specialist teachers, educational psychologists and other specialists, including occupational therapy and physiotherapy colleagues – and, of course, SLT colleagues with specific specialist expertise, as needed. Finally, the place-based principle opens the possibilities of functional application of therapy interventions in context, whether that be classroom-based facilitation or supporting interactions in social spaces such as mealtimes and the playground.

Learning points 2.5

- *Strategic*: Understanding the relative needs of each school, based on data and the identified caseload, supports allocation of resource to schools in a link model. The SENCO or ASN lead liaison supports the identification process which in turn impacts on waiting lists as children are discussed regularly and where a referral is not necessary, support can be put in place through school systems.
- *Operational*: Deploying resources to schools is efficient and effective.
- *Practitioner*: Place-based working allows collaboration with colleagues in a functional context. Working with children and young people in their everyday context opens possibilities for application of speech, language and communication skills in functional contexts alongside their peers.

A robust targeted offer

The Balanced System® high-level outcomes across family and young person support, environment, workforce, identification and intervention are also articulated across the universal, targeted and specialist levels. In a whole system approach to the population, it is therefore essential to ensure that all these strands and levels are being considered when planning and delivering provision. The continuum of support from the universal offer, through targeted and to specialist levels, is key. Where there is a lack of a robust targeted offer across any of the strands, the consequence is that any child or young person with a need that cannot be met by the universal offer has no alternative other than to be directed to the specialist level. This in turn creates the waiting list pressures that have already been referred to, and so,

30 *Supporting Children's Speech, Language and Communication Needs*

along with easy access and being place-based, the need for the targeted offer as the third of the central delivery principles becomes clear.

The targeted offer is defined as high-frequency interventions or activities to support frequently occurring SLCN which may be delivered by SLTs directly, or alongside wider system colleagues, with the potential for wider system colleagues to deliver interventions at a targeted level independently with the appropriate training, coaching and support. Since the introduction of the concept of the universal, targeted and specialist continuum of support (Gascoigne, 2006), various interpretations have arisen which, in some instances have led to a confusion that 'targeted' = 'delivered by school or setting staff'. This is not the case and was never the intention. A targeted intervention may be delivered by school or setting colleagues, but the place-based SLT will be key to ensuring that the system around a practitioner will enable the targeted intervention to be delivered with fidelity and achieve the intended outcomes. Equally, many interventions delivered by an SLT might be described as 'targeted'.

The importance of the targeted offer in the continuum of support is how it relates to the analysis of the population need in a whole system. Figure 2.5 illustrates how, for a population-defined context (school, setting, ward, Local Authority area), what might be thought of as a targeted offer in one context might be needed by so many children, young people and families as to become universally available. This is particularly relevant when considering the expectations of mainstream schools around the 'ordinarily available provision' to support inclusion and children and young people with additional needs. In some areas, based on the prediction of need, the 'ordinarily available provision' may need to be at a higher specification than in other areas. Another example of the need to consider the context would be the continuum of support in special schools and provisions. In this situation, the expectation of what might be targeted 'ordinarily available provision' in a mainstream school might be expected to be part of the universal offer in a special school.

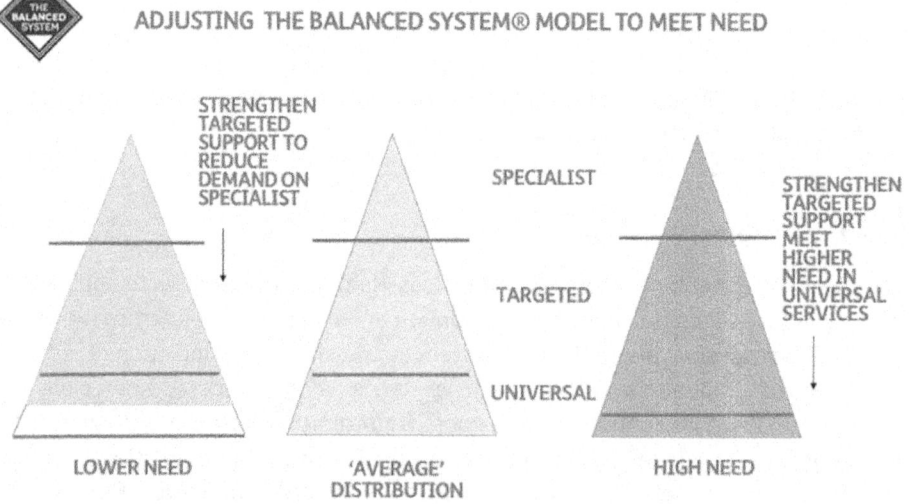

Figure 2.5 Illustrating how the universal, targeted and specialist offer might differ in response to population need

A 'whole system' approach to SLCN 31

> **Learning points 2.6**
>
> - *Strategic*: The targeted level is potentially the highest risk of duplication of effort, misunderstanding and tension between organisations and teams in a local area. It also presents the greatest opportunity for ensuring high impact for children and young people if the planning and delivery can be agreed strategically.
> - *Operational*: The targeted level is the highest frequency area for activity. It also has the potential to be impactful for significant numbers of children and young people and therefore requires development. The challenge is the perception in some parts of the system that this is 'lesser' than using SLT time at the specialist level. The key is in evidencing the impact of supporting the targeted offer which also plays a part in every child or young person requiring additional specialist level support.
> - *Practitioner*: The targeted offer provides opportunity for direct work with children and young people alongside colleagues where some element of workforce development is also being supported. It requires confidence to work alongside others and to offer coaching and modelling support as well as working with children and young people directly in their functional context.

Danny's story

To conclude, a case study (see Figure 2.6). Thanks to Emma Jordan, Speech and Language Therapy Team Lead for Worcestershire, for providing an example of a child's journey through a system like that described in this chapter.

Danny attends his local mainstream school. The school is a large primary school and has a team of link SLTs and assistant practitioner support on a weekly basis.

Danny was in Year 1 when his parent expressed concerns about his talking and understanding. His Mum attended a *drop-in* session with the SLT and school staff. It was agreed that Danny needed some further assessment. A referral was made to speech and language therapy. The therapist gave Mum and the class teacher some initial *advice*.

Danny's language skills were supported in class. Classrooms are already *communication-friendly* with visual support available. Several *universal interventions* are already in use across the school, for example, Teaching Children to Listen and Word Aware. All teachers and teaching assistants have received *training* in these areas in the past.

Four weeks after the meeting with Danny's Mum, the SLT carried out an *assessment* with Danny, observing him in class and carrying out some assessment on a 1:1 basis. The therapist identified moderate to severe receptive and expressive language difficulties (with scores ranging from 2nd to 9th percentile). These difficulties were impacting on Danny's understanding in lessons, his access to the curriculum and confidence talking both at home and at school. Danny's needs were discussed with his Mum and class teacher and next steps were agreed.

Danny attended *targeted interventions* delivered by trained teaching assistants at school. These interventions were set up and supported by the Speech and Language

32 *Supporting Children's Speech, Language and Communication Needs*

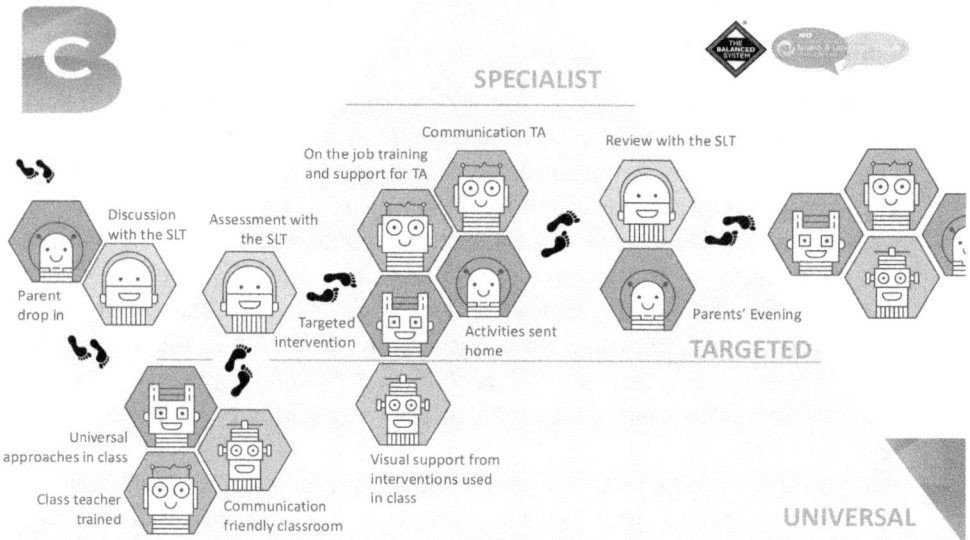

Figure 2.6 Danny's journey

Therapy Team, alongside support being available from one of the school's Communication Teaching Assistants. The SLT team coordinated the intervention plan for each year group each term, ensuring resources were available and school staff were appropriately supported.

Danny accessed this support on a weekly basis over an academic year. These interventions were supported back in class and activities and ideas were sent home to help Danny to use his new skills both back in class and in his home environment. Danny's progress was monitored by the speech and language team throughout the year.

Danny's progress was reviewed at the start of Year 2 by the SLT. He was seen in class and on an individual basis. His progress was discussed with school staff. Danny's parents attended *Parents' Evening* during the same term to discuss his progress and ongoing needs. Danny had made good progress in class and on assessment. Some ongoing expressive vocabulary difficulties were *identified*, and next steps were agreed. Danny has started to attend some further *targeted* intervention delivered by trained teaching assistants at school. This is being supported in class as the whole school uses a *universal* approach to teaching vocabulary.

Eleven months following his initial assessment with the SLT, Danny had made good progress:

- ✓ Functional impact evident in classroom:
    - ○ engaged and participating across the curriculum
    - ○ able to assert himself in class
    - ○ now able to tell mum about his school day
    - ○ more able to engage in conversations at home
    - ○ parents and teacher reporting good progress and increase in confidence

- ✓ Formal assessment of receptive language (Following Directions CELF-P) score moved from age equivalent score of 3 years 11 months to 5 years 8 months
- ✓ Formal assessment of receptive language (Sentence Structure CELF-P), percentile rank scores moved from the 9th to the 25th percentile
- ✓ Moved from Level A-B of Language for Thinking questions to Level C
- ✓ On assessment of expressive language using the Renfrew Action Picture Test, Danny moved from scores below 3 years 6-11 months range to a score within the 6 years 6 months to 7 years 5 months range for information and above 8 years 0 to 5 months for grammatical content.

Summary

This chapter provides a methodology for understanding population need, to develop whole system approaches. The learning points at each stage are directed to the different professional audiences as the 'whole system' is not just a whole system across organisational and operational boundaries but a 'whole system' within a professional area or service. For the practitioner or student practitioner, the key messages are to understand the child or young person you are supporting (in the context of their family, their immediate environment, their community, where they learn and have leisure) and to plan your support taking those contexts and their individual characteristics and needs into account. Other chapters will focus on specific profiles of need or diagnoses. This chapter provides a context into which all the specific examples can be related, as even the most complex profile of need requires good universal and targeted provision in the wider system to maximise impact.

Recommended resources

The Balanced System®: www.thebalancedsystem.org

References

Bronfenbrenner, U. (1979) *The Ecology of Human Development: Experiments by Nature and Design.* Cambridge, MA: Harvard University Press.

Gascoigne, M. (2006) 'Supporting children with speech, language and communication needs within integrated children's services'. Available at: https://www.bettercommunication.org.uk/downloads/ (accessed 27 March 2025).

Gascoigne, M. (2015) 'Commissioning for speech, language and communication needs: Using the evidence from the Better Communication Research Programme'. Available at: https://www.bettercommunication.org.uk/downloads/ (accessed 27 March 2025).

Gascoigne, M. (2021) 'Equity for all: Children's speech and language therapy services in Scotland'. Available at: https://www.bettercommunication.org.uk/downloads/ (accessed 27 March 2025).

Gascoigne, M. (2024) 'Meeting speech, language and communication needs: A whole-systems, population-based approach', *Paediatrics and Child Health*, 34(7), 201-210. https://doi.org/10.1016/j.paed.2024.04.001

Gascoigne, M. and Gross, J. (2017) 'Talking about a generation: Current policy, evidence and practice for speech, language and communication'. Available at: https://www.bettercommunication.org.uk/tct_talkingaboutageneration_report_online_update.pdf (accessed 27 March 2025).

Gascoigne, M., Nield, C., Jordan, E. and Moore, A. (2023) 'Easy access: An alternative to the "refer-assess-treat" paradigm for supporting children and families to access speech and language therapy advice and support in the early years'. Paper presented at Royal College of Speech and

Language Therapists conference, November 2023. Available at: https://www.thebalancedsystem.org/downloads/rcslt-conference-presentation-2023/ (accessed 27 March 2025).

Law, J. and Charlton, J. (2022) 'Interventions to promote language development in typical and atypical populations', in J. Law, S. Reilly and C. McKean (eds), *Language development: Individual differences in a social context*. Cambridge: Cambridge University Press, pp. 470–494.

Law, J., Rush, R., Schoon, I. and Parsons, S. (2009) 'Modeling developmental language difficulties from school entry into adulthood: Literacy, mental health, and employment outcomes', *Journal of Speech, Language and Hearing Research*, 52(6), 1401–1416. https://pubs.asha.org/doi/10.1044/1092-4388%282009/08-0142%29

Moss, G. and Washbrook, L (2016) 'Understanding the gender gap in language and literacy development'. Available at: https://www.bristol.ac.uk/media-library/sites/education/documents/bristol-working-papers-in-education/Understanding%20the%20Gender%20Gap%20working%20paper.pdf (accessed 27 March 2025).

Norbury, C.F., Gooch, D., Wray, C., Baird, G., Charman, T., Simonoff, E., Vamvakas, G. and Pickles, A. (2016) 'The impact of nonverbal ability on prevalence and clinical presentation of language disorder: evidence from a population study', *Journal of Child Psychology and Psychiatry*, 57(11), 1247–1257. https://acamh.onlinelibrary.wiley.com/doi/10.1111/jcpp.12573

Reilly, S., Cook, F., Bavin, E.L., Bretherton, L., Cahir, P., Eadie, P., Gold, L., Mensah, F., Papadopoullos, S. and Wake, S. (2018) 'Cohort profile: The Early Language in Victoria Study (ELVS)', *International Journal of Epidemiololgy*, 47(1), 11–20. https://academic.oup.com/ije/article/47/1/11/3868353

Save the Children (2016) 'Early language development and children's primary school attainment in English and maths: New research findings'. Available at: https://i.stci.uk/dam/early-language-development-and-childrens-primary-school-attainment.pdf-ch11234005.pdf/3avd35265cren41ss02q12fh7car5av2.pdf (accessed 27 March 2025).

3 Inclusive communication

Kim Hartley Kean

What you'll learn in this chapter

- What inclusive communication is and who benefits from it
- Why inclusive communication is important
- How to identify support needs in this area of practice
- How to implement inclusive communication good practice.

Key information about inclusive communication

Communication diversity is the norm in every community. Individuals within any group will need or prefer to use different ways, channels and situations to communicate. Inclusive communication includes as many people as possible in any verbal or non-verbal communication in person, online, on the phone or on paper at any time, place or situation. Inclusive-communication good practice can change people's everyday lives.

Inclusive communication environments embed inclusive communication good practice. They benefit everyone by removing or reducing the communication disadvantages arising from diversity. That includes children, parents, carers, staff, colleagues, organisations and communities.

Inclusive communication helps to build equal, positive relationships and partnerships and so it supports individual and organisational change and development. It is fundamental to equity, diversity, inclusion and enjoyment of human rights. It enables as many people as possible to enjoy equal access to health, education, employment, justice and all other services and opportunities.

Implementing inclusive communication good practice requires sustained, systemic action. A one-off training workshop is not enough. Staff need a supportive organisational infrastructure to consistently implement good practice. Speech and language therapists (SLTs) have a unique and expert leadership role in the development of inclusive communication environments. SLT services themselves must lead by example. Inclusive communication is an innovative, growth area of SLT practice. It offers significant potential for improved outcomes for individuals, services, society and the profession.

What is inclusive communication?

Inclusive communication means enabling people to understand and express themselves:

- in the ways they need or prefer
- on channels they can use or prefer
- in situations they need or prefer
- at every step of a communication journey.

Ways people understand information and express themselves

All human beings use a range of ways to understand what is going on around them and to express themselves. These include:

- reading, writing, speech, sign language
- photographs, drawings, cartoons, symbols, icons
- objects, eye pointing, eye contact, facial expressions, gestures
- routines, touch, body movements, natural human sounds.

Some of these ways such as complex speech, reading and writing, take most people years to develop. These ways of communicating are harder to learn and use. If an organisation (or environment) only uses these harder ways to communicate, they include fewer people and exclude more people.

Other ways, such as use of pictures, icons, gestures and objects are commonly developed at an early age by almost everyone. These are easier to learn and use. If an organisation (or environment) uses these ways to communicate, they include more people and exclude fewer people.

Inclusive communication good practice means offering people a range of ways to understand information and express themselves. People tend to prefer the ways of communicating which they find easy (Communication Inclusion People, 2024).

Channels of communication

There are essentially four channels of communication:

- in-person communication – either remote or face-to-face
- online, including websites, emails, social media
- on the phone voice calls
- on paper, including letters, leaflets, guidelines, posters, forms and door signs.

Each channel enables people to use different ways to communicate. In-person interaction allows people to use all ways of understanding and expressing themselves. Phone voice calls, however, only allow people to understand and express themselves through speech. Smartphones offer a lot of online channels as well as 'in-person remote' opportunities.

Inclusive communication good practice means offering people a choice of communication channels. People tend to prefer to use the channels they find easy.

Situational factors

Time

The day of the week and time of day can influence people's ability to prepare, turn up for and meaningfully engage in an interaction. So does the time available to take information in and get their point across before, during or after an interaction.

Inclusive-communication good practice means:

- communicating with people on days and at times that work for them
- providing inclusive information well before an interaction
- giving people time to understand and express themselves during an interaction
- providing inclusive information after an interaction to help people remember and follow up any advice given.

Place

If it is easy for a person to travel to a building, find it, access it, and find their way around it, they are more likely to attend and be ready and able to communicate more effectively during a meeting. Inclusive communication good practice means providing services in a person's home or another familiar community setting, or in buildings that:

- are easy to reach by public transport and have family and disabled parking
- have accessible doors, rooms, child-friendly areas and toilet facilities
- have inclusive signs outside and inside
- provide quiet, light and comfortable space for interactions.

People

Some people are comfortable communicating in small or large groups. Others prefer to interact with only one or two people at a time. Cultural norms and life experiences may influence who people prefer to communicate with and how. Inclusive communication good practice means giving people the choice of who and how many people they communicate with.

Specialist communication supports

Some people need specialist communication support, for example, sign language interpreting and translation, Braille, large print, audio, video and Easy Read. Inclusive communication good practice means providing these supports if people ask for them.

Costs

Communicating with service providers can incur costs for individuals, families and supporters, for example, travel, phone and childcare costs. Inclusive communication good practice means eliminating these costs and/or providing people with the means to cover these costs.

The communication journey

A 'communication event' happens whenever someone needs to understand information or express themselves. A series of events forms a 'communication journey'. Communication events are often aligned with steps in a care pathway. A typical communication journey of a parent/SLT consultation may include:

- Event 1: Parent reads the information about the SLT service.
- Event 2: Parent contacts the SLT service; SLT service interacts with parent.
- Event 3: SLT sends appointment information to the parent; parent reads the information and plans to attend.
- Event 4: Parent and SLT meet to discuss the child
- Event 5: Parent understands advice and acts on it.

Inclusive communication good practice is essential at every step on this journey. If it is not, Event 5 may never happen. Inclusive communication ensures optimum impact for the child, parent and service.

What are inclusive communication environments?

Our environment is everything around us. It includes:

- physical factors, such as building design, furniture, signs
- social factors, such as relationships, attitudes, institutional systems, policies, and laws.

The interaction between a person's abilities and these factors determines the person's functioning within that environment.

The 'communication environment' is the physical and social context of any communication. It influences communication functioning. Inclusive communication environments embed inclusive communication good practice, as described above.

Who needs inclusive communication?

Everyone can benefit from inclusive communication, including service users, families, carers, colleagues and the public. Few people want communication to be harder than it needs to be! Everyone can experience communication disadvantages and exclusion at some time. Inclusive communication good practice removes or reduces these.

People tend to be less able to pay attention, understand, think and express themselves clearly when they are tired, upset, stressed, ill, distracted or in unfamiliar situations. People who do not have or cannot use a phone, smartphone or computer are excluded from services which only use these channels. This includes people without the funds or technology for internet connection, phone connection, phone credit and those without computer skills or confidence.

Many disabilities, long-term conditions and illnesses are associated with communication disability or differences. They may be hidden; they are not necessarily declared. For example, sensory loss, mental illness, drug and alcohol dependency, neurodivergence, attention deficit hyperactive disorder (ADHD); developmental language disorder (DLD); literacy or numeracy difficulties; dyslexia; learning disability or head injury.

People in some life circumstances and/or who have had certain experiences are more likely than the general population to encounter communication disadvantages, which often go unrecognised. Examples include people living in poverty; those not in education, employment or training; those who have had adverse childhood experiences (ACEs) or care experience; non-English speakers; Gypsy Travellers or those who have been a victim, witness to or perpetrator of a crime.

Evidence indicates an intergenerational cycle of communication disadvantage. Children whose parents experience communication disadvantages are more likely to experience communication disadvantages throughout their own lives (RCSLT, 2016a).

Why is inclusive communication important?

Every group includes people with diverse communication needs and preferences. Inclusive communication environments acknowledge and proactively respond to this diversity. They remove avoidable barriers to effective communication for everyone. It is fundamental to equality of access to services, person-centred care, increased participation and social interaction (Communication Inclusion People, 2024).

Inclusive communication can change the lives of people who communicate in different ways

Inclusive communication is life-changing for many, including those who access SLT services, parents, carers and colleagues. It enables people, possibly for the first time, to join in and feel part of a conversation, community or activity as an equal, respected and valued person. Some quotes from users:

> Inclusive communication would help me feel like a person without a disability. Just to be treated like everyone else. So that it is equal. People will listen to me and respect what I say.
>
> (woman who speaks using a communication aid)

> Inclusive communication will make it easier to understand many of the communications we get sent from school or the council.
>
> (mother of an autistic son)

> Inclusive communication means being able to communicate how I need to, when I need to, without fear of prejudice or exclusion. It means acceptance, accessibility, inclusion, belonging, safety. And it would mean improved mental and physical well-being.
>
> (woman who identifies as neurodivergent)

Service users want inclusive communication

Surveys show that many people experience communication exclusion (Health and Social Care Alliance Scotland, 2024), and that they want services to implement inclusive communication approaches (Healthcare Improvement Scotland, 2018; Independent Care Review, 2020).

Benefits for all parents, especially vulnerable parents

Parents' health has an impact on the health of their child, in utero, at birth and throughout life (Stoiber et al., 2024). Evidence indicates an intergenerational cycle of communication disadvantage, described as follows.

Parents' own communication capacity determines their access to health-enhancing services and opportunities pre-conception and pre-birth. Once their baby is born, parents who experience communication disadvantages can find it harder than other parents to access advice and support to stimulate their child's speech, language and communication development. Their children are therefore more likely to arrive at school with less developed speech, language and communication skills in comparison to their peers.

Evidence indicates communication disadvantage at age 5 follows children through school and into adulthood. This determines their access to health-enhancing services and opportunities. These young people then become parents themselves and so the cycle may be repeated.

Implementing inclusive communication good practice at every stage of this cycle, from pre-conception onwards, offers vulnerable parents and services the opportunity to break the intergenerational cycle of communication disadvantage (RCSLT, 2016a). Communication inclusive advice helps all parents to be the parents they want to be. It enables them to be the best possible communication partners for their children.

Responding to children's current communication strengths

The communication environment influences the functionality of children's current speech, language and communication skills. Inclusive communication environments optimise a child's communication functionality. Inclusive environments motivate a child to communicate and learn, impacting their current and future communication capacity.

> Inclusive communication will give my daughter more choice and control over her life. She will be enabled to understand her choices, make them, and know what the consequences will be.
>
> (parent of child with additional support needs)

> Inclusive communication will make it easier for my son to know what his rights are and allow him to choose the way to communicate any of his needs in the way he feels comfortable with rather than forcing 1-1 verbal communication at all times.
>
> (mother of an autistic child)

Benefits for SLT and public services

Inclusive communication good practice makes services more person-centred, kinder and fairer. It underpins the effectiveness of universal, targeted and specialist level SLT services.

It can make services more efficient by improving the reach and impact of provision. SLT services can have a greater impact on more people while reducing demand for specialist level SLT services.

Services save time and avoid the financial and human costs of communication breakdown. Successful communication the first time reduces the need for crisis interventions. Independent assessment of the impact of inclusive communication has found the benefits make investment in inclusive communications cost neutral or cost saving to the public sector in the medium to long term (Fraser of Allander Institute, University of Strathclyde, 2021).

Professional values, ethics and standards of practice

SLTs recognise, respect and equally value all forms of communication. Achieving communication is more important than how it is done. Inclusive communication good practice is the practical expression of this core value. The SLT professional body (UK) expects inclusive communication to be integral to all speech and language therapists' work (RCSLT, 2024a).

The SLT Professional Development Framework (UK) aspires to 'A profession that works proactively to reduce health inequalities and the impact of socioeconomic disadvantage on service users' (RCSLT, 2024b). Inclusive communication good practice is a proactive response to health inequalities and socioeconomic disadvantage.

Professional standards of conduct, performance and ethics require SLTs to take all practicable steps to meet service users' and carers' language and communication needs (HCPC, 2024a). For proficiency, SLTs must 'modify their own means of communication to address the individual communication needs and preferences of service users and carers and remove any barriers to communication where possible' (HCPC, 2024b).

The law

Inclusive communication environments enable everyone to enjoy their human rights and greater equality. They visibly demonstrate implementation of equality, diversity and inclusion law and policy.

Article 12 of the United Nations Convention on the Rights of the Child (2022) states: 'the child who can form his or her own views [has] the right to express those views freely . . .'. Article 13 states:

> The child shall have the right to freedom of expression; this right shall include freedom to seek, receive and impart information and ideas . . ., either orally, in writing or in print, in the form of art, or through any other media of the child's choice.
>
> (United Nations, 2022)

The Human Rights Act (1998) states everyone has the right to freedom of expression. The Equality Act (2010) requires service providers to take reasonable steps to provide accessible information. Additionally, the Public Sector Bodies (Websites and Mobile Applications) Accessibility Regulations (2018) require public sector bodies to ensure websites, apps and other online channels are accessible.

How to identify support needs in this area of practice

Communication diversity is the norm across any population or group. It is not necessary, therefore, to assess need before implementing inclusive communication good practice. However, there is value in finding out about communication needs and preferences at population and individual levels.

Communication needs and preferences data can do the following:

- prove that communication diversity exists in a population
- help to make the case for adoption of inclusive communication good practice
- show the level of demand and trends in needs and preferences in a population
- show the diversity (or not) of people accessing a service
- help organisations to work out the best ways, channels, and situations to use to reach a particular population and to design services accordingly
- help organisations to work out the budget required to pay for specialist communication support needs.

Finding out about needs at a population level

The likelihood of communication disadvantage, exclusion, needs, and preferences can be inferred from population data, much of which is regularly updated, public and freely available. For example, census data on ethnicity can indicate preferred spoken and written languages. Income and educational attainment data can indicate the likelihood of disability, physical and mental health, communication disadvantage associated with life circumstances or experiences, and financial capacity to pay costs, such as technology, transport and childcare. Health equity and inequalities audit tools also support reflection and analysis of population needs (Office for Health Improvement and Disparities, UK Government, n.d.; RCSLT, 2024c).

Finding out about needs at an individual level

Service providers should ideally find out about an individual's communication needs and preferences as early as possible in the service pathway or communication journey. Relevant questions can be incorporated into referral forms, client registration systems or initial conversations. Health records may also hold some relevant data. Various tools are available to help identify an individual's communication needs and preferences. These are called, for example, communication passports, digital passports or communication profiling tools (PAMIS, n.d.).

Implementing inclusive communication good practice: supporting three levels of good practice

Multiple interdependent influences shape inclusive communication environments, illustrated in the three levels in Figure 3.1.

The logic of this model is:

- Level C: Laws, policies, strategies and budgets enable -->
- Level B: Organisations to build the assets they need to enable -->

Inclusive communication 43

- Level A: Staff to implement inclusive communication good practice in their individual and population-level communications.

Inclusive communication good practice subsequently delivers equitable, diverse, affirmative and inclusive services, which in turn impact on child, family, community and service outcomes. Establishing inclusive communication environments involves more than a one-off or occasional training workshop for front-line staff. Sustained impact requires collaborative, strategic, systemic, and ongoing action (NHS England, 2022a).

A key purpose of the SLT service is to use their unique, expert knowledge of human-to-human communication to prevent, reduce or remove communication disadvantages. Facilitating inclusive communication good practice is therefore core to all SLT professional practice. SLT success in this area of practice, as in so many other areas, involves skilled collaboration and change management. Individual SLTs and SLT services play crucial leadership roles at all three levels of inclusive communication, as shown in Tables 3.1, 3.2 and 3.3. The need to implement inclusive communication good practice especially applies to SLT services themselves. Most speech and language therapists engage in some form of inclusive communication activity (RCSLT, 2016b). SLTs must lead by example if they are to secure a credible leadership position in respect of communication equity, diversity and inclusion.

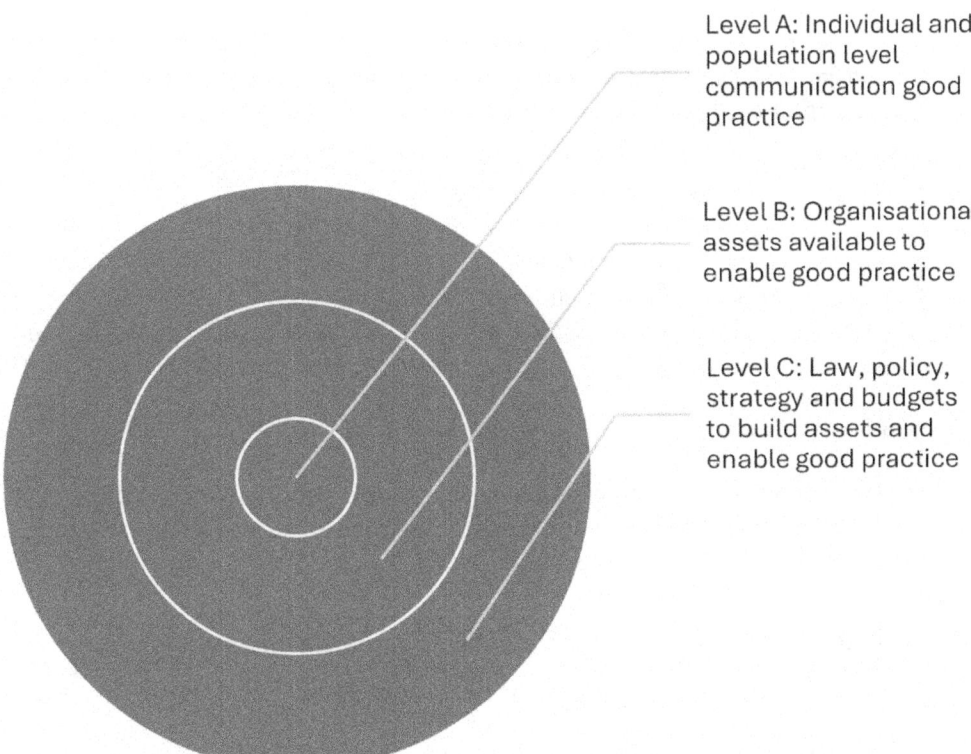

Figure 3.1 Three levels influencing inclusive communication good practice

Level A: Inclusive communication good practice at population and individual levels

Services communicate with individuals on two levels:

1. *Community, population or universal level communication* is generally managed by an organisation's communication team or leaders. It is designed to reach lots of people, many of them unknown to the organisation. It may have standard content, be permanent and available every day, all day. It includes, for example, standardised responses at a reception desk, answering machine messages, web pages, printed leaflets, standard appointment letters, advice sheets, and external and internal door signs.
2. *Individual level communication* is managed by individual staff. It is personal and targeted to a known person. It is specific to an interaction. It can be unique in content and 'bespoke' to an individual's needs and preferences. It includes, for example, communication during individual appointments, personal phone calls, letters, reports, emails, and client-specific advice.

Inclusive communication good practice must apply at both levels. If communication exclusion occurs at the population level, then individual level communication may never happen.

Multiple standards, principles and good practice guides have been published (Communication Access UK, 2024; RCSLT, 2013; Scottish Government, 2011). They share common elements, summarised below and in Table 3.1 as four elements of good practice essential to achieve inclusive communication.

Good practice 1: Recognise that every community includes diverse communication needs and preferences

At the population level, education, health and other child services communication teams and leaders:

- demonstrate an awareness of communication
- demonstrate an awareness of communication disadvantage and exclusion and a focused commitment to mainstreaming inclusive communication good practice across the organisation.

Individual staff in education, health and other child services:

- demonstrate a similar awareness of communication disadvantage and exclusion and a focused commitment to inclusive communication good practice in all their communications.

Good practice 2: Find out about communication needs and preferences

At the population level, communication teams and leaders:

- use data on the target populations to assess the risk of communication exclusion, diversity and inequity

- ask people about their communication needs and preferences for population-level activity, such as parents' events, meetings, and consultations.

Individual staff:

- ask people about their communication needs and preferences as soon as they can in a relationship
- access permitted information about people's communication needs and preferences.

Good practice 3: Act on communication needs and preferences

At the population level, communication teams and leaders:

- deliver the same quality of information and services on different channels, at flexible times, in physically and communication accessible buildings
- offer free specialist communication supports if people ask for them
- speak in a communication-inclusive way at community events, such as school assembly, parents' meetings and workshops
- write in a communication-inclusive way in forms, leaflets, waiting room posters and webpages
- provide communication-inclusive activities throughout the environment, on posters and display walls, and at events.

Individual staff:

- provide communication partners with a choice of two-way communication on different channels, at flexible times, in physically and communication accessible buildings
- arrange and use specialist communication supports if people ask for them
- provide inclusive information before, during and after contacts
- speak in a communication-inclusive way while teaching, during therapy sessions, and parent workshops
- write in a communication-inclusive way in all teaching and therapy materials, emails, text, letters, reports, notes, advice sheets for communication partners
- use communication-inclusive activities in the classroom and therapy sessions.

Good practice 4: Check and improve inclusive communication practice

At the population level communication teams and leaders:

- ask people what they think about the organisation's communication and how to improve it – and then act on these suggestions.

Individual staff:

- ask people what they think about their communication and how to improve it – and then act on these suggestions.

Good practice 1: Recognise every community includes diverse communication needs and preferences
- Establish positive, proactive attitudes towards communication equity, diversity and inclusion, not least by demonstrating through their own practice that it is desirable and 'doable'

Good practice 2: Find out about those needs and preferences
- Source and analyse data to help identify the relative risk of communication exclusion, diversity and inequity in a population
- Provide and support use of communication profiling across organisations
- Identify communication needs and preferences of individuals and populations

Good practice 3: Act on communication needs and preferences
- Provide advice, guidance, training, mentoring, coaching, supervision and practical resources to enable organisations and individual staff to do the following:
  o speak and write in a communication inclusive way
  o use communication inclusive activities throughout schools
  o improve communication accessibility of websites
  o set up communication accessible buildings and rooms
- use specialist communication support services

Good practice 4: Check and improve inclusive communication practice
- Support organisations and individual staff to evaluate, plan and implement inclusive communication improvements

Table 3.1 SLT roles at Level A: Establishing inclusive communication good practice

Level B: Organisational assets required to implement good practice

Inclusive communication good practice is more likely, and easier for staff to do, if five kinds of organisational assets are in place (Communication Inclusion People, 2024). They are described below and summarised in Table 3.2.

Asset 1: Leadership and ownership of inclusive communication

- Leaders and individual staff across services understand the impact of communication disadvantage on child and service outcomes
- They have an inclusive communication development plan, backed up by an adequate budget and realistic timelines (Independent Care Review, 2020).

Asset 2: Involvement of people who communicate in different ways

'Nothing about us without us' expresses the simple truth that services are better at meeting the needs of diverse service users if they are involved in the design, development, monitoring, delivery and evaluation of that service (Munro and RCSLT, n.d.; NHS England, 2022b; Patient Information Forum, 2023). Individuals who communicate in different ways are experts in identifying communication barriers and advising on ways to overcome those barriers.

- People who communicate in varied ways participate in service development, delivery and evaluation.
- Services have a budget to involve people who communicate in diverse ways.

Asset 3: Inclusive communication policy, standards, communication journeys

The design of service pathways or communication journeys can help or hinder inclusion. Policy and practice standards shape service design and thus service users' experience.

- Organisations have an inclusive communication policy and standards.
- Services give people a choice of ways, channels, and situations for communicating throughout a communication journey. Therefore, services flexibly respond to the needs and preferences of users, not the other way around.
- There is an easy-to-use system to record communication needs and preferences. Staff can access permitted information as required.
- Inclusive communication good practice is a standard requirement in all job descriptions.
- Inclusive communication practice is evaluated as part of the quality assurance process.

Asset 4: Attitudes, knowledge and skills (competencies)

All staff need knowledge of inclusive communication good practice and skills to implement it effectively (Disabled Children and Young People Advisory Group, 2023; Independent Care Review, 2020). This requires:

- a shared list of the competencies (attitudes, knowledge and skills) employees require to implement inclusive communication good practice
- an ongoing, team-wide competency development programme
- in-house champions to support sustained improvements
- a shared, open bank of user-friendly guidelines on how to speak, write and set up a room in an inclusive way.

Asset 5: Practical resources

Staff are more likely to implement their inclusive communication competencies if the practical resources they need are easy to access and use (Independent Care Review, 2020). This requires:

- inclusive spaces outside and throughout the environment
- a bank of communication-inclusive document templates set up with inclusive styles, spacing, icons, layout, and so on
- a bank of symbols and photographs representing common vocabulary for different settings and activities
- an easy system for booking specialist communication support services.

Asset 1: Leadership and ownership of inclusive communication • Raise awareness of communication disadvantage and exclusion and the impacts on outcomes for individuals, communities and services • Build a commitment to inclusive communication good practice from leaders and staff across child services • Jointly assess current practice and the organisational assets available to a service or school • Co-produce an inclusive communication development plan including timelines, budget estimates
Asset 2: Involvement of people who communicate in different ways • Help services to involve people who communicate in diverse ways in processes such as service development, delivery and evaluation
Asset 3: Inclusive communication policy, standards, communication journeys • Co-produce, agree and communicate inclusive communication policy and standards based on good practice set out above. A policy may be as simple as 'All staff in (this place) will implement inclusive communication good practice standards in communications with (these people).' • Co-audit communication journeys experienced by children and parents. For example, the journey for joining in a parents' group, school club or participating in parents' evenings. • Provide advice on service designs which implement standards of good practice at each stage of communication journeys.
Asset 4: Attitudes, knowledge and skills (competencies) • Model inclusive communication good practice in their own communication • Provide a competency framework for inclusive communication good practice • Co-assess competencies. This may involve staff self-assessment and observations by SLTs, children and their communication partners. Co-produce and deliver sustainable knowledge and skills programmes. This may include workshops, online learning modules, coaching and mentoring staff and developing a network of inclusive communication champions.

Asset 5: Practical resources
• Provide user-friendly, co-produced material:
  o Communication profiling tools or questions for forms
  o Communication inclusive templates, for example for letters, worksheets and posters
  o Checklists for setting up inclusive places
  o Icons and photo banks
• Help to connect schools with locally available specialist communication support services

Table 3.2 SLT roles at Level B: Developing organisational assets
Source: (RCSLT, 2016b; 2024b).

Level C: Law, policy, strategy and budgets

Laws, policies, strategies, and available budgets influence the interest and capacity of service providers to build the assets they need to enable staff to implement inclusive communication good practice. SLTs have a leading role in shaping these influences, in partnership with other leaders, the public and politicians. Table 3.3 presents roles for SLTs at Level C.

Participate in campaigns led by professional bodies or service user organisations Respond to national and local government consultations Provide case studies and data on the costs and benefits of inclusive communication good practice

Table 3.3 Indicative SLT roles at Level C: Influencing law, policy and standards

Good practice example: a communication-inclusive classroom

The whole school, inside and outside, should be communication-inclusive. That includes classrooms, meeting rooms, corridors, reception, gym, lunch halls, displays and the playground. Table 3.4 shows features of a communication-inclusive classroom.

Examples

Example 1: This project aims to reduce pupil anxiety during transitions between activities. Object signifiers were used to explain to pupils what was happening. Teaching staff noticed that pupils were generally calmer at times of transition. Staff reported increased confidence with supporting pupil cognition. Available at: https://www.rcslt.org/wp-content/uploads/media/Project/case-study-4-whole-school.pdf (accessed 3 December 2024).

Example 2: This service uses communication passports to tell hospital staff about children's communication needs and preferences. Children also receive photograph information about the hospital before they go. The service has received very positive feedback from children, families and from hospital staff. Available at: https://www.rcslt.org/wp-content/uploads/media/Project/case-study-6-smooth-transitions.pdf (accessed 3 December 2024).

Example 3: This project used 'Talking Mats' (a visual tool used to elicit opinions or choices) to identify children's priorities for their own education and health care plans. Talking Mats empowered students to make meaningful decisions about their future, communicate where they would like further support and discuss likes and dislikes. Available at: https://www.talkingmats.com/ehc-plans-with-the-talking-mats-app/ (accessed 3 December 2024).

---

1. A clear inclusive sign on the door with a large 'classroom symbol', a photograph of the teacher and the teacher's name in large print
2. A bright, naturally lit room with the teacher illuminated from the front
3. As 'low arousal' sound and sight environment as possible, including matt walls, strong colour contrast between walls and furniture, and soft furnishing to reduce echo
4. A box of 'fidget' toys
5. Child-sized desks and chairs in small groups or pairs, positioned so that all pupils can easily see and hear the teacher and information without twisting round
6. A quiet space with one or two chairs for quiet time or 1-to-1 work
7. A visual timetable on the wall, and individual visual timetables available
8. Labels with object signifiers, symbols or photographs, large, simple text on cupboards, zones, pupils' chairs, boxes or lockers
9. A few display boards, at child height, with muted backing paper to avoid overwhelming some pupils
10. 'Talkie tins' so pupils can record what the display is about, and pre-readers can understand it. And the option of adding laminated 'thumbs up' to comment on the display.
11. Staff who use different ways to communicate
12. Staff who are responsive to the different ways learners communicate
13. Worksheets with communication-inclusive writing – simple sentences, in a logical order, spaced layout, accessible font and symbols and/or photographs
14. A bank of object signifiers, symbols and / or photographs covering various topics for use on timetables, choice making, white or black boards, etc.
15. A library with books to read or listen to online. And age-appropriate toys.

Table 3.4 Fifteen features of a communication-inclusive classroom

Summary

Communication diversity is the norm in every community or group. Inclusive communication means including as many people as possible in any communication. Inclusive communication environments embed inclusive communication good practice. In doing so, they remove or reduce disadvantages or exclusion caused by communication diversity. Such environments encompass ways of communicating, channels of communications and situational factors. Inclusive communication is important at every stage of a communication journey. Inclusive communication helps everyone. It is essential for many people with and without communication disability. There is a strong ethical, clinical, legal, social and business case for implementing inclusive communication good practice. Multiple interdependent influences shape inclusive communication environments. Finding out about and acting on communication needs and preferences is fundamental to inclusive communication good practice.

SLTs have a key leadership role in establishing inclusive communication good practice. It is a growing area of SLT practice which offers significant opportunities to children, families, communities, society, and the SLT profession.

Recommended resources

This list is a snapshot of resources at the time of writing. Sharing tried and tested resources among children's services could enhance practice considerably.

Contacts and networks

Communication Inclusion People: https://www.communicationinclusionpeople.com/
RCSLT Inclusive Communication Overview (extra content including networks available to members): https://www.rcslt.org/speech-and-language-therapy/inclusive-communication-overview/

Creating accessible documents

https://abilitynet.org.uk/sites/abilitynet.org.uk/files/Creating-accessible-documents-Easy-Read.pdf?utm_source=Website0&utm_medium=CreatingAccessibleDocsEasyReadPDF&utm_campaign=EasyRead

Creating a communication supportive educational environment (Speech and Language UK)

https://speechandlanguage.org.uk/educators-and-professionals/resource-library-for-educators/creating-a-communication-supportive-environment-primary/

Communication profiling tools

https://www.communicationpassports.org.uk/Home/index.php#:~:text=Personal%20Communication%20Passports.%20For%20anyone%20who%20needs%20help%20to%20communicate

Symbols/visual resources

Microsoft 365: https://support.microsoft.com/en-gb/office/insert-icons-in-microsoft-365-e2459f17-3996-4795-996e-b9a13486fa79
Symbol sets: https://inclusivecommunication.scot/symbol-sets
Talking Mats: https://www.talkingmats.com/

References

Communication Access UK (2024) Let's talk about communication. Available at: https://communication-access.co.uk/ (accessed 2 December 2024).

Communication Inclusion People (2024) Is your organisation communication inclusive? Available at: http://communicationinclusionpeople.com (accessed 29 November 2024).

Disabled Children and Young People Advisory Group (2023) '"Seen, Heard, Included" Report: Supporting meaningful engagement and participation'. Available at: https://www.alliance-scotland.org.uk/blog/resources/seen-heard-included-report/ (accessed 2 December 2024).

Equality Act (2010) Available at: https://www.legislation.gov.uk/ukpga/2010/15/contents (accessed 4 December 2024).

Fraser of Allander Institute, University of Strathclyde (2021) 'The financial case for inclusive communications: A report for the Royal College of Speech and Language Therapists (RCSLT) and Camphill Scotland'. Available at: http://rcslt.org/wp-content/uploads/2021/04/The-Financial-Case-for-the-Inclusive-CommunicationsBill-Final-002.pdf (accessed 29 November 2024).

Health and Care Professions Council (2024a) 'Standards of Conduct, Performance and Ethics'. Available at: https://www.hcpc-uk.org/standards/standards-of-conduct-performance-and-ethics/ (accessed 4 December2024).

Health and Care Professions Council (2024b) 'Standards of Proficiency for Speech and Language Therapists'. Available at: https://www.hcpc-uk.org/standards/standards-of-proficiency/speech-and-language-therapists/ (accessed 4 December 2024).

Health and Social Care Alliance Scotland (2024) 'ALLIANCE Literature review: Children and young people's experiences of social care'. Available at: http://alliance-scotland.org.uk/blog/news/alliance-literature-review-children-and-young-peoples-experiences-of-social-care/ (accessed 29 November 2024).

Healthcare Improvement Scotland (2018) 'Your Voice Citizens' Panel: Survey on HIV awareness, mental health and wellbeing and inclusive communication'. Available at: https://www.hisengage.scot/media/1165/fourth_citizens_panel_report_may18.pdf (accessed 2 December 2024).

Human Rights Act (1998) Available at: https://www.legislation.gov.uk/ukpga/1998/42/contents (accessed 4 December 2024).

Independent Care Review (2020) 'The Promise'. Available at: http://thepromise.scot/resources/2020/the-promise.pdf (accessed 29 November 2024).

Munro, S. and Royal College of Speech and Language Therapists (n.d.) 'Case study: Communication champions in Tayside save 295 hours of SLT time'. Available at: https://www.rcslt.org/wp-content/uploads/media/Project/case-study-7-comms-champions.pdf (accessed 2 December 2024).

NHS England (2022a) 'Tackling inequalities in healthcare access, experience, and outcomes: Actionable insights'. Available at: https://www.england.nhs.uk/wp-content/uploads/2022/07/B1779-Actionable-Insights-Tackling-inequalities-in-healthcare-access-experience-and-outcomes-guidance-July-202.pdf (accessed 2 December 2024).

NHS England (2022b) 'The benefits of partnership with people and communities'. Available at: https://www.england.nhs.uk/wp-content/uploads/2022/09/benefits-of-partnership.jpg (accessed 2 December 2024).

Office for Health Improvement and Disparities, UK Government (n.d.) 'Health Equity Assessment Tool (HEAT): What it is and how to use it'. Available at: https://www.gov.uk/government/publications/health-equity-assessment-tool-heat/health-equity-assessment-tool-heat-executive-summary(accessed 2 December 2024).

PAMIS (Promoting a More Inclusive Society) (n.d.) 'Digital passports: Supporting inclusive communication'. Available at: https://pamis.org.uk/services/digital-passports/ (accessed 2 December 2024).

Patient Information Forum (2023) 'Co-production: Involving users in developing health information'. Available at: https://pifonline.org.uk/resources/involving-users/(accessed 2 December 2024).

Public Sector Bodies (Websites and Mobile Applications) Accessibility Regulations (2018) Available at: https://www.legislation.gov.uk/uksi/2018/952/contents (accessed 4 December 2024).

RCSLT (Royal College of Speech and Language Therapists) (2013) 'Five good communication standards'. Available at: https://www.rcslt.org/wp-content/uploads/media/Project/RCSLT/good-comm-standards.pdf#:~:text=The%20five%20good%20communication%20standards:%20Standard%201:%20There%20is%20a (accessed 2 December 2024).

RCSLT (Royal College of Speech and Language Therapists) (2016a) 'Speech, Language and Communication Capacity. A national asset: The intergenerational cycle of speech, language and communication outcomes and risks'. Available at: http://rcslt.org/wp-content/uploads/media/Project/RCSLT/rcslt-communication-capacity-factsheet.pdf (accessed 29 November 2024).

RCSLT (Royal College of Speech and Language Therapists) (2016b) 'Position paper: Inclusive communication and the role of speech and language therapy'. Available at: https://www.rcslt.org/wp-content/uploads/2021/02/20162209_InclusiveComms_final.pdf (accessed 2 December 2024).

RCSLT (Royal College of Speech and Language Therapists) (2024a) 'Inclusive communication overview'. Available at: http://rcslt.org/speech-and-language-therapy/inclusive-communication-overview/(accessed 29 November 2024).

RCSLT (Royal College of Speech and Language Therapists) (2024b) 'The professional development framework'. Available at: http://rcslt.org/professional-development-framework/(accessed 29 November 2024).

RCSLT (Royal College of Speech and Language Therapists) (2024c) 'Health inequalities resources and references'. Available at: http://rcslt.org/learning/diversity-inclusion-and-anit-racism/health-inequalities/resources/(accessed 29 November 2024).

Scottish Government (2011) 'Principles of inclusive communication: An information and self-assessment tool for public authorities'. Available at: https://www.gov.scot/publications/principles-inclusive-communication-information-self-assessment-tool-public-authorities/pages/9/ (accessed 2 December 2024).

Stoiber, K.C., Ruehl, C.A., Landry, K.K., Smith, A.A. and Brosig, C.L. (2024) 'Enhancing interprofessional interagency collaboration for minoritized and low income children with chronic illnesses', *School Psychology*, 39(4), 395–406. https://doi.org/10.1037/spq000632

United Nations (2022) 'Convention on the Rights of the Child'. Available at: https://www.unicef.org.uk/what-we-do/un-convention-child-rights/ (accessed 4 December 2024).

4 Augmentative and Alternative Communication (AAC)

Janice Murray

What you'll learn in this chapter

This chapter will support you to consider how AAC impacts clinical decision-making and intervention across a range of speech, language and communication diagnoses in children. Specifically, it will explore:

- AAC user identity
- AAC service structures and provision
- AAC terminology
- AAC assessment and recommendation processes
- AAC intervention and management
- Awareness of professional AAC skills, knowledge and clinical competencies.

Key information about AAC

Identity: why AAC is relevant to children with a range of SLCN

Across the lifespan, children and young people may have varying reasons to use augmentative and alternative communication (AAC) techniques, strategies or systems. Reasons may mean occasional AAC use, permanent AAC use or AAC use over a specific period of time. Individuals may be described as AAC users or not. How such labels are applied will be influenced by several things. It is important to stop and think about why certain AAC labels are being used at any point in time. These labels may be influenced by diagnosis, educational and social contexts, perceptions of ability, and attitudes towards the individual. Most importantly, the child or young person's perception of self will impact on how AAC approaches are introduced and described.

There are very few instances of speech, language and communication needs (SLCN) in children and young people where an AAC strategy, technique or system could not be of value. The core influence of AAC will be summarised in this chapter and demonstrated across the rest of this book.

How are AAC services organised in the UK?

Before considering the theoretical and practical field of AAC, it is helpful to understand how services and AAC resources are made available according to the area of the UK where you

DOI: 10.4324/9781003671626-6

live. The four nations of the UK recognise the need to support children and young people who may benefit from AAC. However, there are differences in the policy, service structure and delivery in each nation, reflected in their referral processes and how people can access AAC services. These are long-established differences in service provision. This is detailed in the recently updated RCSLT Clinical Guidance in AAC (RCSLT, 2024). For ease, aspects of service structure are summarised here, with a link in the key online resources section to current policy documentation provided by the RCSLT (2024).

England offers a hub-and-spoke structure, where the 14 specialist services act as hubs covering 10% of the AAC population who meet strict referral criteria. The remaining 90% of AAC users are supported at a spoke (local) level through statutory or independent assessment and by accessing various funding sources.

In Northern Ireland, there are five Health and Social Care Trusts and one Regional Specialist AAC service. There are specific referral criteria for the specialist service. SLTs in the five Trusts work collaboratively with the regional team to support AAC users.

Scotland has two national AAC services for children. They support 12 of the 14 health boards The remaining two health boards have local (commissioned) specialist services. All tertiary services work collaboratively with the local services. There are no specific referral criteria.

Wales has one national AAC service offering assessment and provision for electronic AAC. The seven Health Boards provide a range of non-powered solutions via local specialist SLT services. There are criteria for referral to both local and national services. All funding routes are via NHS-Wales.

Defining AAC for children

There are numerous debates about the terminology that is or should be used to describe types of AAC. The key elements are defined here with more extensive descriptions available from many online sources. Two key UK sources of AAC terminology can be found on the Communication Matters website and in the RCSLT clinical guidelines in AAC. Hyperlinks for both sources are included in the Recommended Resources section at the end of this chapter. Further terminology considerations can be found in the textbook in the 'Working with' series, *Working with AAC* (Robinson, 2025).

AAC is often conceptualised as only meaning electronic communication devices. This is inaccurate and belies the complexity of the field of AAC. AAC can more accurately describe differing tools, devices, techniques and strategies used to enhance speech, language and communication where the individual cannot always rely on their own speech to convey their message.

There are two broad types of AAC: unaided and aided methods of communication:

> *Unaided communication* refers to the use of methods involving the user's body, such as body movements, facial expressions, gestures, key word signing, sign languages, eye-pointing, fixed gaze and vocalisations. One form of unaided communication includes a familiar person 're-voicing' the AAC users' speech. Even with compromised physical abilities, unaided methods of communication can be quick and effective for many AAC users.
> (RCSLT, 2024)

Aided communication involves the use of physical tools and techniques. These can include paper-based materials as well as electronic devices. Aided communication methods are rarely as quick as an unaided method but for many can offer more communication autonomy.

(RCSLT, 2024)

Another point of terminology confusion arises from the inaccurate use of the term non-verbal. This is often used inappropriately to describe anyone who uses AAC as their main way of communicating. When the term non-verbal is used accurately, there may be some specific meaning intended by the child, but most signals used rely on the *communication partner's linguistic (verbal) abilities* or knowledge of the child to interpret. The types of AAC in use when someone could be described as non-verbal would include skills like vocalisations with intonation, laughter, crying, body movements and gestures as well as eye movements and gaze direction. All other forms of AAC require the user to have verbal (or linguistic) knowledge, therefore they should not be described as non-verbal just because the user cannot speak. In these instances, the AAC user will communicate their language skills via anything from pictures, symbol-graphics to the written word, or a combination. To complicate things a little further, verbal skills can be demonstrated using unaided forms of AAC (e.g., sign vocabularies and sign languages), or aided forms of AAC (e.g., paper-based communication charts or folders, and electronic communication). Incidentally, AAC users, like all of us, rarely employ just one form of AAC, for example, they may use their eyes and vocalisations in combination with a communication device.

It is worth noting that the vocabulary you can make available on paper-based AAC systems can be as extensive and as complex as many electronic communication aids, busting another myth that you are more intellectually able if you use electronic devices. In fact, you could have the vocabulary App used on an electronic device printed off and replicated in a paper-based folder. Why might you do that? Well, battery-powered devices can be less reliable, or it may be helpful for the AAC user to be able to see all pages in their folder to learn how to navigate to the vocabulary on their electronic device. We'll return to reasons for choosing different vocabulary set-up and navigation options later in this chapter. One key benefit of an electronic device is that it usually offers the user a range of outputs, i.e., different spoken voices, picture, symbol-graphic and/or the written word. You may be surprised that I have reached this point and not named any AAC device or system. This is for two reasons: (1) names and types change all the time, so, it would quickly date this book in an unhelpful way, and (2) what you need to be able to do is describe and understand the attributes of any AAC system or device. The terms provided in this chapter, and the online links to further descriptions, will allow you to always appraise any new system or device.

Important points about SLT practice and AAC

The principles underpinning AAC introduction include recognition of the unique needs of the individual and how their needs vary across the contexts they inhabit (see Chapter 3). Communication abilities, challenges or differences may relate to physical, sensory, neurodivergent perspectives, learning or cognitive abilities. AAC systems must always be customised to match the characteristics of the child or young person, but as they are on a trajectory of change (usually developing), identifying the right AAC system for now that will still be right in five- and ten-years' time is critical.

Opting to include AAC resources in any therapy management plan is likely to mean that you have considered the different attributes of the AAC system chosen and its relevance to the presenting characteristics of the child (Murray et al., 2019). For example, an AAC system can help a child to organise their thoughts and ideas, support their understanding of a context, develop speech, language and communication skills, build relationships and gain a sense of their identity. In some instances, the child may have established speech and language but is losing these skills. Key to all of this is working out what is most important to the young person and those around them. The impact of communication partners is considered in detail in Chapter 5 but the introduction of AAC will always involve training communication partners. It is important to remember here that partners vary tremendously. Who are those partners? Across the day for the child, it could include paid staff, family members, classmates, friends and the general public. Remaining mindful of who the partners are will result in differing training content.

Understanding the need to use AAC

Having considered some of the attributes of AAC tools and systems, the most critical aspect of getting a good match between a child and an AAC system is comprehensive assessment. How you approach assessment does not need to be from a deficit perspective, such as unintelligible speech, but can readily be from a more functional, dynamic and positive perspective, for example, speech is intelligible to some people in most contexts. The process of assessing a child's speech, language and communication skills where AAC is a consideration should be as comprehensive and robust as it might be for a child with developmental language disorder (DLD) where AAC is *not* being considered.

Comprehensive assessment processes

An AAC assessment should include speech, language and communication appraisal. It will differ in how the assessment may be conducted, especially as the child may have difficulty pointing or speaking a response to an assessment item (i.e., the most typical types of assessment responses required). Unfortunately, there are limited standardised measures for children or young people who could benefit from AAC. In the absence of such assessments, we can and should use standardised measures but use them descriptively. Several clinical cases are described where standard measures have been used with minor adaptations, for example, by placing standardised picture material on an Eye-Transfer (E-Tran) frame (https://www.rcslt.org/members/clinical-guidance/augmentative-and-alternative-communication/augmentative-and-alternative-communication-guidance/#section-4) and using gaze as the method of indicating a choice (Robinson, 2025: Smith, 2023). Importantly, taking this practical and pragmatic approach to assessment enables you to describe abilities and note changes at a point in time, logging speech, language and communication details that will allow you to demonstrate changes in abilities over time (Lynch et al., 2019; Murray et al., 2019).

In addition to standardised assessments, there is a plethora of observational, descriptive and dynamic resources in the form of checklists, profiles, and scales. These are mostly ordered in what is regarded as a typical developmental trajectory, for example, language comprehension checklists, speech and communication scales, pragmatic profiles. These can also add to the detailed description of the child's current abilities.

AAC-specific resources

A few AAC-specific assessment tools are in regular use in the UK. This section is a summary of what is detailed in the assessment section of the RCSLT AAC clinical guidance and included in a link in the online resources section (RCSLT, 2024; Robinson, 2025).

- *Communication Competence*: This framework is strongly embedded in AAC clinical practice (e.g., Light, 1989). It describes four key elements of competence in an AAC user (operational, linguistic, strategic and social). It focuses on the AAC users' competence but does not really consider the competencies of the communication partner. More recently, the framework has been extended to include context of use (Light et al., 2019). It has a bias towards electronic rather than paper-based AAC systems.
- *Identifying Appropriate Symbol Communication (I-ASC)*: A more recent UK- developed framework that has already gained traction in the clinical field is the I-ASC Explanatory Model of clinical decision making (Lynch et al., 2019; Murray et al., 2019; https://iasc.mmu.ac.uk/i-asc-explanatory-model-of-aac-decision-making/). It specifically considers children and explores the holistic elements of an AAC assessment and recommendation process, for example, beyond the child to include levels of support, attitudes and skills, and periods of transition.
- *Means, Reasons and Opportunities*: This model is useful for exploring what vocabulary an AAC system might include (https://agrainofsalt1.wordpress.com/author/agrainofsalt123/).
- *The Participation Model*: This comprehensive model focuses on assessment as a dynamic process that needs continual revisiting as people learn new skills (Beukelman and Mirenda, 2013). It considers four components of the support process: (1) identification of complex challenges, (2) access and opportunity barriers affecting participation, (3) the scope of intervention, and (4) monitoring progress.
- *The Communication Matrix*: This helps you identify how a child communicates currently to inform the development of intervention-communication goals (Rowland et al., 2016; https://www.communicationmatrix.org/uploads/pdfs/handbook.pdf). Originally designed to explore the expressive communication skills of children with profound and multiple disabilities, it covers communication most often emerging between 0 and 24 months of age.

Also, embedded in the UK assessment or AAC decision-making processes are two resources that support AAC users, family members and staff to identify what is important to the user. These are Talking Mats (Murphy and Boa, 2013) and Personal Communication Passports (Millar and Aitken, 2003).

All assessment resources and the reports they contribute to will inform an AAC system recommendation and intervention plan. Recommendation reports should include insights into the following:

- the perspectives, preferences and aspirations of the child who will use AAC, their family members and supporters
- the multimodal aspects of communication and the range of AAC systems that may be helpful to an individual user, e.g., an individual's AAC package may include objects of reference, key word sign and a tablet device
- recognition of unaided forms of communication as core to the user's identity, e.g., gesture, vocalisation, facial expression
- the range of vocabulary that an AAC system should offer the user
- the way that vocabulary should be (visually) represented for the individual (e.g. written, graphic, photographic and/or real object)
- how the vocabulary can be organised (e.g., columns may best suit some, rather than rows)
- the preferred or possible method/s of accessing any aided AAC (e.g., direct or indirect access)
- the use of voice output or animation options
- how the chosen vocabulary should be able to support the individual as they develop or lose language abilities.

This bullet point summary is adapted from the AAC guidelines (RCSLT, 2024).

Supporting children's needs in AAC

AAC is used to enable language learning, enhanced communication and access to education. This section outlines key intervention considerations.

The decision to introduce any AAC tool, technique or strategy will be part of an intervention plan. Merely creating or acquiring the AAC resource is always the start of the process, not its conclusion. Let me give you an analogy of what you are aiming to achieve: merely acquiring the piano will not make a child a concert pianist or even a Grade 2 pianist. Input and time are required. Typically, AAC interventions need to be completed over many years, especially when related to children developing and attaining ever more complex language and communication skills. While I have used this example already, I revisit it here specific to SLT interventions: if you were working with a child with a diagnosis of DLD, you'd expect to be involved and planning intervention developments for years. The same expectation should apply to those using any aspect of AAC. It is the exception, rather than the rule, that you provide the AAC system and then discharge from SLT services. You should expect to provide on-going episodes of care over many years for most users of any type of AAC (Smith, 2023: Smith and Murray, 2016).

Implementation considerations specific to AAC must consider three foci of intervention: (1) the organisation of the vocabulary, (2) AAC-specific teaching and learning, and (3) non-AAC specific interventions that resonate with AAC. There are other elements that will impact on intervention, e.g., access to methods training, staffing support resources. Across these three areas, however, this chapter focuses on the key role for any SLT, and this is language, not technology, focused.

Vocabulary organisation relates to the options you have for arranging vocabulary on whatever system is used, i.e., paper-based or electronic. Some organisational arrangements are determined by the choice of symbol-graphic or representation system/s chosen. Theoretically organisational systems would be described as encoded, semantic/schematic, taxonomic and/or semantic (Beukelman and Mirenda, 2013; Smith and Murray, 2016). That said, you are more likely to be aware of their related description terms, e.g., semantic compaction, core and fringe vocabulary, visual scene display, phrase-based display, pragmatic organisation and grid displays. More information about the evidence base for any of these organisational features can be found on the RCSLT website guidance pages (RCSLT, 2024). Detailed considerations are also given in Sadiku et al. (2022), Smith (2023), Smith and Murray (2016), and Robinson (2025).

AAC-specific teaching and learning methods of intervention offer you a range of strategies to enhance learning and skills development in AAC system use. Theoretically, they can be summarised as language interventions, motor patterning approaches, cause and effect strategies, partner-assisted intervention approaches, and person-centred participatory approaches. In addition, there are several lesson-plan outlines available on various AAC supplier websites. Communication Matters' website provides up-to-date information about current AAC suppliers (see Recommended resources). These intervention approaches have been appraised for their evidence base as part of the RCSLT AAC guidance and include specific examples, such as aided language stimulation, conversational scaffolds, narrative therapy, language acquisition through motor planning (LAMP), intensive interaction, Picture Exchange Communication System, (PECS) (RCSLT, 2024). Considerations are also given in Smith (2023) and Robinson (2025).

Non-AAC-specific teaching and learning methods that are relevant to AAC intervention plans include approaches that emerge from theoretical concepts of person-centred design and participatory interventions, or linguistic approaches related to the teaching of grammar. Specifically, these could include traditional language intervention approaches, cultural awareness methods, parent-child interaction methods, and DLD interventions (detailed in RCSLT, 2024).

In summary, there are many approaches to AAC intervention and remaining aware of different intervention strategies can usefully inform your clinical decision-making. These AAC elements will be expanded, as appropriate, in other chapters of this book.

Examples

For some specific examples of AAC intervention processes, consider looking up the following chapters from Smith's (2023) clinical cases textbook:

- Gita and decisions around her AAC needs (Chapter 2 by Lynch and Murray).
- Emerging communicators' journey of development (Chapter 3 by McCleary and Lynch).
- Bridging the gaps of potential – from speech intelligibility to representation of language

ability (Chapter 4 by Harrington et al.).
- Language and literacy learning in AAC (Chapter 5 by Clendon and Erikson).
- Autism spectrum disorder and AAC considerations (Chapter 6 by White et al.; Chapter 7 by Allen et al.).
- Personal perspectives from a parent and young person (Chapter 8 by Fitzpatrick et al.).

Defining your own AAC knowledge and skills

And a final word, as an SLT, there is courage to be found in understanding your current and aspirational knowledge and skills in AAC. A resource to support you understand what you know now and what you might want to develop is Informing and Profiling Augmentative and Alternative Communication (AAC) Knowledge and Skills (IPAACKS, https://www.aacscotland.org.uk/files/cm/files/ipaacks.pdf). Among many other elements and uses of this resource, there are four levels of knowledge to support SLTs to appraise where they are in their AAC career, and it offers a means of planning for your own AAC professional development.

Summary

This chapter has introduced you to key considerations in the application of AAC techniques, tools and systems. In particular, you are asked to remain mindful of the range of ways in which children and young people may regard themselves as AAC users, or users of AAC techniques. Their sense of identity may be influenced by people, contexts and experiences.

Wherever you work in the UK, you need to consider that AAC service structures and provisions vary. The range of current and historical terminology used to describe aspects of AAC varies tremendously. It is important to be aware of the many AAC synonyms in use. It is critical to be clear about ways of describing AAC users and recognise when the descriptions being used are not accurate.

AAC assessment and recommendation processes should be detailed and will take time. It is important to complete a comprehensive assessment of current language and communication skills prior to any AAC recommendation. Recommendation and provision of AAC are the beginning of the process.

AAC intervention and management are likely to be required for a considerable period of time to support the young person to develop their language and communication skills. This is analogous to the time expected to support a child with DLD and no AAC needs.

And, finally, there are resources available to help you appraise your current and aspirational AAC skills, knowledge and clinical competencies.

Acknowledgements

Grateful thanks to the author team for the RCSLT AAC Clinical guidance: Sinead Barker, Bronagh Blaney, Claire Cardador, Mary Dunningham, Gillian Hazell, Jenny Herd, Catherine Martin, Beth Moulam, Jamie Preece, Katie Radtke, Katherine Small, Emma Sullivan, Helen Whittle with Janice Murray.

Recommended resources

ACE Centre. Available at: https://acecentre.org.uk/resources
CALL Scotland. Available at: https://www.callscotland.org.uk/
Communication Matrix. Available at: https://www.communicationmatrix.org/
Communication Matters. Available at: https://www.communicationmatters.org.uk/
Identifying Appropriate Symbol Communication (I-ASC, 2019). Available at: https://iasc.mmu.ac.uk/i-asc-explanatory-model-of-aac-decision-making/
NHS Education Scotland. 'Informing and Profiling AAC Knowledge and Skills (IPAACKs)'. Available at: https://www.aacscotland.org.uk/files/cm/files/ipaacks.pdf
Means, Reasons and Opportunities. Available at: https://agrainofsalt1.wordpress.com/author/agrainofsalt123/
RCSLT (Royal College of Speech and Language Therapists) (2024) 'AAC (Augmentative and alternative communication) guidance'. Available at: https://www.rcslt.org/members/clinical-guidance/augmentative-and-alternative-communication/augmentative-and-alternative-communication-guidance

References

Beukelman, D. and Mirenda, P. (2013) *Augmentative and Alternative Communication: Supporting Children and Adults with Complex Communication Needs*. 4th edn. Baltimore, MD: Paul H. Brookes.
Light, J. (1989) 'Toward a definition of communicative competence for individuals using augmentative and alternative communication systems', *Augmentative and Alternative Communication*, 5(2), 137-144.
Light, J., McNaughton, D. and Caron, J. (2019) 'New and emerging AAC technology supports for children with complex communication needs and their communication partners: State of the science and future research directions', *Augmentative and Alternative Communication*, 35(1), 26-41.
Lynch, Y., Murray, J., Moulam, L., Meredith, S., Goldbart, J., Smith, M., Batorowicz, B., Randall, N. and Judge, S. (2019) 'Decision-making in communication aid recommendations in the UK: Cultural and contextual influencers', *Augmentative and Alternative Communication*, 35(3), 180-192.
Millar, S. and Aitken, S. (2003) *Personal Communication Passports: Guidelines For Good Practice*. Edinburgh: CALL Centre.
Murphy, J. and Boa, S. (2013) *A critical Appraisal of Existing Methods of Measuring Outcomes in Relation to Augmentative and Alternative Communication*. Edinburgh: NHS Education for Scotland.
Murray, J., Lynch, Y., Meredith, S., Moulam, L., Goldbart, J., Smith, M., Randall, N. and Judge, S. (2019) 'Professionals' decision making in recommending communication aids in the UK: Competing considerations', *Augmentative and Alternative Communication*, 35(3), 167-179.
RCSLT (Royal College of Speech and Language Therapists) (2024) 'AAC (Augmentative and alternative communication) guidance'. Available at: https://www.rcslt.org/members/clinical-guidance/augmentative-and-alternative-communication/augmentative-and-alternative-communication-guidance
Robinson, H. (2025) *Working with AAC: A Guide for Supporting Augmentative and Alternative Communication Users*. London: Routledge.
Rowland, C., Fried-Oken, M., Bowser, G., Granlund, M., Lollar, D., Phelps, R., Simeonsson, R.J. and Steiner, S.A. (2016) 'The Communication Supports Inventory-Children and Youth (CSI-CY): A new instrument based on the ICF-CY', *Disability and Rehabilitation*, 38(19), 1909-1917.
Sadiku, L., Small, K. and Martin, S. (2022) 'Augmentative and alternative communication', in S. Pert (ed.), *Working with Children Experiencing Speech and Language Disorders in s Bilingual Context: A Home Language Approach*. London: Routledge, pp. 182-196.
Smith, M.M. (ed.). (2023) *Clinical Cases in Augmentative and Alternative Communication*. London: Routledge. https://doi.org/10.4324/9781003106739
Smith, M.M. and Murray, J. (eds) (2016) *The Silent Partner? Language, Interaction and Aided Communication*. Guildford: J&R Press Limited.

5 Communication partners

Hayley Moroke

What you'll learn in this chapter

- What a communication partner is, and what they can do
- Why it is important for speech and language therapists (SLTs) to work with communication partners
- How communication partners can contribute to understanding children's speech, language and communication needs (SLCN)
- Why communication partners' needs and preferences are important
- How to support children's SLCN *together with* communication partners
- Possible challenges and how to overcome them.

Key information about communication partners

Who are communication partners? A communication partner is someone who supports the two-way interaction between themselves and another person. They should help communication to be successful and inclusive by making the appropriate adaptations within different interactions. Communication partners are fundamental in supporting children's SLCN. Essentially, communication partners can be anyone who is interacting with the child or young person on a regular basis and is supporting their communication.

Here is a list with some examples of communication partners. This list is not exhaustive:

- parent/carers
- teachers
- nursery staff
- family members
- childminders
- social workers

Often, SLTs work indirectly. This means that they try to ensure that the people and places around a child are effective in meeting their communication support needs. For many children, indirect support will be the main (or indeed the only) way that SLT intervention is delivered. Communication partners are central to the success of the indirect approach.

Even when direct therapy forms part of the response to a child's needs, it is usual also to promote conditions which optimally support a child's communication during the bulk of their time that is not spent with the SLT. Children's communication partners are key to ensuring these communication-facilitating environments.

When direct therapy is offered, it is common for one or more of a child's communication partners to become their therapy partner. A therapy partner is someone who attends therapy appointments with the child and supports the therapy process. The terms are sometimes used interchangeably. Very frequently, however, key communication partners are not the therapy partner. For example, at school, the class teacher may be a communication partner within the classroom and the wider school environment, but they are unlikely to be attending weekly therapy sessions with the child. Therefore, the SLT must be mindful that the information they are sharing to upskill therapy partners is also making its way to the teacher (in this case) and any other communication partners. In the initial stages of contact between the SLT and therapy partner, who is to pass on the information gained from the sessions should be decided.

What can communication partners do?

Communication partners can give important insight into the child's or young person's life which will help aid decision making, ensuring the most appropriate therapy plan and goals. They are usually someone who has a close relationship with the child or young person and spends a lot of time with them, such as a parent. Parents are considered the experts on their own children (MacKean et al., 2012) and so their input and expertise from the very beginning are essential to delivering the best care.

If the therapy plan is indirect, the SLT relies solely on the communication partners to implement the recommended strategies. If offering direct therapy for a child or young person, the SLT relies on the therapy partner accompanying them to the appointment but also continuing therapy activities and implementing communication support strategies beyond the therapy sessions.

Recommended strategies will vary depending on the child's needs and may involve the communication partner in making adaptations to the communication environment. This may be the physical environment (such as reducing background noise) or it may involve the social-communicative environment (such as creating more opportunities for conversation and ensuring more favourable conditions by making sure there is space for everyone to have a turn). If a child uses Alternative and Augmentative Communication (AAC), the communication partner may be supported to promote and facilitate its use. Strategies may directly support the child's communication experience, for example, through communication partners speaking in shorter chunks with simpler language and longer pauses; or, alternatively, using techniques to expand or recast what the child says. Communication partners who are also therapy partners may also be equipped to use specific task-management, prompting, cueing, and feedback techniques to support aspects of the child's speech, language or communication at agreed times.

Important points about communication partners

Working collaboratively with communication partners is governed by professional standards. In the UK, an example of this would be the Health and Care Professions Council (HCPC, 2023)

Standards of Proficiency which state that professionals should work in partnership with clients and caregivers. The specific policy context is dependent on the country the SLT is working in. Regardless, the message is based on the same principle, which is that this is simply good practice.

Communication partners are fundamental to the development of a child's speech, language and communication. When babies and children learn language, they do so in a 'learn as you go' process. To learn language, exposure is key. If there is no exposure, there is no language (Yehuda, 2016). A child learns language and communication skills from the people they are with most, such as parents and caregivers. Therefore, supporting and jointly working with communication partners are paramount.

Communication partners spend a lot of time around the child so they can use the strategies suggested by the SLT very frequently, thus creating an environment that will promote the child's communication development and naturally increase the 'dosage' of communication support. The evidence surrounding dosage for indirect support to be effective remain limited (Ebbels et al., 2019) and more research would be welcome. Typically, however, and based on clinical experience, there is consensus that increased dosage of effective input results in better outcomes. Communication partners are therefore valuable members of the therapy team around the child. They complement and add to the input from other team members, including SLTs. In doing so, they boost the capacity of stretched SLT provisions and can extend the benefits of communication support all day, every day. They can offer much more regular communication support than a visiting SLT service.

Crucially, though, communication is an act of connecting with other human beings. To develop communication, a child needs to connect or communicate with other people. That communication needs to be useful and rewarding for the child if it is to develop effectively. Development requires a need, motivation, and an ability to communicate. Communication partners are the people who have the closest and/or the most impactful relationships with the child or young person. Equipping them with the skills and strategies to enable effective communication will support everyday interactions. Not only will this enable the child to participate more fully and beneficially in their daily activities, but it will also strengthen and enrich the relationships within which people thrive and grow.

Understanding children's needs with communication partners

There are many tools which can be used to assess the support needs of children in collaboration with the communication partner. These include checklists, interviews with parents and observations. Completing these together can be an important part of building a positive relationship with communication partners. Filling out communication checklists together helps generate useful insights into relevant aspects of the child's everyday communication and their needs for support. The conversations involved in this joint activity can also enable sharing of information about how the communication partner communicates with the child and the ways in which they have tried to support communication already.

For example, within the Hanen More than Words™ programme, there is a checklist which is completed jointly at the start of the programme. This helps the SLT identify the child's level and style of communication, but also it helps the parent understand those aspects as well. There are specific targets and strategies which can be used for each communication stage.

By following this process, the parents have clear suggestions and strategies which are in line with the child's development. For example, a parent may have been focusing on the child saying words, when developmentally the child should still be working on making choices by reaching out and picking an object.

Additionally, SLTs must be mindful that communication partners are also likely to have their own communication preferences. This should be explored at the earliest opportunity to ensure that the therapy plan is created with this in mind (see Chapter 3). SLTs must ensure they are gauging input at the correct communication level for the communication partner. SLTs should use their skills to make sure the communication partner is able to follow what is being said. This can be checked very simply, by asking the communication partner to feedback what has been discussed, in their own words.

Extra care is advised when communication partners are a child's parents or other family members. SLCN can often be inherited (Barry, Yasin and Bishop, 2007), meaning that if an SLT is working with a child with SLCN, then there is a possibility that family members may also have SLCN. SLTs may find this out while taking a case history, in which case they can explore the communication partner's communication needs and preferences. Furthermore, if a communication partner had SLT input themselves previously, it would be beneficial for the SLT to find out what this was like, and what their views were of their own experiences. This will help to manage expectations, as the delivery of SLT services may have changed since the communication partner's experience. It may also alleviate any anxiety they may be feeling because of negative experiences they may have had in the past.

If an appointed communication partner is from within the educational establishment, or indeed any other setting, their skills and preferences must be also taken into consideration, the same way that a parent's (or those of any family member) are considered.

Supporting children's needs together with communication partners

Once all the relevant information has been gathered and the support needs of the child and the communication partner have been identified, this then leads to a coaching process between the SLT and the communication partner. The SLT's role is to establish, develop and maintain positive collaborative partnerships with communication partners. The steps to achieving this will be outlined in this section.

Explore and set expectations

Regardless of any communication partner's relationship with the child, it is helpful to discuss expectations as early as possible to avoid any confusion or disappointment. Sometimes prospective communication partners may be hoping for direct therapy provided exclusively by an SLT. They may be surprised to learn that a different approach is indicated, far less any expectation that they themselves may have a significant role in supporting the child's SLCN. Open discussion at the earliest opportunity could avoid frustration or confusion later. Levickis et al. (2020) looked at parental expectations in parent-child interaction programmes and demonstrated that parental engagement is increased if parental expectations are managed and supported from the initial contact.

Therapists must also be transparent about service delivery policies and constraints. This is particularly true in the case of therapy partners, where SLTs should discuss the service's expectations about participation in the child's appointments and continuing input beyond the sessions. This will give prospective therapy partners a chance to consider whether they can commit or not. For example, if parents are not able to commit to being therapy partners, other possibilities can be explored, such as grandparents, or someone from the child's school. Otherwise, there is a risk of disengagement, and potentially the need to discharge the child from the service, depending on the local policies. It must be kept in mind that a therapy partner must be someone who will see the child frequently.

Goal-setting with communication partners and the children themselves

Once an appropriate communication partner has been identified, the next thing therapists must consider is goal-setting. A collaborative approach to goal-setting should be a focus for the SLT. The SLT may have an idea in their mind what the goal should be, but all relevant parties should be consulted. Participation of the child's parents is usually important here. Parental involvement is said to lead to better decision making (Stevens et al., 2013). Additionally, parents will be able to share what is important to their family in relation to goals and what they will be able to manage (Baylor and Darling-White, 2020). This creates an opportunity for the SLT to create a plan specifically tailored not only to the needs of the child, but also to the needs of the family. If initial goals between therapist and communication partners differ, then this should be discussed openly, to arrive at a realistic agreement which will work best for the child's interests.

If communication partners feel like they have been included in each step of the journey, it takes away the power dynamic between them and the therapist and creates equal experts with shared goals. In return, the communication partners are much more likely to try the recommended strategies. If the goals do not hold equal concern for all parties, the communication partner may not see the point in adopting the strategies in all environments. Therefore, they will not see beneficial outcomes and can lose trust in the SLT.

When considering goals, it is also important, where possible, to consult the child about what is important to them. For example, in cases where the SLT is choosing a goal for speech work, they should discuss with the child how much they are concerned about their speech. If they are not bothered, then it is unlikely that they will put the strategies into practice. Or, if the focus of support is around the communication partner adapting their communication style, then again, the child should be consulted, if possible, to find out what is most important to them and what changes they feel would support them best. The SLT and communication partner may think that using visuals in the environment is the most important strategy to implement, for instance, but the child may be more concerned with the adult reducing the number of instructions in one utterance. This does not mean the views of the SLT and the communication partner should not be considered; it is not one or the other. More than one goal can be decided, with collaboration and good communication between all parties.

Supporting the child to be included in the decisions around their own communication support is not only good practice but also fits with a rights-based approach (Macrae, 2025). The

United Nations Convention on the Rights of the Child (UNCRC) Article 12 states that children have the right to be listened to and have their views considered when adults are making decisions about them (UN, 1989). Article 12 also explains that children should be supported to make their views heard. The Laura Lundy model takes this slightly further, stating that giving a child a voice is not enough. She explains that a child should be given a safe space to discuss matters which are important to them. They must be given a voice, and an audience to listen to their views, and – importantly – their views should hold influence and be acted upon in a meaningful way (Lundy, 2007).

SLTs are exceptionally well placed to do this do this in comparison to other professionals, as they can use their unique skillset to help give children a voice. They are also able to ensure the environment is safe and communication inclusive, listen to the views expressed, and act accordingly. The SLT should decide to do this in a way they feel will support the child best. In some cases, a facilitated conversation at the child's language level may be enough. In other situations, the SLT may opt to use an approach such as Talking Mats to help the child express their views on things such as therapy targets, how they feel about their own communication, and how they feel about the ways in which other people communicate with them. This should inform the SLT about how best to proceed.

Include, involve and upskill the communication partner

There are many ways of providing SLCN intervention for a child or young person and their family, and communication partners are integral in all these methods. This section outlines how SLTs can empower and equip communication partners.

Yehuda (2016) explains that the conditions in a child's environment must be facilitative to ensure that the process of speech, language and communication development proceeds smoothly. Quantity of communication exchanges is not enough; qualitative aspects are integral to optimum development. It is up to the SLT to work collaboratively with communication partners to help them understand all aspects of their potential role in supporting the child.

Communication partners can implement small but meaningful changes within the communication environment with the guidance of the SLT. For example, this may involve reducing noise levels or managing turn-taking to support everyone's participation. Or it may involve having a choice board on the fridge at home to help a child select and convey what they would like to eat. Equally, it may involve using a visual timetable in the classroom to help the young person understand expectations and organise themselves (ICAN communication-friendly checklist: https://speechandlanguage.org.uk/wp-content/uploads/2023/12/communication_friendly_environments_checklist_updated.pdf).

SLTs should support communication partners and upskill them so they can support the child's SLCN effectively. This may mean helping them to understand the child's individual needs and how to implement strategies to support them. SLTs need to explain to the communication partner *why* they are suggesting, for example, expanding vocabulary, or using shorter (or indeed longer) utterances. It may be helpful to justify strategies in the wider context of the child's readiness for school transitions, learning capacity and behaviour support. This may help the communication partners understand why it is important for them to adapt their own communication for the benefit of the child's communication development.

The SLT must work with communication partners in a way that recognises and responds to the communication strengths of both the communication partner and the child. This can mean, for example, coaching the communication partner to use language functions or strategies they might not ordinarily use. The SLT must therefore be confident enough to support the communication partner to reflect on their communication. At times, this may involve gentle challenge, within the context of a warm and understanding working relationship. The SLT should check in frequently with the communication partner to determine the extent to which joint goals are being met or if more support is needed. Therapists must be able, where necessary, to adapt their own language and use inclusive communication practices to adjust for the communication partner's level of understanding.

A child's parents are often key communication partners. Klatte et al. (2020) explain that taking a family-centred approach to supporting a child's SLCN is essential and that collaboration between SLTs and parents is a crucial element in family centred approaches. Including families in the decision-making and therapy process has been shown to have positive outcomes. The use of parent-child interaction (PCI) programmes has increased over recent years. These are delivered by the therapist directly to someone who spends a lot of time with a child. Typically, participants are the children's parent(s), although this is not exclusively the case. Grandparents, foster carers and others have successfully completed these programmes. The aim is to equip the participant to be the 'agent of change' by adapting the ways they promote and support the child's communication development in everyday routines and interactions (Pickles et al., 2016). PCI programmes often deliver a combination of information, support and practical upskilling. The latter aspect is often approached through video-recording the participant's interaction with the child. Then, the SLT and the participant view the recording together so the SLT can support them to identify personalised goals and strategies that both resonate with them and build on their strengths.

The Hanen Centre is an example of an organisation that has created several different PCI programmes. It describes the whole family as the client, rather than just the child. There are programmes focusing on different age ranges; and targeting children with various language, literacy and communication differences. These include 'Late Talkers', young children with language delays, and autistic children. One example is Hanen's More than Words™ programme, which is aimed at the parents of young children who are autistic or who would benefit from social communication support. In this programme, there are group sessions for parents and caregivers (in-person or online) offering relevant information. Group sessions also offer natural opportunities for social support from other parents going through the same process. Parents are supported to understand their child's communication cues and preferences, and to use fun everyday interactions to build connection and communication. There are also two scheduled video sessions (usually home-based) where the SLT will video the programme participant(s) interacting with the child. They will then review the video together and look at what went well, what the child responded to, and how that could be built upon.

SLTs also work frequently with educators, aiming to equip them to support children's communication. Sometimes the aim is to upskill educators in supporting the communication of all learners, and sometimes the focus is on specific groups or individuals identified as having communication support needs. Some programmes have been developed to guide this work. For example, Elklan is an organisation that trains SLTs and others to deliver various programmes targeted at a range of audiences, including educators. Often, though, SLTs design and deliver bespoke professional development packages to suit the needs of their local contexts.

As well as those approaches where the SLT is helping others to support the child's communication, there are also occasions when the SLT provides direct therapy to a child, together with a communication partner who is also acting as a therapy partner. In such circumstances, therapy partners should not just be observers in the sessions. SLTs should involve and include the therapy partner, giving them an opportunity to 'be the SLT' in that session. An example of this is if a therapist is completing a minimal pairs task with a child. The therapy partner should be included, both taking part in the task and taking a turn at 'being the SLT' in the session. This creates the opportunity to coach the therapy partner in how best to carry out this task beyond the session. The SLT can gently make suggestions on how best to go about the therapy tasks, including the use of prompts or cues, adapting levels of challenge, and providing feedback to the child. Participating in this way helps therapy partners to see and discuss where exactly the child may be experiencing challenge. Often therapy partners will comment that they did not realise how a task that might initially look like 'just play' has a lot of complexity, including structure and scaffolding to get the balance of challenge 'just right'.

Therapists must be mindful of how they offer feedback to a therapy partner, ensuring they are not perceived as criticising their best attempts. This can be done by highlighting aspects that went well. Therapists can also ask the therapy partner to reflect how they thought it went, and what they found easy or tricky. It is important to encourage them to feel confident to ask questions, and to make suggestions of their own as equal partners. Phrases like 'I wonder if you could try . . . ' or 'Do you think trying x, y, z would help?' are softer and less likely to make the therapy partner feel under attack or criticised.

Once the therapy partner has seen and participated in the direct therapy, they can then carry this on into the child's everyday contexts. For parents, this may mean finding times to carry out therapy-focused tasks at home. If the therapy partner is from education, they can incorporate it into the child's school day. This higher dosage of therapy input will help support better outcomes (Kaipa and Peterson, 2016).

Possible challenges and how to overcome them

Challenges for parents

Therapists should be working with families in a way that works best for them, rather than a way that works best for the service, and this is underpinned by professional standards such as the HCPC Standards of Proficiency. This does not come without its challenges, and those will be explored in this section.

Klatte and Roulstone (2016) researched how SLTs felt about working with parents to enhance their approaches to supporting their children's SLCN. They identified four critical components: parental engagement, parental understanding, parental reflection, and therapist skills. It could be argued that the four key elements are all interlinked, and that therapist skills underpin good practice in this area. Inclusive communication good practice (see Chapter 3) is key to achieving all these most effectively and with the largest number of parents.

Parental engagement can be difficult to achieve and sustain, for a variety of reasons. If parents themselves do not understand the need for the input, it will be difficult for them to see the point in engaging. Exploring parents' hopes and expectations for their child may help the SLT to tailor their approach. It may be beneficial for the SLT to explain that by helping with the communication concern, it can also help with other aspects of the child's life, for example, educational attainment, social interaction with peers and overall mental well-being.

If parents do not understand advice, or if they lack the confidence to ask questions, they may disengage (or not engage as they had intended to) out of confusion, shame or embarrassment. Some parents will require additional support with the language, communication or relational demands of communication partner strategies or parent-mediated interventions. Parents with SLCN are less likely to ask for clarification than those without (Lanz., 2009). This is where therapists should become more flexible and creative to support parents. SLTs could focus less on using verbal ways of conveying information by supplementing talk-based activities with accessible, appealing methods such as videos and infographics. Using Talking Mats could be one possibility to consider with parents, as appropriate, to work towards shared understandings of key elements of the intervention. Handled with sensitivity, and with clear explanation and justification, this approach would be unintrusive and does not rely solely on the parents' verbal language. Overall, it is the SLT's job to make sure that intervention has been delivered with skill and sensitivity, using inclusive communication good practice.

While most research on parent mediated interventions has shown that this type of input is effective and leads to positive outcomes for families, there can be challenges for parents. Some parents have reported feeling overwhelmed, undervalued and stressed. Some report that the SLT came across as the expert, and not the parent (Jurek et al., 2023). This is why it is so important to see parents as equal partners in the therapy process. If a parent does not yet have the self-awareness and self-observation skills to reflect on their own communication, it could be difficult for them to adapt their communication style. They may struggle to describe what they feel went well and what did not. Therapists should use their full skillset to ensure that parents are appropriately supported and encouraged, within a strengths-based coaching relationship.

There can be practical problems too. Parents may have hectic lives. Logistical challenges can occur if their availability is not in line with what the SLT can offer. SLT services may face constraints on availability of suitable clinical accommodation, and there may be pressure to demonstrate quick throughput of cases. Research has shown, however, that engagement can be better if services are flexible towards families' needs (Kokorelias et al., 2019). SLTs may therefore have to advocate strongly for the importance of this work, and the need to approach it in truly family-centred ways. This could be by providing input somewhere which is accessible to families and/or providing the input at a time that works best. They could also use different channels to communicate such as WhatsApp or online meetings. Moreover, parents have reported that it can be difficult finding time to implement strategies or to carry out set tasks (Divan et al., 2015). This could be avoided if parents are helped to understand the time involved from the beginning, and if the SLT works collaboratively with them in joint problem-solving to reach workable compromises.

Challenges for educators

Often, educators would like to help and can see how input SLT input would benefit the child. In some circumstances, they may agree to be therapy partners in place of the parents, to avoid children being discharged. While this can work well, having someone from the child's educational establishment act as a therapy partner comes with its own unique challenges. Most schools are happy to have the support of SLTs but again may struggle to find suitable space to accommodate them if the appointment is to be held in school. Schools are complex organisations and even with the best goodwill, communication can break down at times. SLTs may therefore find themselves in school for an organised appointment and the class have left to go on a trip or there is a special assembly or school event which means they cannot see the child that day. Education establishments have their own difficulties in terms of staffing and balancing the needs of multiple children. They may not fully understand the commitment when they initially agree. Having agreed, they may then find they cannot commit to the number of therapy sessions or consolidation activities recommended by the SLT, due to situations arising outwith their control. This can be mitigated by the SLT communicating clearly and explicitly at the start about the expectations on education. Additionally, therapists may want to consider a contracting arrangement between the SLT department and the educational establishment, outlining what is expected. Although a contract like this would not necessarily be legally binding, it sets a precedent and will clearly outline what education should be doing.

Daisy's story

Daisy is a 2½-year-old girl who was referred to speech and language therapy with concerns over her language development. The SLT relied on Daisy's mum explaining how Daisy communicates and sharing the family dynamics for the SLT to get a true insight into what Daisy's communication environment is like. Daisy's mother was a carer for her own parent who was needing end-of-life care. She was not able to commit to weekly sessions due to her caring responsibilities but was very eager to learn how to support Daisy.

After a discussion with Daisy's mum and the nursery it was agreed that Daisy's Key Worker would attend the appointments and the SLT would organise these appointments to take place within the nursery. Being a therapy partner equipped the Key Worker with the confidence to use therapy techniques and activities both during and beyond therapy sessions.

The SLT would send a short video message to Daisy's mum at the end of each session to let her know what had been covered and what strategies she could try at home. This meant strategies were implemented both within the nursery environment and at home. Daisy's mum reported that although she was unable to attend appointments she felt included from the start and knew she could contact the SLT if she needed further clarification from the videos. Daisy's mum shared the strategies with other family members so they could also support Daisy's language development.

After a period of using these strategies consistently, Daisy's language began to show progress. She began to use more single words and later began to put some words together. All parties worked together collaboratively, which resulted in positive outcomes for all.

Building on the positive experience, the Key Worker also completed Teacher Talk™ training, delivered by a suitably trained Early Years Educator from the local area. This helped the Key Worker to implement evidence-based techniques to promote language, literacy and interaction development of all the children in the nursery. The Key Worker felt more confident supporting both Daisy's communication development and that of other children within the nursery whom she felt may have needed some extra support.

Summary

This chapter has explained the significant role of communication partners in supporting a child's SLCN. Some communication partners take on additional, specific roles. These include parents (or others) being coached to be agents of change via parent-child interaction therapy approaches. Other roles include being therapy partners, who accompany children to direct therapy sessions and learn how to carry out therapy activities beyond the sessions. Communication partners contribute meaningfully to a rounded understanding of a child's SLCN. It is important for the SLT to consider the communication partners' needs and preferences, to establish shared expectations, and to involve the communication partners in goal-setting. Communication partners benefit from strengths-based coaching, and from a flexible solution-focused approach.

Recommended resources

https://www.hanen.org/programs/more-than-words
https://www.hanen.org/programs/teacher-talk
https://www.talkingmats.com/

References

Barry, J.G., Yasin, I., and Bishop, D.V. (2007) 'Heritable risk factors associated with language impairments', *Genes, Brain, and Behavior*, 6(1), 66-76. https://doi.org/10.1111/j.1601-183X.2006.00232.x

Baylor, C. and Darling-White, M. (2020) 'Achieving participation-focused intervention through shared decision making: Proposal of an age- and disorder-generic framework', *American Journal of Speech-Language Pathology*, 29(3), 1335-1360. https://doi.org/10.1044/2020_AJSLP-19-00043

Divan, G., Hamdani, U., Vajartkar, V., Minhas, A., Taylor, C., Aldred, C., Leadbitter, K., Rahman, A., Green, J. and Patel, V. (2015) 'Adapting an evidence-based intervention for autism spectrum disorder for scaling up in resource-constrained settings: The development of the PASS intervention in South Asia', *Global Health Action*, 8(1). doi: 10.3402/gha.v8.27278.

Ebbels, S.H., McCartney, E., Slonims, V., Dockrell, J.E. and Norbury, C.F. (2019) 'Evidence-based pathways to intervention for children with language disorders', *International Journal of Language and Communication Disorders*, 54(1), 3-19. https://doi.org/10.1111/1460-6984.12387

HCPC (Health and Care Professions Council) (2023) *Standards of proficiency: Speech and Language Therapists*. Available at: https://www.hcpc-uk.org/standards/standards-of-proficiency/speech-and-language-therapists/

Jurek, L., Leadbitter, K. and Geoffray, M-M. (2023) 'Parental experience of parent-mediated intervention for children with ASD: A systematic review and qualitative evidence synthesis', *Autism: The International Journal of Research and Practice*, 27(3), 647-666. https://doi.org/10.1177/13623613221112204

Kaipa, R. and Peterson, A.M. (2016) 'A systematic review of treatment intensity in speech disorders', *International Journal of Speech-Language Pathology*, 18(6), 507–520. https://doi.org/10.3109/17549507.2015.1126640

Klatte, I.S., Lyons, R., Davies, K., Harding, S., Marshall, J., McKean, C. and Roulstone, S. (2020) 'Collaboration between parents and SLTs produces optimal outcomes for children attending speech and language therapy: Gathering the evidence', *International Journal of Language and Communication Disorders*, 55(4), 618–628. https://doi.org/10.1111/1460-6984.12538

Klatte, I.S., and Roulstone, S. (2016) 'The practical side of working with parent–child interaction therapy with preschool children with language impairments', *Child Language Teaching and Therapy*, 32(3), 345–359. https://doi.org/10.1177/0265659016641999

Kokorelias, K.M., Gignac, M.A.M., Naglie, G., and Cameron, J. (2019) 'Towards a universal model of family centered care: A scoping review', *BMC Health Services Research*, 19(1), 564. https://doi.org/10.1186/s12913-019-4394-5

Lanz, R. (2009) 'SLT within the Milton Keynes YOT', Milton Keynes: Youth Offending Team.

Levickis, P., McKean, C., Wiles, A. and Law, J. (2020) 'Expectations and experiences of parents taking part in parent-child interaction programmes to promote child language: A qualitative interview study', *International Journal of Language and Communication Disorders*, 55: 603–617. https://doi.org/10.1111/1460-6984.12543

Lundy, L. (2007) '"Voice" is not enough: Conceptualising Article 12 of the United Nations Convention on the Rights of the Child', *British Educational Research Journal*, 33: 927–942. https://doi.org/10.1080/01411920701657033

MacKean, G., Spragins, W., L'Heureux, L., Popp, J. and Wilkes, C. (2012) 'Advancing family-centred care in child and adolescent mental health: A critical review of the literature', *Healthcare Quarterly (Toronto, Ont.)*, 15 (Spec No 4), 64–75. https://doi.org/10.12927/hcq.2013.22939

Macrae, A. (2025) 'Giving voice to all of Scotland's children: Respecting, protecting and fulfilling the language and communication rights of children'. Available at: https://www.rcslt.org/wp-content/uploads/2025/03/Giving-a-voice-to-all-children-in-Scotland.pdf (accessed 26 March 2025).

Pickles, A., Le Couteur, A., Leadbitter, K., Salomone, E., Cole-Fletcher, R, Tobin, H. . . . Green, J. (2016) 'Parent-mediated social communication therapy for young children with autism (PACT): Long-term follow-up of a randomised controlled trial', *Lancet*. Doi: 10.1016/S0140-6736(16)31229-6.

Stevens, A., Beurskens, A., van der Weijden, T. and Koke, A. (2013) 'The use of patient-specific measurement instruments in the process of goal setting: A systematic review of available instruments and their feasibility', *Clinical Rehabilitation*, 27(11), 1005–1019.

UN (United Nations) (1989) Convention on the Rights of the Child, Treaty no. 27531. United Nations Treaty Series, 1577, pp. 3–178.

Yehuda, N. (2016). *Communicating Trauma: Clinical Presentations and Interventions with Traumatized Children*. London: Routledge.

6 So what? And prove it!
Evidencing impact

Marie Gascoigne

What you'll learn in this chapter

- How to build impact measurement into your everyday practice
- Why it is crucial to understand the difference between doing something and knowing that it was useful
- How to use impact measurement for reflective practice and service development including articulating your own 'prove it' statements.

Introduction

In Chapter 2, the importance of taking a whole system approach to understanding and meeting children's speech, language and communication needs (SLCN) was outlined. This chapter will focus on the 'so what?': considering what we do as practitioners, in the whole system, to enable children to meet their speech, language and communication outcomes. It will also review the evidence for impact that allows us to 'prove it'.

The Balanced System® methodology outlined in Chapter 2 has system-level outcomes at its core. The integrated delivery model outlines the relative contributions of each part of the specialist and wider system to achieving those outcomes. The 'Prove It!' element challenges all those working with children to evidence the impact of their activity.

The Balanced System® Outcomes Framework and Balanced System® Prove It! tools are underpinned by the Friedman Results Based Accountability Framework (Friedman, 2005) and Realistic Evaluation (Pawson and Tilley, 1997).

Measure what you value

The challenge of choosing appropriate metrics to measure impact is one that reaches across industry, public sector organisations, and policy at local and national government levels. Hauser and Katz (1998) illustrate that whenever metrics are used to measure performance, those leading the organisation will determine how the service is to be delivered based on 'doing well' relative to those metrics. However, this drive to 'meet the metrics' can potentially have unintended and negative consequences on the core goals of the organisation if these are not properly aligned.

DOI: 10.4324/9781003671626-8

We can apply this thinking to common pressures in children's services for SLCN. If the metric of being a 'good service' is to have no child waiting longer than x weeks to be seen, that will drive service design and activity to make sure that metric is achieved. However, this does not necessarily equate to delivering impactful support to the same children if the system then struggles to follow through. Paradoxically, then, the 'industry' of taking children 'off the waiting list' can drive less effective intervention. Similarly, most speech and language therapy (SLT) services have traditionally been measured through 'activity data', with targets being set for a set number of 'face-to-face' contacts. In that model, all other forms of activity are classified as 'non-patient-related' or 'indirect', with the implication that those other activities are of less value. These examples are real and highly pertinent at the time of writing. However, they also reflect an outdated medical deficit model of need and provision.

This thinking prompts us to consider whether the 'overall goals' for a system supporting children with SLCN have been properly articulated. Rousltone et al. (2012) identified that children valued SLT outcomes that related to their relationships with friends, family, and those around them. Parents valued outcomes that related to their children developing 'independence, acceptance and inclusion'. Academic skills such as literacy and numeracy were valued in the context of future independence but not singularly as primary ambitions. Roulstone (2015) explored this further, in considering the relationship between the children's and the parents' desired outcomes alongside the SLT expert view and the research evidence. The conclusion is as follows:

> Parents and children value functional outcomes and positive experiences; these are not routinely measured in research or practice. Therapy is perceived positively by most parents; however, some are ambivalent and less clear about the rationale. Commonly used interventions are supported by evidence, but there are gaps regarding some critical therapy components.
>
> (Roulstone, 2015, p. 211)

The 'so what?' is evidently sometimes unclear to parents and children. Practitioners are relying on research evidence that has, in the main, been generated through the lens of impairment-focused remediation, without always presenting a direct link to the longer-term goal of functional ability in everyday life.

Learning points 6.1

- *Strategic*: Consider whether the metrics that you are valuing in your service provision are directly measuring impact for children. If not, who do you need to influence and how?
- *Operational*: Can you build impact measurement into operational service delivery and support teams to make evaluation part of everyday practice?
- *Practitioner*: Can you reflect on the evidence you have to show impact of what you do with a child?

Using outcome measures to drive system change

As set out in Chapter 2, the Balanced System® is not based on a medical model or premise. Therefore, the 'overall goal' is not based on traditional activity metrics but in building an outcomes framework that facilitates the whole system and all its resources to be deployed to effect maximum impact for the population of children with SLCN. This section will describe the different kinds of outcome data that might be collected. It will explain how these can be used as evidence of impact at several different levels, including the child and their family, but also at a group or cohort level, such as a class or school, and even at a population level in any given geography. The difference in focus between child outcomes and population outcomes brings in the element of timeframe, and this parameter will also be considered.

Let's begin then with the theoretical perspectives that underpin the Results Based Accountability (RBA) framework (Friedman, 2005) that has been widely used in public policy for more than 20 years. The drivers behind the RBA methodology are to encourage public services (in particular) to use data to 'turn the curve' on challenging service delivery problems in the context of whole systems.

The core RBA approach separates population results from performance results. To explain this a little more, population results might include aspirational targets such as those set by the government, for example, increase school readiness of the population. Performance results, however, are the results that need to be identified and measured at a service level within a system with a long-term goal of improving the population result. The difficulty sits in identifying and capturing the performance results that will be most useful and ceasing to chase those results that are not actually providing the necessary data. The performance results part of the RBA framework fits well with the Balanced System® ethos of a whole system with contributions from different elements of the system to a set of common outcomes. For this reason, the Balanced System® Outcomes Framework is based on the structure of the RBA model. Figure 6.1 shows the

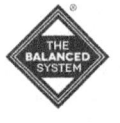
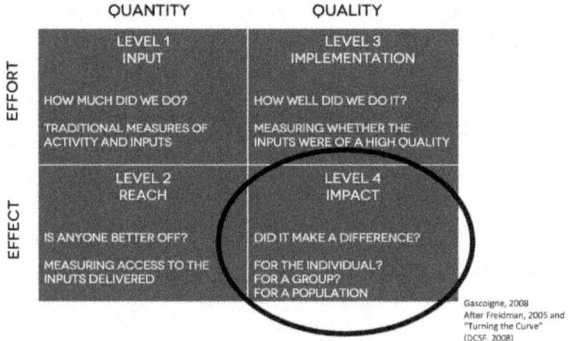

Figure 6.1 The Balanced System® Outcomes Framework

So what? And prove it!: Evidencing impact 77

Balanced System® Outcomes Framework taking the columns and rows of the Friedman RBA but then reinterpreting the content to the children's services and therapies systems and potentially moving from individual to population level outcomes within the same framework.

The structure of the grid essentially has quantitative measures and qualitative measures in one dimension and effort and effect in the other. To apply these distinctions to the measures that are relevant to speech, language and communication and other wider children's services, the four 'boxes' that emerge in the grid have been named as follows:

Level 1 Input: quantitative measures of effort (how much did we do?)
Level 2 Reach: quantitative measures of effect (how far towards our target did we reach?)
Level 3 Implementation: qualitative measures of effort (was it done well? Was it a high quality activity or intervention?)
Level 4 Impact: qualitative measures of effect (did it make a difference?).

Where we extend from the core RBA model here is that we can interpret Level 4 (Impact) at an individual level, at the level of a cohort (class, group, school or setting), and at population level, with the timelines appropriately adjusted. Let's consider some examples.

Level 1: Input

The traditional face-to-face activity data recorded for a session with a child or family is an input measure. It sits in the 'quantitative x effort' box in that it is a measure of 'an event that happened'. As a measure, it assures that contacts with children and families occurred and cumulatively tells us about the number, frequency and even duration. It rarely provides a contextual indication of the extent of the need (so, one 'contact' out of how many that might be necessary) or the location for the delivery of the contact.

Input data in relation to SLT activity is often limited to that face-to-face, direct contact. Data relating to the amount of liaison, training, and providing more general advice and guidance is unlikely to be captured in many systems (even though if it were, it would still only provide information to say that events happened).

The limitations of input data are therefore clear. They tell us that events occurred but provide no insight into the effectiveness or change for the child or the system that supports them.

Level 2: Reach

The input measure of number of face-to-face contacts could be turned into a reach measure if those contacts were analysed as a percentage of a target. This adds a level of analysis to the metric, as we now know that there was an intended number of contacts to be achieved and that a percentage of those (counted) have been achieved. It remains the case, however, that from these data alone we have no idea if there was any positive benefit from this activity in terms of child, family or system outcome.

Reach measures can be valuable, for instance, in capturing the extent of the roll-out of a training programme for staff in schools to enable them to deliver an intervention. Understanding the number of schools that have received the training relative to the total or target number is a useful metric of measurement of delivery. However, if our interest is in the *impact*, the '*so what?*', of the training programme for the children who will receive the intervention, the reach measure does not tell us anything useful.

Reach measures are widely used in relation to training and workforce development as a metric. A good example in relation to speech, language and communication skills is the raft of training available for various targeted school-based interventions, sometimes commissioned locally but sometimes funded nationally. Understanding the Level 1 and Level 2 data alone on the delivery of the training, the number of learners receiving the training, and so on, provides no information about the difference that the training has made.

Level 3: Implementation

Moving to the qualitative dimension of the outcomes grid, let's consider quality and effort. Evaluating the quality of an intervention, or training, or specific therapy session is good practice and to be encouraged. However, while it's a key baseline expectation that we deliver high quality provision, this alone is not the same as having evidence that the quality intervention has made the expected or desired difference. Quality is not the same as impact.

This can be illustrated by a couple of examples. Thinking further about the training programme described above, it would be usual to have an evaluation survey for the participants and perhaps even a before-and-after measure of some key goals of the training, such as confidence in the approach or theoretical knowledge imparted. The evaluation might also ask about the quality of the training experience itself and invite suggestions for improvement. All of these are valuable but do not in and of themselves provide any evidence that the training itself will make a difference to children or the systems in which they operate.

Similarly, a therapist or student therapist might prepare a session with a group of children meticulously and deliver the session with skill but it can happen that for a host of reasons the impact on the day is not realised, perhaps because of external factors in the children's day that means that the planned activity is not going to be effective on this occasion.

Level 4: Impact

An impact measure will be a measure of *quality and effect*. There are three characteristics of a good impact measure. First, that it evidences that something changed. Next, that it identifies what helped that change. And, finally, that it articulates how that change is being demonstrated functionally. That is, how the change is important in the day-to-day life of the child and family.

Impact measurement is important across the whole system. If we are to work as systems around children, impact measures need to be sought from all areas of the system. For example, if an SLT spends time advising on how to make environmental enhancements in a classroom to enable listening, learning and communication (such as, perhaps, visual timetables), there should be an impact measure in place to capture the positive change in the children's engagement and participation.

Thinking about the training and development examples outlined earlier, it is possible to capture changes such as the trained person delivering the associated intervention. There are also opportunities to measure tangible functional outcomes for the children receiving the intervention.

Learning points 6.2

- *Strategic*: How can you embed impact measurement within the culture of the system you are developing? Who needs to be involved in developing the appropriate impact metrics locally?
- *Operational*: Can the language of input, reach, quality and impact be used with teams to ensure that practitioners are evaluating all elements of their support?
- *Practitioner*: For valid baseline measurement, are you considering at the outset the impact measures that best fit the provision you are delivering? These can be within-child but also across the system that you are working within.

How to measure impact? Prove it!

We have identified that measures that capture activity or the quality of effort have a place in outcome measurement. This section will focus on extending outcome measurement in practice to focus on *impact* not only at child level but also across the whole system.

Starting, however, with the individual, when thinking about measuring impact and outcome, the World Health Organization's International Classification of Functioning, Disability and Health (ICF: see Recommended Resources at the end of this chapter) has long provided the paradigm though which to consider not only the 'impairment' or 'disability' element of a person's need but also the impact on 'activity' and 'participation'; and all of these in the context of the environmental and personal factors for the individual. Figure 6.2 summarises this influential model.

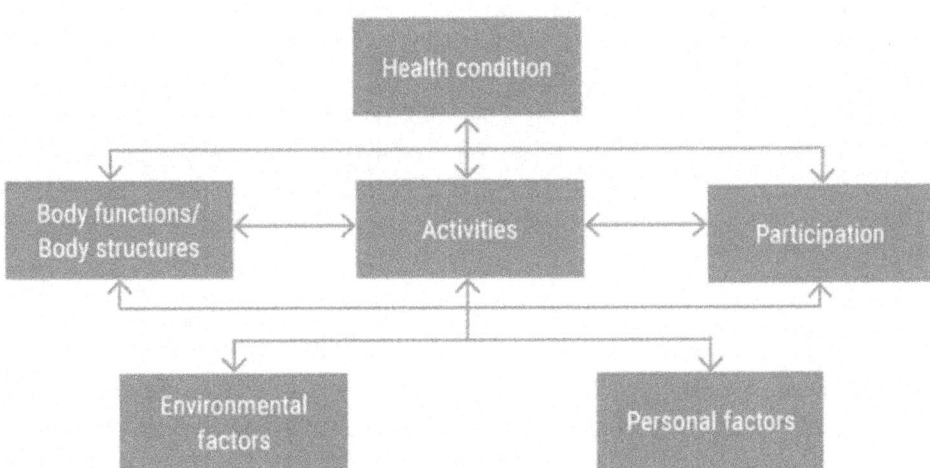

Figure 6.2 Bio-psycho-social Model of Functioning, Disability and Health

This model has been used to inform many outcome measurement tools at the individual level including the Therapy Outcomes Measures (TOMs; Enderby et al., 2006). Tools such as TOMs continue to have a place when thinking about measuring impact for the individual, ensuring a focus on the functional goals of activity and participation that consider the personal and environmental factors around the child. So, an outcome measured through TOMs would be an example of a child-level intervention outcome that could demonstrate impact in that part of the system. Cumulatively, the measures for many children could be used to evidence change at a service level.

However, it is important to think more broadly if we want to understand the role of what has brought about a change and been impactful for a child, especially if we want to evaluate system impact. There are several important additional parameters to consider:

- *The domain of the change we are seeking to evidence.* So, is it a change in performance on an assessment, a change in functionality, a change in participation, or a change in well-being?
- *The context for the change.* This is linked very much to functional outcomes and the importance of place, for example, home, park, leisure centre, school or setting.
- *The factors that have brought about the change.* For example, change to the environment or change to the way others interact with the child or young person.
- *Change in the behaviours, skills and confidence of others in the system,* for example, the training example that we have been thinking about in this chapter.
- *Who is observing and capturing the change.* For example, a parent who observes their child interacting in a different way than previously with other children at the swings in the park and wants to ensure that this impactful example is recorded as part of their child's journey.

Clearly, it is not possible, practical or desirable to capture all these elements all the time. However, we do need to pay attention to evaluation across all areas of the whole system if we are to avoid falling into the trap of only capturing inputs as outlined above.

The first step is to decide what you want to evidence or 'prove'. For example, if you want to prove that an impairment-focused intervention has had an impact on an element of speech, language and communication, you will still use appropriate assessment processes at time intervals to capture change in those specific areas that you have been working on with the child and family. Even in this 'within child' example, you will still want to know about the impact in different contexts, for instance, home vs school. You will also want to hear different views or 'voices' around the child, and of course ideally the views of the child themselves. This is not as complicated as it sounds! Measuring impact can be distilled into four key questions, considered below.

What changed?

The change might be for the child but could also be for someone in the system around them, for example, the class teacher commenting rather than questioning following some coaching from a Link Therapist. Or it might be a change in the atmosphere in a setting following some environmental adaptations recommended in a training session for Early Years practitioners.

So what? And prove it!: Evidencing impact 81

What helped?

This involves asking the child wherever possible, but also those around them, to describe what they believe has been impactful. This is important and answers are often surprising, as the 'focus' of the therapy 'input' may not in fact be reported as the element that was most impactful. For example, a parent may report the most impactful element of the therapy as being the reduced stress of not having to take a child out of school to attend a clinic appointment, knowing that they will be supported in school. That parent may have more confidence that those at school are able to support their child and more time to follow guidance at home as their part of the system support.

How do you know? What is the evidence (worded accessibly for a range of audiences)?

Examples of impact might be a picture of a reorganised classroom with a visual timetable and a word wall. Or a sample recorded on a phone of the child interacting with a grandparent. Or voice notes from a parent who wants to capture a particular moment and share an observation. More traditional evidence can also evidence impact, such as progress on pre- and post-assessments, or more manualised observations and so on.

The Balanced System® Prove It! Platform (see Recommended resources at the end of this chapter) has been developed to help impact measurement across the whole system. The platform invites the user to identify 'what they want to prove' in the context of the Five Strands and Three Levels of the Balanced System® and to capture change data from a range of sources. For example, if a child accesses an intervention, you can ask for evidence of change from any of those around the child and in some instances, of course, ask the child themselves! The Prove It! approach allows a practitioner, a service, a system to consistently capture evidence that can then be used to improve the offer for children and thus influence policy, commissioning and practice.

Learning points 6.3

- *Strategic*: There is significant value of capturing impact data at service and system level and demonstrating why this is more useful than over-emphasis on counting inputs. This may involve challenging the traditional IT (information technology) systems that you are required to use to capture data. Enough challenges from enough system leaders will lead to change – be impactful, in fact!
- *Operational*: Recognise that capturing impact data across the system is still measuring child outcomes and that developing cumulative case studies of children's journeys through the system provides data about impact.
- *Practitioner*: Accept the challenge to question 'so what?' and 'Prove It!' in all that you do for children. Can we do better? Do we use impact evidence to shape the service offer to children and young people? Can good outcomes be at the level of family support, environment and workforce development as well as identification and intervention?

82 *Supporting Children's Speech, Language and Communication Needs*

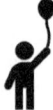

Danny's story

Finally, let's return to Danny and his journey as discussed in Chapter 2, and look at the impact measures along his journey (see Figure 6.3).

Accessing support

Danny's journey begins with his parent accessing a drop-in session with the Link Therapist in the school – no appointment necessary, signposted by the Special Educational Needs Coordinator (SENCO, equivalent to the ASN Coordinator in Scotland).

- *So what?*: The therapist was in place and accessible, no waiting list.
- *Impact?*: The parent was able to seek advice quickly and be reassured. In this case, Danny progressed to some assessment in context. Because of the Link Therapist being part of the school team, the SENCO received feedback on the day and was made aware of the universal offer already in place. Consequently, the class teacher immediately had guidance on appropriate universal approaches to support Danny.
- *Prove it!*: The baseline of where Danny is starting his journey is captured.
  - *Voice 1*: The parent is asked for their view on the impact of being able to access the Link Therapist and then asked at a later point in the journey to reflect on any relevant changes.
  - *Voice 2*: The SENCO and class teacher are asked for their views on how they have been able to immediately use universal approaches to support Danny.

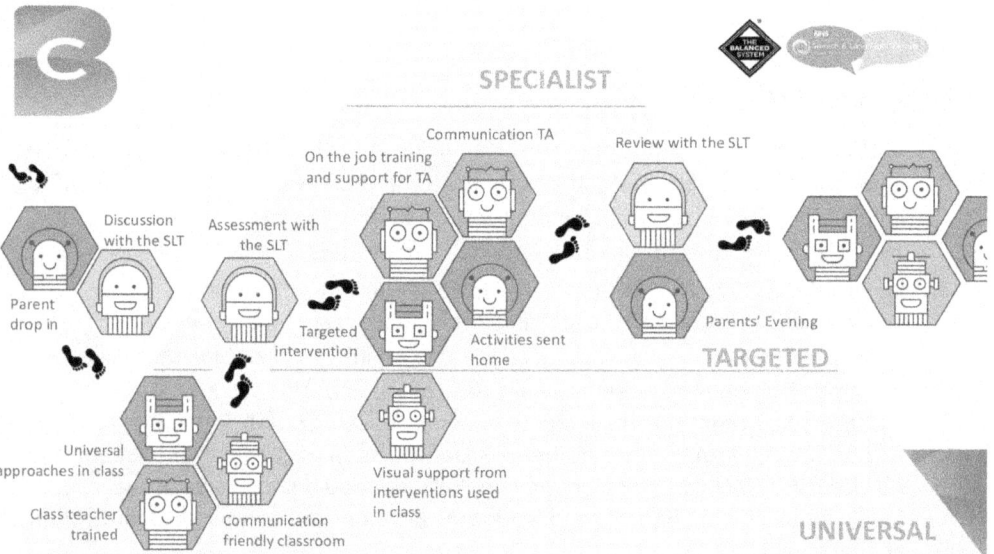

Figure 6.3 Danny's journey (focus on impact)

Universal support

The universal offer has been developed in the school over the time the Link Therapist has been working in a whole school approach. It doesn't have to be 'created' for Danny - it is simply part of the infrastructure, but that is only because the Link Therapist has had time to do that work with the school system.

- *So what?*: The Link Therapist existing in the whole system is a critical part of this impact journey.
- *Impact?*: The Link Therapist has already developed the school infrastructure which will be benefitting all children in the school and possibly preventing some from needing more focused support.
- *Prove it!*: Danny is benefitting from the universal offer in the classroom. This is in place because of the Link Therapist whole-school approach.
    - *Voice 1*: The SENCO is asked for their view on the evidence of change for children in the school, resulting from taking a whole-school strategic view of supporting speech, language and communication.
    - *Voice 2*: The class teacher is asked for their view of using universal approaches in their day-to-day practice.

Targeted support

Following further assessment, the Link Therapist establishes some targeted support for Danny. This includes a targeted intervention which is a small group activity with his peers to enable Danny to develop his language in a functional context. The group is established by the Link Therapist alongside the Teaching Assistant who has had appropriate training as part of the whole-school training plan. It is also supported by the Communication Teaching Assistant (TA) in school. This is an enhanced role that the SLT Service has supported and developed across their Local Authority area. The training for the targeted intervention and the enhanced expertise of the Communication TA are already in place - they do not have to be provided specifically for Danny to access this support.

- *So what?*: If these parts of the offer were not in place, the Link Therapist would have to either spend time setting these up before Danny could benefit or perhaps spend even more time themselves delivering a targeted intervention that could safely and effectively be delivered by the TA. Either of those eventualities would put pressure on the system and prevent the SLT spending time effectively and efficiently supporting other children.
- *Impact?*: Danny can access support quickly and in context alongside his peers.
- *Prove it!*: It isn't essential to capture all these all the time, but the possibilities are illustrated as a learning point.
    - *Voice 1*: Danny's views on how he finds the activities in the targeted group intervention helpful.
    - *Voice 2*: Parents' views on what they see at home in respect of Danny's functional progress.
    - *Voice 3*: TA's view on how Danny is progressing, including specific examples of change.

Reviewing progress

Review of progress in school is carried out by the Link Therapist who does some reassessment against the baseline and reports to parents at the parents' evening.

- *So what?:* There is a before-and-after measure that is captured by the SLT providing objective measurement of progress in Danny's speech, language and communication skills. Parents can speak with the Link Therapist in context at school alongside other school-based practitioners, rather than having to attend a specific meeting elsewhere and thus this provides easy access.
- *Impact?:* Danny shows progress in his speech, language and communication but requires more support at a targeted level which is arranged in school as before. Had he needed more specialist or individualised intervention, the Link Therapist would have provided this in school. Parents have confidence in the system to support Danny, and he is accessing whole-class learning more effectively than before.
- *Prove it!:* A range of measures evaluate change, highlighting functional impact from different viewpoints.
    - *Voice 1*: SLT records the progress on assessment measures and determines next steps.
    - *Voice 2*: Parents' view of change for Danny is captured along with their confidence in the next steps.
    - *Voice 3*: Class teacher reports on Danny's progress with specific examples (prepared for parents' evening, so not an additional burden).

Summary

This chapter focused on the 'so what?'. It considered what we do to enable children to meet impactful speech, language and communication outcomes, whether individually or in populations. It also reviewed the evidence that allows us to 'prove it'. The chapter introduced the four domains of the Balanced System® Outcomes Framework, going beyond the traditional measures of *input* and *reach* to also consider the key complementary aspects of *quality* and *impact*. This prompts SLTs to evaluate whether any activity was done well and whether it had the desired effect. The chapter proposed four key questions for measuring meaningful impact. What changed? What helped? How do you know? What is the evidence? These ideas were illustrated through a case study, showing how the impact of different kinds of communication support could be evaluated in a child's journey through a multi-layered system. It is hoped that having read this chapter the reader will go on to consider the possibilities of impact measurement across the chapters that follow.

Recommended resources

The Balanced System® Prove It Platform: Prove It!: Measuring Impact across the Balanced System, Available at: https://proveit.thebalancedsystem.org

World Health Organization: International Classification of Functioning, Disability and Health (ICF). Available at: https://www.who.int/standards/classifications/international-classification-of-functioning-disability-and-health

References

Enderby, P.M., John, A. and Petheram, B. (2006) *Therapy Outcome Measures for Rehabilitation Professionals: Speech and Language Therapy, Physiotherapy, Occupational Therapy, Rehabilitation Nursing & Hearing Therapists*. 2nd edn. Chichester: John Wiley & Sons.

Friedman, M. (2005) *Trying Hard Is Not Good Enough: How to Produce Measurable Improvements for Customers and Communities*. Bloomington, IN: Trafford Publishing.

Hauser, J. and Katz, G. (1998) 'Metrics: You are what you measure!', *European Management Journal*, 16(5), 517–528. DOI: 10.1016/S0263-2373(98)00029-2

Pawson, R. and Tilley, N. (1997) *Realistic Evaluation*. London: Sage Publications.

Roulstone, S. (2015) 'Exploring the relationship between client perspectives, clinical expertise and research evidence', *International Journal of Speech Language Pathology*, 17(3), 211–221.

Roulstone, S.C., Coad, J., Ayre, A., Hambly, H. and Lindsay, G. (2012) 'The preferred outcomes of children with speech, language and communication needs and their parents'. Available at: https://assets.publishing.service.gov.uk/media/5a7ce59940f0b6629523c764/DFE-RR247-BCRP12.pdf (accessed 10 April 2025).

PART II
Speech

7 Speech Sound Disorders (SSDs)

Joanne Cleland and Helen Stringer

What you'll learn in this chapter

- What Speech Sound Disorders are, and how to describe different subtypes
- How to do a basic differential diagnosis for children with more straightforward presentations of Speech Sound Disorder
- Key intervention choices for children with Speech Sound Disorder.

Key information about Speech Sound Disorder

Speech Sound Disorder (SSD) is a term for any difficulty a child has learning to perceive and/ or produce the speech sounds in their language learning environment. The severity of SSD varies widely from speech that is unintelligible to even close family members, to mild difficulties with only one or two speech sounds such as the consonants /ɹ/ and /s/. Severity is not necessarily correlated with impact: children with difficulty with only one or two speech sounds may have significant social and emotional impacts. SSD is a theory-neutral term; this means that it encompasses a wide range of aetiologies and presentations, and a diagnosis of SSD in itself does not indicate a particular management plan. This requires differential diagnosis of specific SSD subtypes and a full understanding of a child's communication profile.

In some children, SSD is caused by anatomical differences, such as cleft palate +/- lip (see Chapter 16), or is associated with a congenital condition such as Down syndrome. However, for many children the SSD is of (currently) unknown origin. This chapter focuses on these children, but the assessment and treatment principles generally apply across both known and unknown causes. SSD is a high incidence condition, affecting about 3.4-3.8% of children aged 4-8 (Eadie et al., 2015; Wren et al., 2016; Shriberg et al., 2019). In the UK, over 57,000 children are referred for speech and language therapy services annually due to SSD (Broomfield and Dodd, 2004). For most children with an SSD of unknown origin, the prognosis is good, with many children achieving speech like their peers by around 7 years (To et al., 2022). However, when SSD persists into the school years, it can lead to decreased academic performance and negative impacts on social, emotional, and behavioural development (Wren et al., 2021; Wren et al., 2023).

Differential diagnosis of SSD into subtypes is crucial for treatment planning. In many countries SSDs are classified according to a model based on observable features, first

SSD subtype	Definition	Relative incidence
Phonological Delay	Presence of a small number of speech error patterns that are typical of younger children (e.g., in English: stopping of fricatives; deletion of /l, r, w, j/ in stop + continuant clusters; weak syllable deletion). Adapted from (Dodd, 2014).	Most common. 55% (Ttofari Eecen et al., 2019) to 57% (Broomfield and Dodd, 2004) of children with SSD of unknown origin fit this subtype
Consistent Phonological Disorder (CPD)	Consistent use of one or more unusual or non-developmental error patterns (e.g., backing, initial consonant deletion). A child may also display some developmental error patterns that are delayed or not age-appropriate. Children with extensive phoneme collapse, or older children with persistent delayed patterns, may be classified as having CPD. Adapted from Dodd (2014).	Common. 20% (Broomfield and Dodd, 2004; Ttofari Eecen et al., 2019) of children with SSD of unknown origin fit this subtype
Inconsistent Phonological Disorder (IPD)	Multiple phonemic error forms for the same lexical item while having no obvious oro-motor difficulties, with a criterion of ≥40% inconsistency. Children perform better in imitation than spontaneous production. Adapted from Dodd (2014).	Common. 9% (Broomfield, Cleland and Williams, 2022) to 15% (Ttofari Eecen et al., 2019) of children with SSD of unknown origin fit this subtype
Articulation Disorder	Substitutions or distortions of the same sounds in isolation and in all phonetic contexts during imitation, elicitation, and spontaneous speech tasks (e.g., lisp). Child is not stimulable for specific sound(s) at any level. Adapted from Dodd (2014).	Common for children to have some articulatory difficulty but in preschool children it is *uncommon* for the diagnosis to be articulation disorder alone (Ttofari Eecen et al., 2019). Older children may present with residual speech sound errors (usually on /r/ or /s/) that could be classified as this subtype. These are common.
Childhood Apraxia of Speech (CAS)	Inconsistency of consonants or vowels across words and syllables, lengthened and disrupted coarticulatory transitions (e.g., slow/distorted/staccato) AND inappropriate prosody (usually lexical stress). Adapted from (ASHA, 2007).	Rare. 0.2–2.4% of children with SSD have CAS (Broomfield and Dodd, 2004; Baylis and Shriberg, 2019). Greater incidence of CAS in neurodevelopmental conditions, e.g. Down syndrome (Shriberg et al., 2019).

Table 7.1 SSD subtypes and definitions

introduced by Barbara Dodd in 1995 and since updated (Dodd, 2005; 2014). In 2024, the Royal College of Speech and Language Therapists (RCSLT) adopted this model, with some adaptations (Stringer et al., 2024) as standard terminology for the UK. Therefore, SLTs practising in this area should use the classification system and descriptions in Table 7.1 (Royal College of Speech and Language Therapists, 2024). We include incidence figures to help clinicians determine which diagnoses are the most likely for a child presenting with SSD. However, these should be used with caution as they vary by the age of the child and whether the child has any co-occurring diagnoses. For example, a child with a history of consistent phonological disorder may have one or two articulatory errors which persist into later childhood. For more on persistent and residual speech sound errors, see Flipsen (2015). These are relatively common, affecting 1–2% of all adults. Examples of these include lisps or difficulties producing /r/.

Important points about SLT practice in SSD

Although the UK has adopted Dodd's differential diagnosis system for SSD as standard, not all countries have an agreed classification system. A number of different terms are used in practice and research. Clinicians aware of these differences can more accurately access the international evidence base and apply it to their clients.

McLeod and Baker (2017) list 41 different terms to describe SSDs of unknown origin in their textbook. Many of these terms reflect clinician preferences and cultural differences, for example, using the term articulation impairment, rather than articulation disorder. Other differences are for pragmatic reasons. For example, McLeod and Baker (2017) subsume 'phonological delay' and 'consistent phonological disorder' into one label: 'phonological impairment' because the interventions for both are the same (see below). Not all countries use Dodd's differential diagnosis system. For example, the Speech Disorder Classification System (SDCS) was developed in the USA, where it is mainly used (Shriberg et al., 2010), updated in (Shriberg et al., 2019). This classification system is based on aetiology. For example, one SDCS subtype is 'speech delay-otitis media with effusion', reflecting the fact that in many children conductive hearing loss leads to difficulties with intelligible speech. In contrast, in Dodd's model, a child with hearing loss and developmental speech errors might be classified as having phonological delay – even though knowing about the hearing loss is essential to develop a management plan. The SSD subtype of Childhood Dysarthria (Shriberg et al., 2019) is missing from Dodd's model because this condition often arises from a known cause, such as cerebral palsy. Dysarthria is a motor speech disorder cause by neurological impairment characterised by a difficulty controlling and executing speech movements. In some cases of childhood dysarthria augmentative and alternative forms of communication (see Chapter 4) are the most appropriate intervention. For more on speech treatment approaches for childhood dysarthria, see Pennington and Hodge (2021).

One further subtype of SSD missing from Dodd's model is speech motor delay (Shriberg and Wren, 2019). This is potentially a relatively common condition in young children, affecting around 12% of those with SSD of unknown origin (Shriberg and Wren, 2019). It is characterised by a delay in the development of speech motor control. Clinicians will be familiar with children who present as having mild difficulties with speech motor control, but do not meet the definition for CAS (see Table 7.1). Indeed, Ttofari Eecen et al. (2019) suggest that around 10% of children with SSD have atypical speech motor control. In these cases, treatment approaches are likely to involve those suitable for children with articulation disorder or phonological delay/consistent phonological disorder.

For children with complex SSD, a psycholinguistic model can support differential diagnosis and intervention choices (Bates, Titterington and Child Speech Disorder Research Network, 2021). In the UK, the predominant model is Stackhouse and Wells (1993), which is included in the RCSLT recommendations. However, other psycholinguistic models may provide helpful information in areas such as self-monitoring (Terband, Maassen and Maas, 2019). These models provide information about factors contributing to SSD, such as phonological awareness or motor programming, which are important in setting therapy goals. Phonological awareness skills underpin, for example, phonological recognition, phonological representations, motor programming and motor programmes (Stackhouse and Wells, 1997). Difficulties in this area of phonology can have lasting impact on speech, vocabulary learning (Gathercole, 2006) and literacy (Bird, Bishop and Freeman, 1995).

Assessment, diagnosis and therapy for children with SSD, contrary to other types of speech, language and communication needs (SLCN), are often impairment-based. This is especially the case for children with SSD of unknown origin because interventions can be very effective. Intervention is usually at the specialist level with individual sessions carried out by an SLT and extra practice with a carer between sessions.

Understanding children's needs in SSD

SSD can often co-occur with language difficulties and therefore assessment should consider the child holistically. Assessment for SSD should be set in the context of the child's environmental and personal factors, with activity and participation at the core of the assessment process. The languages spoken by the child must also be taken into consideration, although there is a lack of standardised speech assessments in many languages. You can find a useful list of assessments in languages of the world at the Multilingual Children's Speech web resource (McLeod, 2024).

A key aim of assessment is to determine the subtype of SSD (see above). Most interventions for SSD are designed for specific subtypes and therefore an accurate differential diagnosis is crucial for determining a management plan (Stringer et al., 2024). Assessment also helps identify the severity of the SSD and measure progress and outcomes. Population screening for SSD is not recommended. However, a screening process, or triage, to determine the presence or absence of SSD in children observed to have speech difficulties is a useful starting point. If the presence of an SSD is confirmed, then a more detailed assessment, incorporating a full case history alongside the phonetic and phonological profile of the child's speech and assessment of input processing skills and phonological awareness, is needed. At all stages of this assessment, accurate phonetic transcription will be needed.

Cleland et al. (2023) developed a diagnostic protocol with NHS SLTs across the UK. This protocol is designed to align with the SSD subtypes described above and to be suitable for use in the NHS. The protocol suggests using the Diagnostic Evaluation of Articulation and Phonology (DEAP) (Dodd et al., 2002) as the main assessment for this group of children. This assessment is also recommended by the RCSLT. It comprises specific subtests for screening for SSD and for assessing both the phonetic (articulatory) and phonological aspects of a child's speech. It is also standardised on UK children. The DEAP can only be carried out by a SLT (or supervised SLT student) because it requires phonetic transcription skills, knowledge of phonological processes, and knowledge of acquisition norms for specific speech sounds (see McLeod, 2024, for ages of acquisition of consonants in different languages). Assessors new to the DEAP should read the manual carefully, particularly regarding differential diagnosis of subtypes of SSD. The words in the DEAP are carefully chosen to sample English phonology using words familiar to young children in the UK, therefore different word lists will be used in other languages or cultures.

For children with suspected articulation disorder, it is essential to measure stimulability. This is a child's ability to produce consonants and vowels in limited contexts such as a simple consonant-vowel sequence. When a child is not stimulable for speech sounds appropriate to their age, intervention may need to focus on establishing the correct articulation for these sounds.

To measure overall intelligibility, a parent-reported outcome measure such as the Intelligibility in Context Scale (ICS) (McLeod, Harrison and McCormack, 2012) should be used. This parent-reported questionnaire is freely available in over 60 languages. Table 7.2 summarises the key assessments for children with SSD.

It is important to note that this assessment protocol is a minimum. Children with more severe and complex SSD will need additional or different assessments, see Table 7.3. For example, the Newcastle Assessment of Phonological Awareness (NAPA) (Stringer, 2019a) is useful in assessing phonological awareness skills in all children with SSD.

Speech area	Suggested tools for core speech sample
Initial screen	DEAP Diagnostic Screen (Dodd et al., 2002) and the ICS (McLeod, Harrison and McCormack, 2012)
Single Word Naming	DEAP Phonology Assessment or toddler version
Stimulability	Stimulability Assessment (Powell and Miccio, 1996) or DEAP Articulation & Oromotor Assessment, for consonants and vowels absent from the phonetic inventory
Intelligibility	Informal clinician rating based on connected speech from, for example, the Renfrew Action Picture Test (Renfrew, 2016), and the ICS
(In)consistency	DEAP Diagnostic Screen (repeated twice), then the DEAP Inconsistency Assessment if indicated

Table 7.2 Summary of assessment tools for SSD

Source: Cleland et al. (2023).

Assessment area	Example tool
Vowels	Clinical Assessment of Vowels-English Systems CAVES https://sites.marjon.ac.uk/caves/
Polysyllables	Polysyllable Preschool Test (Baker, 2013)
Inconsistency	DEAP Inconsistency Assessment
Oral structure and function	Clinical Assessment of Oropharyngeal Motor Development in Young Children (Robbins & Klee, 1987) or DEAP
DDK	Clinical Assessment of Oropharyngeal Motor Development in Young Children (Robbins & Klee, 1987) or DEAP
Phonological awareness	Newcastle Assessment of Phonological Awareness (Stringer, 2019a)
(Hyper)nasality and resonance	Clinical Assessment of Oropharyngeal Motor Development in Young Children (Robbins & Klee, 1987) or subjective

Table 7.3 Suggested tools for in-depth assessment of areas of difficulty

For children with suspected motor speech disorders, the DEAP Articulation and Oromotor Assessment is helpful in signposting additional assessment. For children with suspected CAS, the Nuffield Dyspraxia Programme Assessment is suggested (Williams and Stephens, 2004). A more detailed oromotor assessment is important for identifying dysarthria, though note many children with dysarthria will have medical diagnoses such as cerebral palsy (Iuzzini-Seigel, Allison and Stoeckel, 2022). Nevertheless, an oromotor assessment is an important part of the clinician's toolkit and necessary for ruling out cleft palate or lip since, for example, children with submucous cleft palate may go undetected or appear similar to children with CAS due to ongoing speech difficulties, including resonance disorders.

Supporting children's needs in Speech Sound Disorder

Clinicians should involve parents/carers and children in the decision-making process about management plans. The overall goal of speech intervention is usually to improve children's intelligibility and this should be measured as the core (main) outcome of intervention using a measure such as the ICS (McLeod, Harrison and McCormack, 2012) and a robust measure of speech production accuracy such as percentage consonants correct (PCC). This can be calculated from the DEAP both before and after intervention. The amount of intervention a child needs will depend on the subtype of SSD, the severity, the impact and any concomitant difficulties. Since most speech interventions are at the specialist level and involve working one-to-one with the child, it is important that children are ready for intervention. Children should have communicative intent, joint attention, and the ability to take turns in an activity. Often sessions can be delivered in shorter durations more frequently, or with additional practice at home by parents/carers, if a child's attention does not allow long sessions. Children with CAS, in particular, may need prolonged and intense intervention, sometimes lasting many years.

There are many different interventions available for children with SSD and it can be difficult to decide which intervention to choose. An umbrella review of interventions for children with SSD identified 46 different interventions for SSD (Harding et al., 2024), but the evidence base for these varies widely. Generally, clinicians think of interventions as falling into two broad categories: phonological interventions and articulatory/motor interventions. As you would expect, phonological interventions are used to treat the various types of phonological SSDs and articulatory/motor interventions are used to treat articulation disorder and CAS.

Phonological interventions are linguistic or cognitive. They presume that a child's difficulty is with the rules of the phonological system of their language and the intervention aims to teach children these rules. For example, a child with the phonological process of final consonant deletion (which will have been identified from the DEAP Phonology Assessment described above) may benefit from an intervention that confronts the child with the homophony in their system by contrasting words which differ only in the presence of a final consonant, for example, 'bee' versus 'beak'. Conventional minimal pair therapy (Baker, 2021) works in this way. You can find lists of minimal pairs online, but you need to ensure that they are suitable for the accent background of the child you are working with. When children have many different phonological processes present in their speech, an approach which targets more than one phonological contrast at a time, such as multiple oppositions, may be more efficient. The Supporting and Understanding Speech Sound Disorder website (Hegarty et al., 2018) has a useful tool for helping choose the right phonological intervention. For children with inconsistent phonological disorder, the underlying difficulty is with selecting and sequencing phonemes. This leads to high levels of inconsistency at a lexical (word) level. Intervention needs to prioritise consistency, rather than accuracy. Core vocabulary therapy (Crosbie, Holm and Dodd, 2021) targets this by focusing on small numbers of words in each intervention session and reinforcing awareness of word structure (syllables and phonemes) and consistent productions.

Articulatory or motor-based interventions focus on helping children learn and sequence the correct speech movements. Often they work in a hierarchical fashion, moving from small units such as consonant-vowel sequences through single syllable words all the way to phrase or conversational level. Where articulatory difficulties seem severe and resistant to change, it may be helpful to revisit their differential diagnosis to rule out submucous cleft palate or CAS. For children with CAS, there are several intervention options. The Nuffield Programme (Williams and Stephens, 2004) and DTTC (Strand, 2021) are recommended for younger children, or those with more severe disorders, while ReST (McCabe et al., 2017) and Integrated Phonological Awareness (McNeill and Gillon, 2021) may be more suitable for older children. Ultrasound biofeedback is useful for establishing new articulations in older children who are not stimulable for specific speech sounds (Cleland and Preston, 2021).

For all speech interventions, practice is key. Interventions delivered with fewer sessions or teaching episodes per session (i.e. the number of times a child practises a target sound within a session) as far less likely to be effective. For children with phonological delay or consistent phonological disorder, over 50 teaching episodes per session are necessary (Williams, 2012), while for children with CAS, over 100 practice opportunities per session are needed (Kaipa and Peterson, 2016). Clinicians should not offer interventions at a dosage which is unlikely to be effective. Table 7.4 details which interventions have the best evidence base for each subtype of SSD.

SSD subtypes	Recommended interventions
Phonological Delay and Consistent Phonological Disorder	Conventional Minimal Pairs (Baker, 2021)
	Multiple oppositions (Williams and Sugden, 2021)
	Complexity approaches (Morrisette, 2021)
Inconsistent Phonological Disorder	Core Vocabulary Intervention (Crosbie, Holm and Dodd, 2021)
Articulation Disorder	Traditional Articulation Therapy (Preston and Leece, 2021)
Childhood Apraxia of Speech	Rapid Syllable Transition Treatment (ReST) (McCabe et al., 2017)
	Nuffield Dyspraxia Programme (Williams and Stephens, 2004)
	Dynamic Temporal and Tactile Cueing (DTTC) (Strand, 2021)
	Integrated Phonological Awareness (McNeill and Gillon, 2021)
	Ultrasound biofeedback (Cleland and Preston, 2021)

Table 7.4 SSD subtypes and recommended interventions

Note: The references given in this table are to recommended reading for clinicians who want to deliver the intervention, rather than to the seminal papers where the intervention was first described or to key empirical studies.

Tom's story

Tom is 4 years 8 months old. He is unintelligible to his family and to strangers. The DEAP Diagnostic Screen indicated further articulation and phonological assessment was necessary. The following sounds were not stimulable: /ʃ, ʧ, ʤ, z/. His Percentage Consonants Correct (PCC) was 25%, giving him a standard score of 3 and placing him in the 1st centile, indicating a severe SSD. Analysis of errors in the DEAP Phonology Assessment revealed 30 instances of final consonant deletion, 20 of cluster reduction, 6 of fronting, stopping and medial consonant deletion and 2 instances of deaffrication and backing. He also showed a phoneme collapse of /f, v, θ, ð, ɹ/ to [w]. His phonological awareness skills were good at syllable level but failed at all phoneme levels. Intervention focused on multiple oppositions (Williams and Sugden, 2021), addressing phoneme collapse and phonological awareness identifying initial and final sounds (Stringer, 2019b). Ten weekly sessions with an SLT with an average of 50 practice items per target were followed up by additional daily practice at home, focusing on a different target each day. Phonological awareness goals were also reinforced at school. On re-assessment, Tom's PCC was 49%, which did not change his standard score or percentile rank. However, his phonological system had changed significantly. There were only nine instances of final consonant deletion which did improve his intelligibility. The nature of cluster reduction changed, with three-part clusters reducing to two-part clusters rather than to just one consonant as previously. Two-part clusters were now realised correctly. The phoneme collapse had now disappeared, replaced by developmental error patterns, for example, fronting (11 instances). His next episode of intervention would therefore focus on a complexity approach for consonant clusters (Morrisette, 2021) and conventional minimal pairs to address fronting and stopping (Baker, 2021). More information about these intervention approaches can be found on the SuSSD website: https://www.ulster.ac.uk/research/topic/nursing-and-health/caring-for-people-with-complex-needs/research-themes/neurodevelopmental/ssd

Summary

Speech Sound Disorder is an umbrella term for difficulties children face in producing or perceiving sounds in their ambient language. Severity ranges from minor mispronunciations to unintelligible speech. Persistent SSD can lead to academic and social challenges. SSD is classified in five different subtypes: Phonological Delay, Consistent Phonological Disorder, Inconsistent Phonological Disorder, Articulation Disorder, and Childhood Apraxia of Speech. Differential diagnosis into these subtypes is crucial to determine the best intervention for a child.

Interventions for SSD are often impairment-based, focusing on improving intelligibility. They are usually delivered at the specialist level by an SLT in collaboration with parents/carers and can be very effective. They are broadly categorised as phonological or motor-based interventions. Phonological therapy teaches children the rules of their language's sound system. Motor-based therapy focuses on practising speech movements, often from simple syllables to more complex speech. For all types of SSD intervention, adequate dosage and consistent practice are key to achieving good outcomes.

Recommended resources

Bates, S., Titterington, J., and Child Speech Disorder Research Network (CSDRN) (2017) 'Good practice guidelines for the analysis of child speech'. Available at: https://www.rcslt.org/wp-content/uploads/2019/11/guidelines-for-analysis-of-childspeech-data.pdf.

Child Speech Disorder Research Network (CSDRN) (2017) 'Good practice guidelines for the transcription of children's speech in clinical practice and research'. Available at: https://www.rcslt.org/wpcontent/uploads/media/docs/clinical-guidance/bsltru-good-practice-guidelinestranscription.pdf

Multilingual Children's Speech. Available at: https://www.csu.edu.au/research/multilingual-speech/home

Royal College of Speech and Language Therapists (2024) *Speech Sound Disorders Guidance*. Available at: https://www.rcslt.org/members/clinical-guidance/speech-sound-disorders/speech-sound-disorders-guidance/

Royal College of Speech and Language Therapists, 'Speech Sound Disorders: Position paper on childhood apraxia of speech'. Available at: https://www.rcslt.org/wp-content/uploads/2024/02/RCSLT-Childhood-Apraxia-of-Speech-CAS-Position-Paper-2024.pdf

SpeechSTAR. Available at: https://speechstar.ac.uk/

SuSSD (Supporting and Understanding Speech Sound Disorder). Available at: https://www.ulster.ac.uk/research/topic/nursing-and-health/caring-for-people-with-complex-needs/research-themes/neurodevelopmental/ssd

References

ASHA (American Speech-Language-Hearing Association) (2007) 'Childhood apraxia of speech' [Technical Report]. Rockville, MD: ASHA.

Baker, E. (2013) *Polysyllable Preschool Test*. Sydney, Australia: Author.

Baker, E. (2021) 'Minimal pairs intervention'. In A.L. Williams, M. Sharynne and J.M. Rebecca (eds), *Interventions for Speech Sound Disorders in Children*. Baltimore, MD: Brookes Publishing, pp. 33–61.

Bates, S., Titterington, J. and Child Speech Disorder Research Network (2021) 'Good practice guidelines for the analysis of child speech'. Ulster: Ulster University.

Baylis, A.L. and Shriberg, L.D. (2019) 'Estimates of the prevalence of speech and motor speech disorders in youth with 22q11.2 deletion syndrome', *American Journal of Speech-Language Pathology*, 28(1), 53–82. http://dx.doi.org/doi:10.1044/2018_AJSLP-18-0037

Bird, J., Bishop, D.V.M. and Freeman, N.H. (1995) 'Phonological awareness and literacy development in children with expressive phonological impairments', *Journal of Speech, Language, and Hearing Research*, 38(2), 446-462. http://dx.doi.org/doi:10.1044/jshr.3802.446.

Broomfield, J., Cleland, J. and Williams, P. (2022) 'What's in a name? Dr Jan Broomfield, Dr Joanne Cleland and Dr Pam Williams make their case for adopting the term "childhood apraxia of speech"', *Bulletin: The Official Magazine of the Royal College of Speech and Language Therapists*, 833, 1-2. Available at: https://strathprints.strath.ac.uk/83091/

Broomfield, J. and Dodd, B. (2004) 'Children with speech and language disability: Caseload characteristics', *International Journal of Language & Communication Disorders*, 39(3), 303-324. http://dx.doi.org/https://doi.org/10.1080/13682820310001625589.

Cleland, J., Burr, S.A., Harding, S.A., Stringer, H. and Wren, Y. (2023) 'Development of an agreed labelling system and protocol for the diagnosis of speech sound disorder subtypes in the United Kingdom'. Available at: osf.io/nm2c6.

Cleland, J. and Preston, J. (2021) 'Biofeedback interventions'. In A.L. Williams, S. McLeod and R.J. McCauley (eds), *Interventions for Speech Sound Disorders in Children*. Baltimore, MD: Pearson, pp. 573-599.

Crosbie, S.L., Holm, A. and Dodd, B. (2021) 'Core vocabulary intervention'. In A.L. Williams, S. McLeod, and R.J. McCauley (eds), *Interventions for Speech Sound Disorders in Children*. 2nd edn. Baltimore, MD: Paul H. Brookes Publishing Co., pp. 225-250.

Dodd, B. (2005) *Differential Diagnosis and Treatment Of Children With Speech Disorder*. Oxford: Wiley-Blackwell.

Dodd, B. (2014) ''Differential diagnosis of pediatric speech sound disorder', *Current Developmental Disorders Reports*, 1(3), 189-196. http://dx.doi.org/10.1007/s40474-014-0017-3.

Dodd, B., Zhu, H., Crosbi, S. and Holm. A. (2002) *Diagnostic Evaluation of Articulation And Phonology (DEAP)*. London: Psychological Corporation.

Eadie, P., Morgan, A., Ukoumunne, O.C., Ttofari Eecen, K., Wake, M. and Reilly, S. (2015) 'Speech sound disorder at 4 years: Prevalence, comorbidities, and predictors in a community cohort of children', *Developmental Medicine & Child Neurology*, 57(6), 578-584. http://dx.doi.org/https://doi.org/10.1111/dmcn.12635.

Flipsen, P., Jr. (2015) 'Emergence and prevalence of persistent and residual speech errors', *Seminars in Speech and Language*, 36(04), 217-223. http://dx.doi.org/10.1055/s-0035-1562905.

Gathercole, S.E. (2006) 'Nonword repetition and word learning: The nature of the relationship'. *Applied Psycholinguistics*, 27(4), 513-543. http://dx.doi.org/10.1017/S0142716406060383.

Harding, S., Burr, S., Cleland, J., Stringer, H. and Wren, Y. (2024) 'Outcome measures for children with speech sound disorder: An umbrella review', *BMJ Open*, 14(4), e081446. http://dx.doi.org/10.1136/bmjopen-2023-081446.

Hegarty, N., Titterington, J., McLeod, S. and Taggart, T. (2018) 'SuSSD: Supporting and Understanding Speech Sound Disorders'. Online resource. Available at: https://www.ulster.ac.uk/research/topic/nursing-and-health/caring-for-people-with-complex-needs/research-themes/neurodevelopmental/ssd/about (Accessed: 16/08/2024).

Iuzzini-Seigel, J., Allison, K.M. and Stoeckel, R. (2022) 'A tool for differential diagnosis of childhood apraxia of speech and dysarthria in children: A tutorial'. *Language, Speech, and Hearing Services in Schools*, 53(4), 926-946. http://dx.doi.org/doi:10.1044/2022_LSHSS-21-00164.

Kaipa, R. and Peterson, A.M. (2016) 'A systematic review of treatment intensity in speech disorders', *International Journal of Speech-Language Pathology*, 18(6), 507-520. http://dx.doi.org/10.3109/17549507.2015.1126640.

McCabe, P., Thomas, D., Murray, E., Crocco, L. and Madill, C. (2017) *Rapid Syllable Transition Treatment – ReST*. Available at: https://rest.sydney.edu.au/ (accessed 16 August 2024).

McLeod, S. (2024) 'Multilingual children's speech'. Available at: https://www.csu.edu.au/research/multilingual-speech/home (accessed 26 February 2025).

McLeod, S. and Baker, E. (2017) *Children's speech: An evidence-based approach to assessment and intervention*. Harlow: Pearson.

McLeod, S., Harrison, L.J. and McCormack, J. (2012) 'The Intelligibility in Context Scale: Validity and reliability of a subjective rating measure', *Journal of Speech, Language, and Hearing Research*, 55(2), 648-656. http://dx.doi.org/doi:10.1044/1092-4388(2011/10-0130).

McNeill, B. and Gillon, G. (2021) 'Integrated phonological awareness'. In A.L. Williams, M. Sharynne and J.M. Rebecca (eds), *Interventions for Speech Sound Disorders in Children*. Baltimore, MD: Brookes Publishing, pp. 111-139.

Morrisette, M.L. (2021) 'Complexity approach'. In A.L. Williams, M. Sharynne and J.M. Rebecca (eds), *Interventions for Speech Sound Disorders in Children*. Baltimore, MD: Brookes Publishing, pp. 91–110.

Pennington, L. and Hodge, M. (2021) 'Intervention strategies for developmental dysarthria'. In A.L. Williams, M. Sharynne and J.M. Rebecca (eds), *Interventions for Speech Sound Disorders in Children*. Baltimore, MD: Brookes Publishing, pp. 601–625.

Powell, T.W. and Miccio, A.W. (1996) 'Stimulability: A useful clinical tool', *Journal of Communication Disorders*, 29(4), 237–253. http://dx.doi.org/https://doi.org/10.1016/0021-9924(96)00012-3.

Preston, J. and Leece, M.C. (2021) 'Articulation interventions'. In A.L. Williams, M. Sharynne and J.M. Rebecca (eds), *Interventions for Speech Sound Disorders in Children*. Baltimore, MD: Brookes Publishing, pp. 419–445.

Renfrew, C.E. (2016) *The Renfrew Language Scales: Action Picture Test*. Milton Keynes: Speechmark.

Robbins, J. and Klee, T. (1987) 'Clinical assessment of oropharyngeal motor development in young children', *Journal of Speech and Hearing Disorders*, 52(3), 271–277. https://doi-org.proxy.lib.strath.ac.uk/10.1044/jshd.5203.27

Royal College of Speech and Language Therapists (2024) *Speech Sound Disorder Guidance* Available at: https://www.rcslt.org/members/clinical-guidance/speech-sound-disorders/speech-sound-disorders-guidance/ (accessed 31 May 2024).

Shriberg, L.D., Fourakis, M., Hall, S.D., Karlsson, H.B., Lohmeier, H.L., McSweeny, J.L., Potter, N.L., Scheer-Cohen, A.R., Strand, E.A., Tilkens, C.M. and Wilson, D.L. (2010) 'Extensions to the Speech Disorders Classification System (SDCS)', *Clinical Linguistics & Phonetics*, 24(10), 795–824. http://dx.doi.org/10.3109/02699206.2010.503006.

Shriberg, L.D., Strand, E.A., Jakielski, K.J. and Mabie, H.L. (2019) 'Estimates of the prevalence of speech and motor speech disorders in persons with complex neurodevelopmental disorders', *Clinical Linguistics & Phonetics*, 33(8), 707–736. http://dx.doi.org/10.1080/02699206.2019.1595732.

Shriberg, L.D. and Wren, Y.E. (2019) 'A frequent acoustic sign of speech motor delay (SMD)', *Clinical Linguistics & Phonetics*, 33(8), 757–771. http://dx.doi.org/10.1080/02699206.2019.1595734.

Stackhouse, J. and Wells, B. (1993) 'Psycholinguistic assessment of developmental speech disorders', *European Journal of Disorders of Communication*, 28(4), 331–348. http://dx.doi.org/10.3109/13682829309041469.

Stackhouse, J. and Wells, B. (1997) *Children's Speech and Literacy Difficulties: A Psycholinguistic Framework*. Chichester: Wiley.

Strand, E.A. (2021) 'Dynamic temporal and tactile cueing'. In A.L. Williams, M. Sharynne and J.M. Rebecca (eds), *Interventions for Speech Sound Disorders in Children*. Baltimore, MD: Brookes Publishing, pp. 587–571.

Stringer, H. (2019a) *Newcastle Assessment for Phonological Awareness (NAPA)*. Available at: https://research.ncl.ac.uk/phonologicalawareness/.

Stringer, H. (2019b) *Newcastle Intervention for Phonological Awareness (NIPA)*. Available at: https://research.ncl.ac.uk/phonologicalawareness/assessmentandintervention/.

Stringer, H., Cleland, J., Wren, Y., Rees, R. and Williams, P. (2024) 'Speech sound disorder or DLD (phonology)? Towards a consensus agreement on terminology', *International Journal of Language & Communication Disorders*, 59(6), 2131–2145. http://dx.doi.org/https://doi.org/10.1111/1460-6984.12989.

Terband, H., Maassen, B. and Maas, E. (2019) 'A psycholinguistic framework for diagnosis and treatment planning of developmental speech disorders', *Folia Phoniatrica et Logopaedica*, 71(5-6), 216–227. http://dx.doi.org/10.1159/000499426.

To, C.K.S., McLeod, S., Sam, K.L. and Law, P. (2022) 'Predicting which children will normalize without intervention for speech sound disorders', *Journal of Speech, Language, and Hearing Research*, 65(5), 1724–1741. http://dx.doi.org/doi:10.1044/2022_JSLHR-21-00444.

Ttofari Eecen, K., Eadie, P., Morgan, A.T. and Reilly, S. (2019) 'Validation of Dodd's model for differential diagnosis of childhood speech sound disorders: A longitudinal community cohort study', *Developmental Medicine & Child Neurology*, 61(6), 689–696. http://dx.doi.org/https://doi.org/10.1111/dmcn.13993.

Williams, A.L. (2012) 'Intensity in phonological intervention: Is there a prescribed amount?' *International Journal of Speech-Language Pathology*, 14(5), 456–461. http://dx.doi.org/10.3109/17549507.2012.688866.

Williams, A.L. and Sugden, E. (2021) 'Multiple oppositions'. In A.L. Williams, M. Sharynne and J.M. Rebecca (eds), *Interventions for Speech Sound Disorders in Children*. Bltimore, MD: Brookes Publishing, pp. 61–89.

Williams, P. and Stephens, H. (2004) *Nuffield Centre Dyspraxia Programme*. Miracle Factory.

Wren, Y., Miller, L.L., Peters, T.J., Emond, A. and Roulstone, S. (2016) 'Prevalence and predictors of persistent speech sound disorder at eight years old: Findings from a population cohort study', *Journal of Speech, Language, and Hearing Research*, 59(4), 647–673. http://dx.doi.org/doi:10.1044/2015_JSLHR-S-14-0282.

Wren, Y., Pagnamenta, E., Orchard, F., Peters, T.J., Emond, A., Northstone, K., Miller, L.L. and Roulstone, S. (2023) 'Social, emotional and behavioural difficulties associated with persistent speech disorder in children: A prospective population study', *Journal of Child Psychology and Psychiatry Advances*, 3(1), e12126. http://dx.doi.org/https://doi.org/10.1002/jcv2.12126.

Wren, Y., Pagnamenta, E., Peters, T.J., Emond, A., Northstone, K., Miller, L.L. and Roulstone, S. (2021) 'Educational outcomes associated with persistent speech disorder', *International Journal of Language & Communication Disorders*, 56(2), 299–312. http://dx.doi.org/https://doi.org/10.1111/1460-6984.12599.

8 Voice

Wendy Cohen

What you'll learn in this chapter

- How voice is produced
- How the complex mechanisms involved in producing voice can go wrong, leading to voice disorder
- How speech and language therapists (SLTs) can assess children with voice disorders
- How SLTs can support children with voice disorders.

Key information about voice disorders in children

Speech consists of sounds produced, while language is how words and sentences are used or understood. Both are assumed to occur with normal laryngeal function. Where there is any disorder of laryngeal function, this leads to a voice disorder (sometimes called hoarseness or dysphonia).

Vocalisation requires the effortless coordination of respiratory, phonatory and resonatory systems. Subglottic air pressure during respiration moves through the larynx, causing the vocal folds to vibrate at high speed. This vibration results in sound – phonation – which moves through the supraglottic airway and vocal tract where discrete movements within the vocal tract alter phonation (resonance). If one (or more) of these systems is operating sub-optimally, this leads to a change in the quality, pitch or loudness of the voice. These changes may only be perceived by the speaker or by the listener or by both. Dysphonia is defined as occurring when there is a change in the quality, pitch or loudness of the voice that is different from what is expected for someone of similar age, gender, cultural background or geographical location (Lee et al., 2004; Boone et al., 2009; Aronson and Bless, 2014). The ICD-11 (World Health Organization, 2022) describes voice disturbances (including dysphonia, aphonia, hypernasality and hyponasality) as relating to the production of various sounds by the passage of air through the larynx.

As these three systems are involved in vocalisation, it might be deduced that any anatomical or physiological differences will impact on voice, however, speakers frequently compensate for minor changes without vocal impact. Furthermore, due to the anatomical changes from infancy to adulthood, only considering respiratory, phonatory and resonatory systems is oversimplistic.

DOI: 10.4324/9781003671626-11

102 *Supporting Children's Speech, Language and Communication Needs*

Full assessment of the voice involves visualisation of the larynx which occurs in a medical setting; thus many published classification systems are derived from a medical perspective. These systems, summarised in Figure 8.1 provide anything from two to nine categories (*Voice Disorders*, n.d.; Mathieson, 2001; Verdolini Abbott et al., 2006; Sapienza and Hoffman, 2022) and differentiate between a congenital (e.g. congenital laryngeal web) and an acquired disorder (e.g. muscle tension dysphonia).

The Royal College of Speech and Language Therapists in the UK (RCSLT, n.d.) recommends we take a more flexible approach, describing voice disorders under four categories: inflammation, neoplastic/structural, muscle tension imbalance and neuromuscular. This model acknowledges that the person's voice disorder might fit into one or more category depending on how long they have had a voice problem and if/how they have changed their own voice production using compensatory manoeuvres.

For example, where the diagnosis is vocal fold nodules (VFN) following Ear Nose and Throat (ENT) investigation, these are defined as small, benign lumps acquired on the vocal folds, classified as *structural* or *organic*. As something abnormal on the vocal folds, either of these classifications is appropriate. However, how VFN arise is multifactorial: they occur due to a physiological response to how the vocal folds are used (i.e. from talking overly loudly all the time or shouting a lot) which is *functional*, and/or the influence of laryngopharyngeal reflux, which is *inflammatory* or *systemic*, so which should we use? In this example, it is <u>how</u> the vocal folds have been used or *how any changes in their use* occur (e.g. in response to inflammation) that causes VFN, and this is more useful information for the SLT. By understanding multifactorial aetiologies, we can help the speaker counteract compensatory behaviours during remediation. This does not detract from needing to know the ENT diagnosis (or classification), as this helps us prepare for any eventuality, and it is important to be familiar with one or more of these classification systems. I recommend whichever your multi-disciplinary team

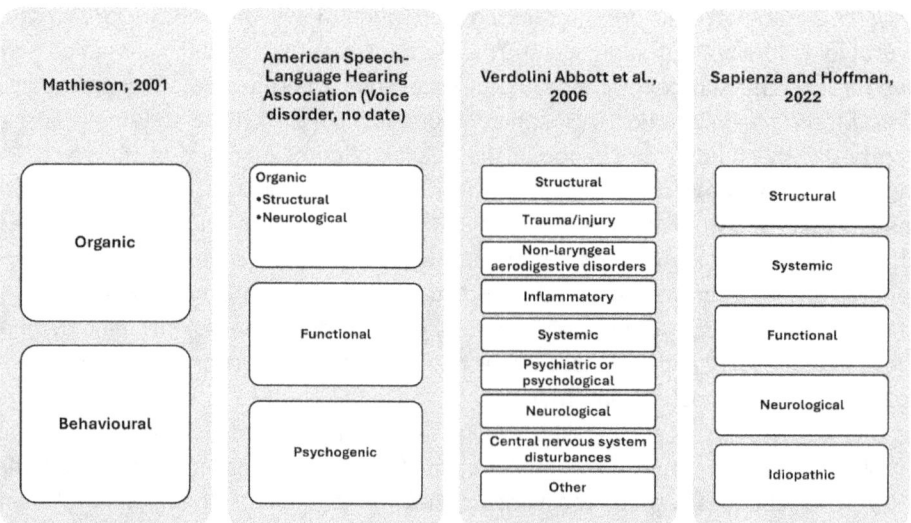

Figure 8.1 Overview of categories in some commonly used voice classifications

(MDT) uses. This allows for a deeper and shared understanding of the various diagnoses and the ability to anticipate what the child's needs might be.

Prevalence of voice disorders in children is between 6-11%, depending on whether the judgement is made by the parent or clinician (Carding, Roulstone and Northstone, 2006). A frequent reason for short-term hoarseness in children is acute viral laryngitis and VFN can occur when hoarseness persists beyond recovery from an upper respiratory tract infection. There is higher prevalence in boys (males) compared to girls (females) (Akif Kiliç et al., 2004; Tavares et al., 2011; Mudd and Noelke, 2018). VFN occur more in the primary school years (5-10 years) with nodules usually shrinking post male puberty though they can persist in females (De Bodt et al., 2007). Other benign vocal fold lesions make up the next most common diagnoses: polyps and cysts (Tavares et al., 2011; Martins et al., 2012). Clinicians need to rule out the rarer juvenile onset recurrent respiratory papillomatosis (RRP), caused by the Human Papilloma Virus (HPV), which usually appears in affected children by 2-4 years though there is evidence that the introduction of the HPV vaccine has contributed to a decline in RRP incidence in countries where the vaccine is widely used.

Benign vocal fold lesions occur as a direct result of phonotraumatic behaviours: that is, there has been repetitive traumatic movement of the vocal folds, sometimes referred to as vocal abuse and misuse. Physiologically, children's vocal folds have not developed the three-layer structure found in adults which provides a shock-absorbing mechanism. Thus, when a child engages in frequent yelling, screaming, talking overly loud, excessive throat clearing or coughing, speaking in too high or too low a pitch (e.g. mimicking cartoon character voices), their vocal folds are more susceptible to (reversible) damage. When combined with the propensity for children to have lower levels of self-control, it can be more challenging for some children to regulate their emotions and vocal output to some situations. Additional risk factors include environmental characteristics (e.g. ventilation, noise, dust, mould, poor temperature regulation); family characteristics (e.g. noise, number of siblings) and individual characteristics (e.g. history of asthma or exposure to irritants; chronic respiratory symptoms and/or infections; personality; participation in extracurricular activities, such as singing, summer camps, sports; dietary effects that may increase likelihood of reflux such as spicy food or dairy produce which can thicken secretions); or children with ADHD who may be more talkative or impulsive, leading to increased phonotrauma through tantrums, yelling and screaming.

While the most common explanation for persistent hoarseness in children is VFN, symptoms of hoarseness may be a sign of another condition, so we should not assume that a child with voice disorder has VFN. Some children may have vocal fold paralysis (unilateral or bilaterial) which may arise following birth trauma or surgical history (iatrogenic); or be neurological or idiopathic in nature. Children with other conditions might also present with hoarseness (e.g. Downs syndrome, Pompe disease, cleft lip/palate). We also provide advice and support to children with voice disorders from more complex but rarer presentations. Examples include those who have had extensive laryngeal reconstruction surgery due to congenital malformation of the larynx (e.g. airway reconstruction surgery), children with RRP, and cases of paradoxical vocal fold movement disorder (PVFMD) (now often described as inducible laryngeal obstruction (ILO)). We should also be mindful of the impact of heavy voice use in young performers. The SLT working with children with voice problems is part of a MDT depending on the child's other needs.

Important points about SLT practice in voice disorders in children

The SLT focuses on behavioural management of voice disorders; however, given the various potential diagnoses, we cannot do this without knowing the underlying aetiological factors. Thus, it is important to ensure that any child with a voice disorder has been evaluated by ENT. This means that, unlike other speech, language and communication needs, paediatric voice therapy can feel more aligned to a medical rather than social model of healthcare, particularly where there is an underlying medical aetiology. Often these children will first present to medical teams who will support the child's presenting medical needs. In some cases (e.g. one risk factor of neonatal cardiac surgery is damage to the recurrent laryngeal nerve causing iatrogenic VFP), a medically unstable infant is primarily supported in relation to safe respiration and feeding. The SLT in a paediatric acute hospital is part of the MDT supporting these vulnerable infants, focusing on feeding and early communication development, rather than voice. In others, some children might present with symptoms of asthma, and it is only if that child is unresponsive to routine asthma treatment that wider MDT evaluation might be considered, potentially revealing PVFMD/ILO. The community-based SLT needs to check the medical background to understand a child with voice disorder's needs - both historically and current - even though these diagnoses are less common than benign vocal fold lesions.

As discussed earlier, benign vocal fold lesions are something on the vocal folds, but how they got there relates to how the child is using their voice. This dynamic relationship between diagnosis and aetiology means we need to support long-term lifestyle change. Children with benign vocal fold lesions need a holistic approach so they alter how they vocalise for the lesions to reduce or resolve. This includes working with parents, siblings and other individuals who have a strong presence in a child's environment, such as teachers.

Identification of children who should be assessed (and/or supported) requires someone in that child's environment to notice there is a problem and act on that observation. Some studies reveal that parents might not be aware of their child's voice care needs unless specifically asked (e.g. Stojanović et al., 2021). The same can be said of teachers, who despite representing a large population in the adult voice clinic themselves are unaware of referral pathways and support for children with voice disorder. Usually when a parent notices that there is a problem, or if teachers have raised this, the first port of call for the parent will be their General Practitioner who is likely to refer for ENT evaluation prior to SLT involvement.

Understanding children's needs in voice

There are international evidence-based guidelines for hoarseness with recommendations for assessment and treatment principally for the adult population (Dejonckere et al., 2001; Stachler et al., 2018). While these are considered relevant for all ages, adaptations are necessary for paediatric populations. There is no single tool that can capture all the information, so we take a multi-factorial approach to voice evaluation. Our approach to understanding how voice disorder affects an individual can be aligned with the ICF framework (World Health

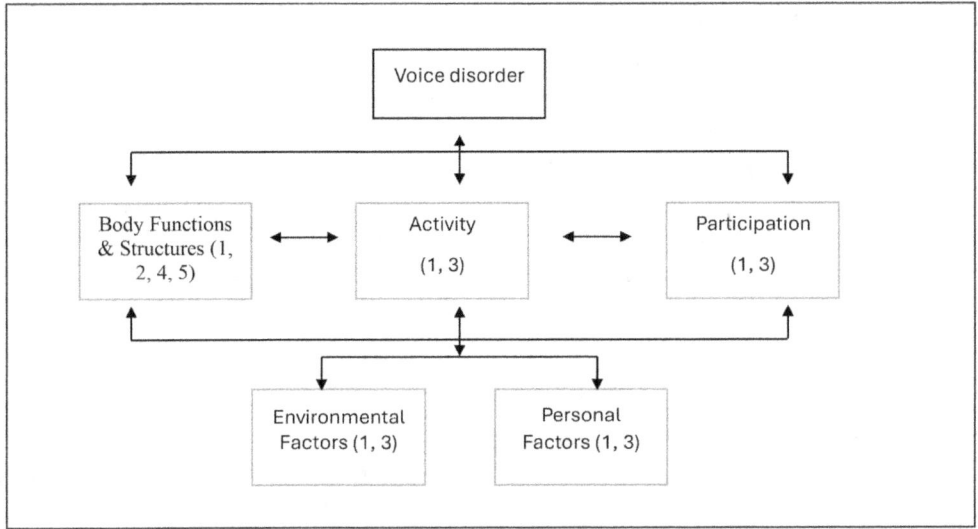

Figure 8.2 ICF framework with numbered reference to voice evaluation for the various domains (1: physical examination of the larynx; 2: detailed case history; 3: self-assessment impact questionnaires; 4: auditory perceptual and acoustic techniques; and 5: aerodynamic performance)

Organization, 2001) as in Figure 8.2, which includes numbered reference to the assessment parameters we need to consider using.

Body functions and structures are evaluated by physical examination of the larynx (usually by ENT) (no. 1 in Figure 8.2), a detailed case history (no. 2), auditory-perceptual and acoustic evaluation (no. 4) and evaluation of aerodynamic performance (no. 5). Activity and Participation along with understanding of the Environmental and Personal factors are through the detailed case history (no. 2) and self-assessment impact questionnaires (no. 3). Each is considered below.

1. Physical examination

Physical examination explores the structure and vibratory function of the larynx. This is possible in children with care and the right equipment, and usually by ENT prior to SLT referral. For children >4 years, careful preparation allows for toleration of flexible or rigid laryngoscopy to visualise laryngeal movement. Children frequently need decongestant and local anaesthetic to tolerate the procedure. Acceptance of awake laryngoscopy remains an issue for some children, and where there are airway or dysphagia concerns, microlaryngobronchoscopy (MLB) is necessary to visualise the larynx under general anaesthetic, without evaluating vocal fold movement. Advances in high-speed ultrasonography are yielding potential for diagnosis, particularly in vocal fold paralysis/paresis and there is emerging evidence of its potential in benign vocal fold lesions (e.g. Ongkasuwan, Ocampo and Tran, 2017) leading to more comfortable physical examination of the larynx.

2. Detailed case history

The case history gathers information about birth and developmental history along with hearing, early feeding and respiratory function. Questions are asked about onset of hoarseness, patterns of hoarseness (e.g. are there times during the day when the voice is better or worse?), hobbies and extra-curricular activities, medical history (e.g. intubation history) and medications (e.g. reflux, asthma) and the impact of the hoarseness on the child's activities and participation. We should take into consideration appropriate developmental expectations or individual variation (e.g. puberty) and what we might anticipate in typical voice for a child of that sex or age.

3. Self-assessment impact questionnaires

The impact of the disordered voice on quality of life (QOL) can be measured using self-assessment questionnaires. These give an indication of the functional impact of voice disorder, providing a self-assessment of severity usually in emotional, physical and functional subdomains. Several are established in adults, with some developed for parental proxy assessment including the 23-item Pediatric Voice Handicap Index (PVHI) (Zur et al., 2007), the 10-item Pediatric Voice Related Quality of Life Survey (PVRQOL) (Boseley et al., 2006) and the 4-item Pediatric Voice Outcome Survey (PVOS) (Hartnick, 2002). A higher PVHI indicates high impact of the voice disorder, while a higher PVRQOL or PVOS conversely indicates a high voice-related QOL. Children without voice disorder typically score close to 100 on the PVRQOL, significantly higher compared to children with known voice disorders. A score <85 is indicative of intervention need (Merati et al., 2008). There is also a version for teachers, the 27-item Teacher-Reported Pediatric Voice Handicap Index (TRVHI) (Yağcıoğlu et al., 2021).

As parental opinion does not always match their child's self-report, two of these instruments have been adapted for children to complete themselves: the PVRQOL has a 10-item child adaptation (Cohen and Wynne, 2015) and the Children's VHI (CVHI) is a 10-item adaptation of the VHI-10 (Ricci-Maccarini et al., 2013). Completing both the parental proxy and child versions of the same instrument yields valuable information for clinical decision-making, particularly as severity of impact does not always correlate with auditory-perceptual severity, and motivation for behavioural change is a necessary requirement for intervention. Therefore, we can make an informed decision about who should be the focus on intervention based on the parental proxy and child self-report.

4. Auditory-perceptual and acoustic techniques

Auditory-perceptual evaluation of voice quality is a clinical subjective skill. There are published protocols to help us judge severity of voice disorder. Commonly used protocols include the GRBAS (Hirano, 1981), the GRBASI (Dejonckere et al., 2001), and the CAPE-V (Kempster et al., 2009). The main difference between these relates to the scaling: the GRBAS/GRBASI use a 4-point ordinal scale and the CAPE-V a 100mm visual analogue scale. Both provide evaluation of overall severity of voice disorder with parameters relating to hoarseness/roughness, breathiness, strain and consistency/instability. The CAPE-V additionally rates pitch and loudness while the GRBAS/GRBASI rates asthenia (vocal weakness). The CAPE-V provides standard stimuli (sustained vowel /a/, six sentences and conversational speech). As there are no set stimuli for the GRBAS/GRABSI, we can use spontaneous speech, sustained vowel production and reading aloud a standard passage or adopt the CAPE-V standard stimuli. The GRBAS was first proposed as a minimum scale for use in the UK (Carding et al., 2006) and is now widely adopted into routine clinical practice. Both protocols were originally designed and validated for use in the adult population, however, there is a useful online resource from the University of Wisconsin-Madison (Connor, n.d.) to supplement development of this clinical skill, and while they are mostly adult scenarios of American-English speakers, there are some paediatric cases for self-study.

SLTs can use acoustic analysis techniques to supplement auditory-perceptual evaluation. Voice offers an ideal opportunity to capture data describing the severity of disturbance in voice production. While there are some specialised acoustic analysis software programs available, most clinicians access the freely available PRAAT software download (Boersma and Weenink, 2025). Standard voice measurements include perturbation measurements (jitter, shimmer and harmonics to noise ratio) giving an indication of the cycle-to-cycle variation of the vocal folds and measuring the Cepstral Peak Prominence (CPP). The reader is directed to a detailed protocol for instrumental evaluation of voice (Patel et al., 2018) and normative data for the age range 4-19 years (Kent, Eichhorn and Vorperian, 2021).

5. Evaluating aerodynamic performance

As the power source for the larynx comes from respiration, it stands to reason that evaluation of respiratory function is helpful. While there are several approaches to measuring respiratory function, these are the domain of the specialist respiratory physiologist, so the SLT uses maximum phonation times (MPT) to gauge the individual's capacity to control and coordinate respiratory function during phonation. These relatively simple tasks are like maximum repetition tasks in motor speech disorders. The child sustains the vowel /a/ and the fricatives /s/ and /z/ for as long as possible at comfortable pitch and volume. Frequent repetition of these tasks has a learning effect, so usual practice is to repeat each three times and record the duration of the longest in seconds. By dividing the longest duration of /s/ by the longest duration of /z/ we determine the S/Z ratio: an indicator of glottal efficiency as the difference between the two sounds is reduced only to voiced or voiceless. Where there is no voice disorder, this ratio should be at or near 1 as phonation of both sounds should be similar. A higher S/Z ratio is suggestive of laryngeal lesion – as phonation of the voiced cognate is more difficult to do, due to the presence of the laryngeal lesion. MPT varies by age, weight and height in the pre-pubertal population with lower typical durations of sustained /a/ of 6;09s (for 4;0-6;0) up to 8.98s (for 10;0-12;0) (see Mendes Tavares et al., 2012). Table 8.1 gives an overview of auditory-perceptual, acoustic and aerodynamic evaluation.

Summary of recommended SLT assessment protocol for voice disorder in children

Figure 8.3 summarises a full paediatric assessment protocol, indicating routine and supplementary items.

Stimulus	Suggested instruction (Any audio recorded data using a microphone in a quiet room can be used for acoustic evaluation)	Auditory-perceptual evaluation	Acoustic evaluation	Aerodynamic performance
Sustained vowel /a/	Try and say the sound /a/ for as long as you can, a bit like this [provide demonstration]. Try not to be too loud or too quiet. Repeat three times.	✓	✓	✓
Sustained fricative /s/	Try and say the sound /s/ for as long as you can, a bit like this [provide demonstration]. Try not to be too loud or too quiet. Repeat three times.			✓
Sustained fricative /z/	Try and say the sound /z/ for as long as you can, a bit like this [provide demonstration]. Try not to be too loud or too quiet. Repeat three times	✓	✓	✓
CAPE-V sentences	Can you read out these sentences? (for younger children ask them to repeat them): 1. The blue spot is on the key again 2. How hard did he hit him? 3. Peter will keep at the peak 4. We eat eggs every Easter 5. We were away a year ago 6. My mama makes lemon muffins	✓	✓	
Spontaneous conversation	Can you tell me what your favourite toy/activity/class at school is [as appropriate to the child's age]?	✓	✓	

Table 8.1 Stimuli, instructions and how these can be used for auditory-perceptual, acoustic and aerodynamic evaluation of voice disorder

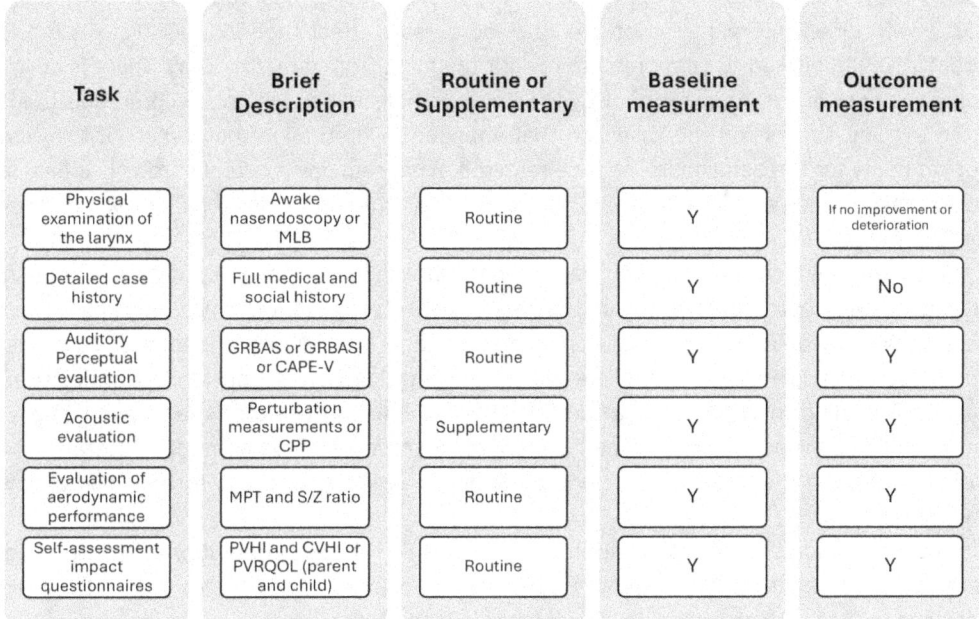

Figure 8.3 Summary of assessment protocol for baseline and outcome measurement

✍ Supporting children's needs in voice

Having gathered a detailed description of the onset, severity and impact of the voice disorder, this helps us decide appropriate management. Management typically includes surgery (phonosurgery) or voice therapy. Phonosurgery is only appropriate in some diagnoses (e.g. cysts, airway reconstruction, injection medialisation laryngoplasty for vocal fold paralysis) and is undertaken by ENT with the SLT an integral part of the MDT. Voice therapy is solely the domain of the SLT, so the focus of this section is how the SLT manages the most common diagnosis where this is the principal approach: VFN. Voice therapy follows modulation of any associated factors (e.g. medication for allergy or reflux). The aim of voice therapy (as in adults) is to change the way that the voice is produced towards that of a healthy, functional voice.

Children might be supported by a hospital or community-based SLT, but the availability of the MDT is important to all SLTs working with voice, particularly if there has been no prior ENT evaluation (which can be the case in some referrals) or if repeat ENT evaluation is indicated due to non-response to therapy. Telepractice is increasing in use with this caseload, with emerging guidelines (e.g. Kelchner, Fredeking and Zacharias, 2021; Myers et al., 2022).

Intervention usually involves a combination of direct strategies (e.g. behavioural modification, resonance training or improving breath support), and indirect strategies (e.g. awareness of vocal hygiene and situations/environments where voice production is modulated for greater protection). There is emerging evidence of the effectiveness of voice therapy: while there is a lack of well-designed research, particularly large-scale RCTs (Adriaansen et al.,

2022), direct and indirect intervention lead to improvement in vocal function (Al-Kadi et al., 2022), with direct intervention generally having greater effect than indirect (Feinstein and Abbott, 2021). Children >8 years tend to benefit the most from direct therapy. There is developing evidence of the importance of satisfactorily established cognition as a prerequisite for voice therapy, supporting the assertion that younger children might not benefit if they are not yet ready for the behavioural change required. What remains less understood is effective dosage (see Braden and Thibeault, 2020) though most studies suggest once weekly therapy for 8-12 weeks.

Voice therapy requires a commitment from the child and their family, with regular attendance and home practice, thus the role of parents and schools in promoting awareness of voice production and maintenance of change cannot be understated. Following multi-factorial voice evaluation, there will be information that supports clinical decision-making, including the parent and child responses to impact questionnaires. Levels of parent and child concern might predict likely engagement in and commitment to therapy and we can use these to focus our attention on either the parent only (e.g. if the child has low impact) or both.

Established adult voice intervention programmes are showing potential in children (e.g. semi-occluded vocal tract exercises) and there are specific programmes that have been designed for use with children (e.g. *Adventures in Voice (AIV) 2.0 - Visions In Voice*, n.d.).

Indirect strategies focus on raising awareness of how the voice works using models and diagrams, talking about how to use the voice healthily in different situations and environments, how to protect the voice from harm, identifying phonotraumatic behaviours and ways to avoid or modify these, discussion and identification of good vs poor voice quality and production. This is sometimes referred to as vocal hygiene. Depending on the needs of the child (as identified from voice evaluation), parents can be advised on diet and hydration, reducing sugary or caffeinated drinks, or suggestions for environmental changes (e.g. improving air quality, reducing shouting), providing an environment conducive to using a quiet voice that is not whispering, talking at a lower volume to reduce strain, and encouraging healthy voice care including short periods of voice rest or steam inhalation to hydrate the larynx.

Direct strategies focus on establishing new patterns of voice production, using motor learning principles and behavioural modelling and/or shaping. Once the child understands how healthy voice is produced, they are supported in using it through games and modelling in CV and CVC productions through to phrases and sentences. Some children respond well to resonance training, which is facilitated by producing a gentle hum where voicing is not forced, followed by [mV] constructions before moving onto single words and phrases. Breath support can be developed through understanding of the different breathing types, using games and models, and practice. Often an eclectic approach is taken - building up the coordination of respiration, phonation and resonance necessary for healthy vocalisation.

The SLT needs to take a holistic approach when working with children with voice disorders - trying out different techniques to find which is most effective alongside establishing a healthy vocal routine. The case study of Tim provides an example of this in practice.

Tim's story

Tim, the youngest of four boys under 14 years, is a 9-year-old boy referred with 'persistent hoarseness' by his GP. He tolerated flexible nasendoscopy which revealed bilateral VFN. Tim's voice problem started when he had an upper respiratory tract infection and has been persistent for 10 months. Tim has no other health or medical issues and is doing well at school, though he is boisterous in classes and doesn't stop talking when he should be focusing on his schoolwork. Tim is busy outside of school: while he goes to Taekwondo once a week, football is his passion, playing in his local football team, training two nights each week and matches every weekend. At home he is often in the garden kicking a ball about or playing online football computer games with his friends. Tim is a picky eater – preferring mostly pasta dishes, usually with cheese. As he is so physically active, his parents give him regular sugary snacks and fizzy drinks. There is noticeable tension in his neck when speaking as he tries to make his voice heard.

Baseline voice evaluation (see Table 8.2) provided the SLT with information supporting both indirect and direct intervention. The added information from the PVRQOL indicated he was motivated for therapy. Had he scored higher on the PVRQOL then the focus of intervention may have been largely with his parents.

Through discussion with Tim and his family, there were several opportunities to improve vocal hygiene. These included exploring a healthier diet and increasing hydration from water rather than fizzy drinks. He took this advice on board when it was presented alongside understanding that professional footballers follow a healthy diet. The family were encouraged to reduce the loudness in the family home by avoiding shouting from room to room, and by speaking to each other in the same room instead. Tim was interested in how the body works and responded well to explanations about healthy breathing for speech and the importance of looking after his larynx in the same way he looks after his body when at football training.

The start of each SLT session involved checking how Tim was implementing these indirect strategies. To help reduce head and neck tension, the SLT introduced direct strategies trying resonant voice exercises using humming. Tim wasn't so keen on these but responded better when semi-occluded vocal tract exercises were used as he enjoyed blowing a straw

Measurement	Baseline	Outcome
Aerodynamic performance	longest sustained [a] = 3s longest sustained [z] = 3s longest sustained [s] = 9s S/Z ratio = 3	longest sustained [a] = 7s longest sustained [z] = 8s longest sustained [s] = 9s S/Z ratio = 1.125
Auditory perceptual evaluation	GRBAS: G2; R2; B1; A0; S0 moderately hoarse, with observable roughness and breathiness	GRBAS: G1; R1; B0; A0; S0 mildly hoarse, with observable roughness
Self-assessment impact questionnaire	Parent PVRQOL score = 42.5 Child PVRQOL score = 75	Parent PVRQOL score = 70 Child PVRQOL score = 95

Table 8.2 Baseline and outcome measurements (Tim aged 9 years)

into a bottle of water while he produced a humming noise. Doing this made Tim think about his breathing and by encouraging him to feel the vibrations on his lips, this focused his mind on reducing laryngeal and mandibular tension. He found this a relatively simple exercise to do and once mastered, the SLT introduced a longer hum and then added in a vowel ([mV]) still using the straw/bottle. Tim practised for 5 minutes twice each day and after three sessions was able to do this comfortably without the straw/bottle in place. At this point, the SLT introduced short phrases with words starting with nasal consonants reminding Tim of the importance of feeling the vibrations from humming in his lips so that he could talk without any residual tension.

After 8 weeks of intervention, Tim had reduced tension in his neck and his hoarseness was decreasing (see Table 8.2). He and his parents were reassured that with continued practice of the indirect and direct strategies his voice should recover completely.

Summary

This chapter provided an overview of how voice is produced and how the complex mechanisms involved in producing voice can go wrong, leading to voice disorder. The reader should have a broad understanding about approaches to classifying voice disorder. By following the description of how to comprehensively evaluate voice disorder it should be possible for the emerging therapist to have some confidence in approaching this in the clinic. Suggestions for voice therapy were provided and illustrated in the case study.

Recommended resources

Connor, N. (n.d.) *Voice Disorders: Simulations*. University of Wisconson-Madison. Available at: https://slpsims.csd.wisc.edu/simulations.html (accessed 16 September 2024).

Praat: Doing Phonetics by Computer (n.d.) Available at: https://www.fon.hum.uva.nl/praat/ (accessed 7 August 2024).

References

Adriaansen, A., Meerschman, I., Van Lierde, K. and D'haeseleer, E. (2022) 'Effects of voice therapy in children with vocal fold nodules: A systematic review', *International Journal of Language & Communication Disorders*, 57(6), 1160-1193. https://doi.org/10.1111/1460-6984.12754.

Adventures in Voice (AIV) 2.0 - Visions in Voice (n.d.) Available at: https://visionsinvoice.com/register/aiv/ (accessed 12 September 2024).

Akif Kiliç, M., Okur, E., Yildirim, I. and Güzelsoy, S. (2004) 'The prevalence of vocal fold nodules in school age children', *International Journal of Pediatric Otorhinolaryngology*, 68(4), 409-412. https://doi.org/10.1016/J.IJPORL.2003.11.005.

Al-Kadi, M., Alfawaz, M.A., Alotaibi, F.Z., Al-Kadi, M., Alfawaz, M. and Alotaibi, F. (2022) 'Impact of voice therapy on pediatric patients with dysphonia and vocal nodules: A systematic review', *Cureus*, 14(4). https://doi.org/10.7759/CUREUS.24433.

American Speech and Hearing Association (n.d.) 'Voice disorders' Available at: https://www.asha.org/practice-portal/clinical-topics/voice-disorders/?srsltid=AfmBOooTFfj1g5d6Wq3oEpvOWPh6-q83J5oVA8Mk8IUv72ZOuQRZVB3r

Aronson, A.E. and Bless, D.M. (2014) *Clinical Voice Disorders*. 4th edn. New York: Thieme.

Boersma, P. and Weenink, D. (2025) 'Praat: Doing phonetics by computer'. University of Amsterdam. Available at: https://www.fon.hum.uva.nl/praat/

Boone, D.R., McFarlane, S.C., Van Berg, S.L. and Zraick, R.I. (2009) *The Voice and Voice Therapy*. 8th edn. London: Allyn & Bacon.

Boseley, M.E., Cunningham, M.J., Volk, M.S. and Hartnick, C.J. (2006) 'Validation of the Pediatric Voice-Related Quality-of-Life survey', *Archives of Otolaryngology-Head and Neck Surgery*, 132(7), 717-720. https://doi.org/10.1001/archotol.132.7.717.

Braden, M. and Thibeault, S.L. (2020) 'Outcomes of voice therapy in children with benign vocal fold lesions', *International Journal of Pediatric Otorhinolaryngology*, 136, 110121. https://doi.org/10.1016/J.IJPORL.2020.110121.

Carding, P.N., Roulstone, S. and Northstone, K. (2006) 'The prevalence of childhood dysphonia: A cross-sectional study', *Journal of Voice*, 20(4), 623-630. https://doi.org/10.1016/j.jvoice.2005.07.004.

Cohen, W. and Wynne, D.M. (2015) 'Parent and child responses to the pediatric voice-related quality-of-life questionnaire', *Journal of Voice*, 29(3). https://doi.org/10.1016/j.jvoice.2014.08.004.

De Bodt, M.S., Ketelslagers, K., Peeters, T., Wuyts, F.L., Mertens, F., Pattyn, J., Heylen, L., Peeters, A., Boudewyns, A. and Van de Heyning, P. (2007) 'Evolution of vocal fold nodules from childhood to adolescence', *Journal of Voice*, 21(2), 151-156. https://doi.org/10.1016/J.JVOICE.2005.11.006.

Dejonckere, P.H., Bradley, P., Clemente, P., Cornut, G., Crevier-Buchman, L., Friedrich, G., Van De Heyning, P., Remacle, M. and Woisard, V. (2001) 'A basic protocol for functional assessment of voice pathology, especially for investigating the efficacy of (phonosurgical) treatments and evaluating new assessment techniques. Guideline elaborated by the Committee on Phoniatrics of the European Laryngological Society (ELS)', *European Archives of Oto-rhino-laryngology*, 258(2), 77-82. https://doi.org/10.1007/S004050000299.

Dejonckere, P.H., Remacle, M., Fresnel-Elbaz, E., Woisard, V., Crevier-Buchman, L. and Millet, B. (1996) 'Differentiated perceptual evaluation of pathological voice quality: reliability and correlations with acoustic measurements', *Revue de laryngologie-otologie-rhinologie*, 117(3), 219-224. http://europepmc.org/abstract/MED/9102729.

Feinstein, H. and Abbott, K.V. (2021) 'Behavioral treatment for benign vocal fold lesions in children: A systematic review', *American Journal of Speech-Language Pathology*, 30(2), 772-788. https://doi.org/10.1044/2020_AJSLP-20-00304.

Hartnick, C.J. (2002) 'Validation of a pediatric voice quality-of-life instrument: The Pediatric Voice Outcome Survey', *Archives of Otolaryngology-Head & Neck Surgery*, 128(8), 919-922. https://doi.org/10.1001/archotol.128.8.919.

Hirano, M. (1981) *Clinical Examination of Voice*. New York: Springer-Verlag.

Kelchner, L.N., Fredeking, J.C. and Zacharias, S.C. (2021) 'Using telepractice to deliver pediatric voice care in a changing world: Breaking down challenges and learning from successes', *Seminars in Speech and Language*, 42(1), 54-63. https://doi.org/10.1055/S-0040-1722320/ID/JR7200009-23/BIB.

Kempster, G.B., Gerratt, B.R., Verdolini Abbott, K., Barkmeier-Kraemer, J. and Hillman, R.E. (2009) 'Consensus auditory-perceptual evaluation of voice: Development of a standardized clinical protocol', *American Journal of Speech-Language Pathology*, 18(2), 124-132. https://doi.org/10.1044/1058-0360(2008/08-0017).

Kent, R.D., Eichhorn, J.T. and Vorperian, H.K. (2021) 'Acoustic parameters of voice in typically developing children ages 4-19 years', *International Journal of Pediatric Otorhinolaryngology*, 142, 110614. https://doi.org/10.1016/J.IJPORL.2021.110614.

Lee, L., Stemple, J.C., Glaze, L. and Keichner, L.N. (2004) 'Quick screen for voice and supplementary documents for identifying pediatric voice disorders', *Language, Speech, and Hearing Services in Schools*, 35(4), 308-319. https://doi.org/10.1044/0161-1461(2004/030).

Martins, R.H.G., Hidalgo Ribeiro, C.B., Fernandes De Mello, B.M.Z., Branco, A. and Tavares, E.L.M. (2012) 'Dysphonia in children', *Journal of Voice*, 26(5), 674.e17-674.e20. https://doi.org/10.1016/J.JVOICE.2012.03.004.

Mathieson, L. (2001) *Greene and Mathieson's the Voice and its Disorders*. 6th edn. Philadelphia, PA: Whurr Publishers.

Mendes Tavares, E.L., Brasolotto, A.G., Rodrigues, S.A., Benito Pessin, A.B. and Garcia Martins, R.H. (2012) 'Maximum phonation time and s/z ratio in a large child cohort', *Journal of Voice*, 26(5), 675.e1-675.e4. https://doi.org/10.1016/J.JVOICE.2012.03.001.

Merati, A.L., Keppel, K., Braun, N.M., Blumin, J.H. and Kerschner, J.E. (2008) 'Pediatric voice-related quality of life: findings in healthy children and in common laryngeal disorders', *Annals of Otology, Rhinology & Laryngology.*, 117(4), 259-262. https://doi.org/10.1177/000348940811700404.

Mudd, P. and Noelke, C. (2018) 'Vocal fold nodules in children', *Current Opinion in Otolaryngology and Head and Neck Surgery*, 26(6), 426-430. https://doi.org/10.1097/MOO.0000000000000496.

Myers, B., Hary, E., Ellerston, J. and Barkmeier-Kraemer, J.M. (2022) 'Telepractice considerations for evaluation and treatment of voice disorders: Tailoring to specific populations', *American Journal of Speech-Language Pathology*, 31(2), 678–688. https://doi.org/10.1044/2021_AJSLP-21-00206.

Ongkasuwan, J., Ocampo, E. and Tran, B. (2017) 'Laryngeal ultrasound and vocal fold movement in the pediatric cardiovascular intensive care unit', *The Laryngoscope*, 127(1), 167–172. https://doi.org/10.1002/LARY.26051.

Patel, R.R., Awan, S.N., Barkmeier-Kraemer, J., Courey, M., Deliyski, D., Eadie, T., Paul, D., Švec, J.G. and Hillman, R. (2018) 'Recommended protocols for instrumental assessment of voice: American Speech-Language-Hearing Association Expert Panel to develop a protocol for instrumental assessment of vocal function', *American Journal of Speech-Language Pathology*, 27(3), 887–905. https://doi.org/10.1044/2018_AJSLP-17-0009.

RCSLT (n.d.). 'Voice'. Available at: https://www.rcslt.org/members/clinical-guidance/voice/ (accessed 24 June 2024).

Ricci-Maccarini, A., De Maio, V., Murry, T. and Schindler, A. (2013) 'Development and Validation of the Children's Voice Handicap Index-10 (CVHI-10)', *Journal of Voice*, 27(2), 258.e23–258.e28. https://doi.org/10.1016/J.JVOICE.2012.10.006.

Sapienza, C.M. and Hoffman, B. (2022) *Voice Disorders*. 4th edn. San Diego, CA: Plural Publishing.

Stachler, R.J., Francis, D.O., Schwartz, S.R., Damask, C.C., Digoy, G.P., Krouse, H.J., McCoy, S.J., Ouellette, D.R., Patel, R.R., Reavis, C.W., Smith, L.J., Smith, M., Strode, S.W., Woo, P. and Nnacheta, L.C. (2018) 'Clinical Practice Guideline: Hoarseness (Dysphonia) (Update)', *Otolaryngology – Head and Neck Surgery (United States)*, 158(1_suppl), S1–S42. https://doi.org/10.1177/0194599817751030.

Stojanović J., Belić B., Erdevički L., Jovanović S., Jovanović M., and Srećković S. (2021) 'Quality of life in dysphonic children measured on pediatric voice-related quality of life questionnaire(PVRQOL) in Serbia', *Acta Clinica Croatia*, 60: 75–81. doi: 10.20471/acc.2021.60.01.11.

Tavares, E.L.M., Brasolotto, A., Santana, M.F., Padovan, C.A. and Martins, R.H.G. (2011) 'Epidemiological study of dysphonia in 4–12-year-old children', *Brazilian Journal of Otorhinolaryngology*, 77(6), 736–746. https://doi.org/10.1590/S1808-86942011000600010.

Verdolini Abbott, K., Rosen, C.A., Branski, R.C., Andrews, M.L. and American Speech-Language-Hearing Association. Special Interest Division 3, Voice and Voice Disorders (2006) *Classification Manual for Voice Disorders-I*. New Jersey: Lawrence Erlbaum.

Voice Disorders (n.d.). Available at: https://www.asha.org/practice-portal/clinical-topics/voice-disorders/#collapse_8 (accessed 24 June 2024).

World Health Organization (2001) *International Classification of Functioning, Disability, And Health : ICF*. Geneva: WHO.

World Health Organization (2022) *ICD-11: International Classification of Diseases*. 11th edn. Geneva: WHO.

Yağcıoğlu, D., Aydınlı, F.E., Aslan, G., Kirazlı, M., Köse, A., Doğan, N., Akbulut, S., Yılmaz, T. and Özcebe, E. (2021) 'Development, validation, and reliability of the Teacher-Reported Pediatric Voice Handicap Index', *Language, Speech, and Hearing Services in Schools*, 53(1), 69–87: https://doi.org/10.1044/2021_LSHSS-21-00033.

Zur, K.B., Cotton, S., Kelchner, L., Baker, S., Weinrich, B. and Lee, L. (2007) 'Pediatric Voice Handicap Index (pVHI): A new tool for evaluating pediatric dysphonia', *International Journal of Pediatric Otorhinolaryngology*, 71(1), 77–82. https://doi.org/10.1016/J.IJPORL.2006.09.004.

PART III
Language

9 Promoting early language development

Sheena Reilly and Cristina McKean

What you'll learn in this chapter

- Why population-level, whole-system approaches are needed to address early language development
- How current evidence can inform models of early language surveillance
- How current evidence can inform models of early preventative interventions
- The characteristics of a population-level, whole-systems approach to early language promotion.

Chapter 2 outlined the importance of a population-based approach to Speech Language and Communication Needs (SLCN). This chapter articulates why whole-system, preventative approaches, involving multiple agencies, are needed to address language development in the early years, that is, the period from birth to 4 years. It begins by outlining the rationale for this approach and then describes a framework for understanding language development and the social determinants that influence the course of language development in the early years and adversely affect life-long outcomes. It describes some of the challenges that exist and then outlines the key principles that underpin the promotion of language in the early years, providing a justification for a framework of early language surveillance and preventative intervention.

Why population-level, whole-system approaches are needed

Language development is a distinguishing evolutionary feature and regarded as one of the most significant developmental accomplishments (Mountford et al., 2022). Language development supports learning throughout childhood and is fundamental to social interaction and to relationships; thus, influential child language researchers have described language as an important indicator of well-being across the life course (Law, Charlton and Asmussen, 2017). While most children develop language effortlessly, approximately 8% do not and will have developmental language disorder (DLD) (Norbury et al., 2016). The rationale for an early years' public health approach to language development is underpinned by several constructs. These include the factors that influence child language development, the social context in which language develops and the impact that early language deficits can have across the life course. Each will be discussed in turn.

DOI: 10.4324/9781003671626-13

Factors that influence child language development

To understand why these concepts are so important, it can be helpful to think about the social and physical environment in which children grow and develop as the social context or ecosystem within which language develops (Law and Charlton, 2022). Bronfenbrenner's bioecological model of human development (adapted in Figure 9.1) illustrates the multiple factors in the ecosystem that can influence language development throughout the early years (Bronfenbrenner, 2005). In this model, the child is at the centre of an ecosystem. The microsystem surrounds the child and represents the infant and young child's immediate environment, capturing the settings in which children are most likely to be raised and the factors within these settings (e.g. the positive early learning environments) that might influence language development. These are known as proximal factors because of how close they are to the child. In the surrounding systems, (e.g. the Exosystem), the factors are further away from the child and are described as distal. It is important to note that these factors depicted are not static; they interact, layer and play out over time, as discussed later in this chapter. Although the model does not explicitly acknowledge the biological endowment, that is, the influence of the genes a child inherits from their parents, there is continuous interaction between biology and early life experience as highlighted earlier. Table 9.1 expands on the structural, material, behavioural and psychosocial factors that interact and influence language development in the early years. All of these factors can interact with each other.

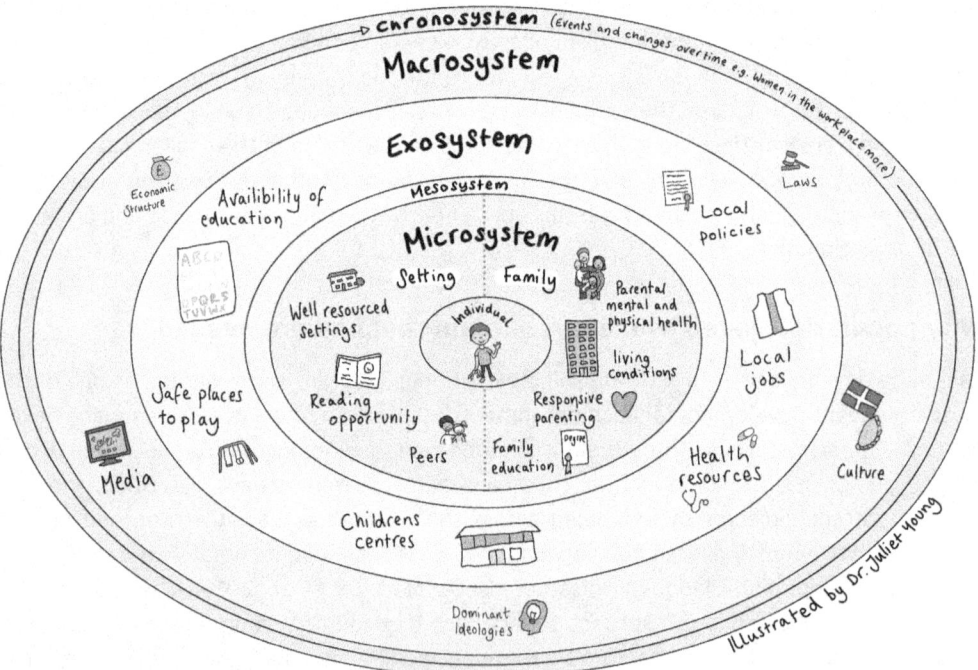

Figure 9.1 Bronfenbrenner's bioecological model adapted to illustrate the family, social and environmental factors that influence child language development

Factors that influence child language development

Structural

- Socioeconomic disadvantage
- Neighbourhood deprivation
- Employment
- Access to services for health and play-based learning activities and exploration

Material	Behavioural	Psychosocial	Other
• Living conditions	• Quality of interaction[1]	• Mental and physical health and wellbeing	• Minority status – isolation
• Poverty	• Shared book reading	• Stress	• Migration
• Crowding	• Screen time		• Language barriers
• Resources, e.g. books, toys			
• Opportunities			

Table 9.1 Illustration of the relationship between the structural, material, behavioural and psychosocial features that influence child language outcomes

Source: adapted from Reilly and McKean (2023).
Note: [1]Parent input, including conceptual, linguistic and interactive,

DLD as a public health problem: the social context of equity and burden

DLD is one of the most prevalent neurodevelopmental disorders. It places a large burden on society and the affected individuals. It is also unfairly distributed across society, thus meeting the criteria for a public health problem. A public health solution is therefore required (see Law, Charlton and Asmussen, 2017; Reilly and McKean, 2023). Several longitudinal population studies have demonstrated the robust association between language outcomes and the circumstances in which a child lives; children living in less advantaged circumstances have poorer longer-term language outcomes (Taylor et al., 2013; McKean et al., 2015; Law et al., 2019; Di Sante and Potvin, 2022). Described as the social gradient (see Box 9.1), this is apparent early, well before entry to formal schooling (Reilly and McKean, 2023).

Box 9.1 The social gradient is associated with levels of language challenge

The social gradient runs from the top to the bottom of the socioeconomic spectrum. The lower an individual's socioeconomic position, the worse their outcomes. For example, children living in less advantaged circumstances with limited family resources (e.g. low income, low maternal education, lack of books in the home, not being read to) are more likely to have:

- poorer language outcomes overall
- persistently poorer language trajectories as opposed to improving or resolving trajectories
- slower rates of language progress
- poorer vocabulary knowledge

Families living in more challenging socio-economic circumstances face many barriers to providing a language-enriching environment. These include work which take parents/carers away from the home at key opportunities in the day for interactions, overcrowding in the home reducing opportunities for responsive interactions, and long-term stress associated with poverty reducing a parent's/caregiver's emotional resource to be able to be available for their child (Dean, 2007; Taylor and Edwards, 2012). Disadvantaged families often are dealing with multiple cumulative and interacting factors which challenge their ability to provide optimal environments for their child's health and development (Christensen, Taylor and Zubrick, 2017; Eadie et al., 2022). Also, in addition to the effects of inequalities in a child's proximal environment, education, health and care systems and services are organised to be less accessible to socially disadvantaged families, further widening the gap.

A life course approach: early preventative intervention for lifelong benefit

While the focus of this chapter is on the early years, it is important to highlight that language development is a continuous process that commences early and continues across the life-course. Further, decades of research have demonstrated that children who experience problems learning language in the early years have a higher risk of poorer outcomes (educational attainment, employment, mental health, quality of life and general well-being) in adolescence and later in adulthood (Dubois et al., 2020). Thus, the foundations for optimal language development are cemented in infancy and early childhood, and what happens in these early years can influence how language develops, and the consequences may reach across the lifespan.

Evidence informing early language surveillance

The imperative to act early to close the gap and reduce what may be long-lasting impacts across the child's life is irrefutable. However, due to individual differences and fluctuation in language trajectories in the early years, complex interactions in early risks, and often inaccessible systems of support, this is not a straightforward task. Approaches to promoting early language in the early years should be set within the context of the child's broader development, an understanding of the social context within which language develops and the need to act early to promote optimal outcomes. Before considering how best to target and support those children and families most in need, it is important to understand some more about the nature and characteristics of language development in the early years.

First, findings from several longitudinal research studies on the individual differences and fluctuation in the early years are described, before moving to consider how risk factors in the child's early ecosystem can influence language development, particularly when multiple risk factors cluster together and accumulate. These insights are particularly important when considering how we might best target and support those most in need.

There is broad agreement that by 4 years of age it can confidently be predicted which children are likely to have developmental language disorder (DLD) although there is a small group of children in whom language disorder may be late to emerge (McKean et al., 2017; McKean, Mensah and Reilly, 2022). There is, however, far less certainty about the early years, when language pathways of both children with typical early development and those with vulnerabilities are known to fluctuate, making it difficult to accurately predict which children will go on to have a DLD. Should we therefore wait until we are certain a child has significant and persisting difficulties to support them? To do so would miss out on the crucial years with greatest brain plasticity and hence potential for change. Opportunities to address the upstream determinants of child outcomes of poverty, maternal mental health, and so on would be lost.

Table 9.2 summarises data from several studies conducted across four different countries. Four main trajectory types (*Stable typical, Fluctuating (Improving and Decreasing), Stable low, Late emerging*) are described, along with the distinguishing features associated with each. Together these findings suggest that children with vulnerable language may be growing up in environments with subtly different features. This is illustrated in Table 9.2 by contrasting the differences between the features associated with the *Fluctuating Improving* and the *Fluctuating Decreasing* trajectories. Research findings in other child development domains (e.g. obesity, mental health) have demonstrated that the presence of a single risk factor, or even a small number of risks that emerge intermittently, might not result in adverse developmental outcomes, whereas the presence of multiple factors can have a much greater influence. Therefore, an important next step was to identify whether risks might cluster (as suggested by the trajectories in Table 9.2) and accumulate over time to influence child language trajectories and outcomes.

In three separate reports, child language researchers (Christensen, Taylor and Zubrick, 2017; Eadie et al., 2022; Taylor, Christensen and Zubrick, 2022) described two main groups of children in their studies: (1) children who were *Developmentally enabled*, with the lowest number of risks, and (2) children with *Vulnerable language profiles*, with not only a higher number of risks but also accumulating risk over time. Within the *Vulnerable group*, several subgroups, with variable features, were described; overall the *Vulnerable* subgroups were characterised by greater socio-economic disadvantage and less than optimal home learning environments. For a more detailed description, readers are referred to Reilly and McKean (2023) and McKean and Reilly (2023).

Trajectory type	Definition	Associated features
Stable typical	Language ability is stable and consistently meets expectations	Well-resourced homes with more highly educated mothers
Fluctuating	Language ability moves between trajectories both improving and decreasing	Improving: greater disadvantage, non-English-speaking background, fewer books in the home, higher levels of maternal vocabulary and education Decreasing: Biological factors such as being male, lower birth weight, increased socioemotional problems, lower family literacy and educational levels
Stable low	Language ability is stable but consistently below expectations	Greater disadvantage, family history of language problems, being male, low language comprehension identified early
Late emerging	Language ability meets expectations in the early years, but difficulties become apparent after school entry or later in childhood.	Familial risk factors

Table 9.2 Types of language trajectories identified in longitudinal population-based studies and the associated factors

Sources: Ukoumunne et al. (2012); Määttä et al. (2012); Zambana et al. (2014); McKean et al., 2015; 2017; Zubrick et al. (2015); Snowling et al. (2016); Christensen et al., 2017

The key findings are summarised as:

- Children in the *Vulnerable group* were 13.7 times more likely to have low language at 7 years (Eadie et al., 2022).
- Children with six or more risk factors (compared to those with two or fewer risk factors) were 17 times more likely to have low language at 7 years (Eadie et al., 2022).
- Compared to the *Developmentally enabled group* the *Vulnerable subgroups* (n=5) lagged on receptive vocabulary growth with the largest delay being up to 26.3 months for one group (Christensen et al., 2017; Taylor et al., 2022).
- When followed up 4 years later, three of the five *Vulnerable groups* demonstrated limited or no catch-up growth in receptive vocabulary (Taylor et al., 2022).

In summary, children's early language development is characterised by several important features that have implications for the way in which we identify children at risk of DLD in the early years. First, fluctuation is a feature of early language development and distinct trajectories or groups have been identified. Second, the trajectories have been shown to be associated with distinct risk profiles; compared to children in the developmentally enabled groups, those in the fluctuating or change groups tend to live in less advantageous circumstances. Third, risks cluster together and as the number of risks accumulates, the likelihood of poorer language outcomes later in childhood also increases. What then are the implications for

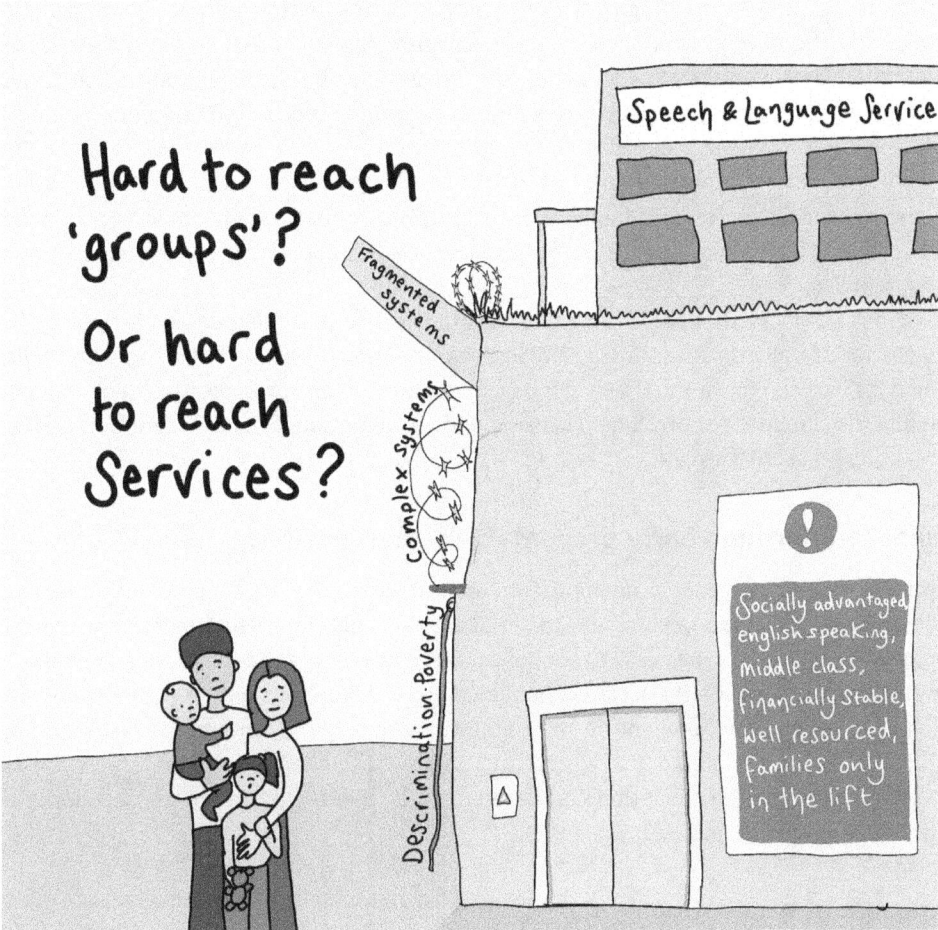

Figure 9.2 Barriers faced in accessing speech and language services

practice and service delivery? Many of the current early years systems would identify children in the stable low trajectories to be at risk for DLD. However, those in the fluctuating or change trajectories might well be missed, depending on when milestones were checked. Further there may be harms associated with wrongly identifying children to be at risk when they are not. These findings contribute to the reasons why there continues to be insufficient evidence to support screening for speech and language in children during the early years (US Preventive Services Task Force, 2024). Focusing on clusters of risks in the child's ecosystem will clearly be important.

There is ample evidence that a family's socio-economic circumstances affect their access to support and the ability to benefit from support. Compared to more advantaged families, those living with disadvantage are less likely to seek support for their child's language (Norbury et al., 2016; Reilly et al., 2018). In one community study, help was sought for only 50% of children up to 5 years with low language (Skeat et al., 2014) and both help-seeking and support were less likely in children living in disadvantages circumstances

(Morgan et al., 2016). McKean and Reilly (2023) discuss these barriers in some detail, highlighting the burden on families to 'join up' services, advocate and negotiate access. Finally, many interventions to support children's language development place a substantial emphasis on supporting parents/caregivers to provide responsive contingent interaction (Law and Charlton, 2022; Levickis et al., 2022). However, it is much more difficult for a family living with multiple challenges to make this change. Hence universal interventions run the risk that children and families with the fewest needs benefit most and vice versa (Mol et al., 2008; Becker, 2011). Figure 9.2 summarises some of the most obvious barriers facing families.

There is no doubt that there are significant barriers to accessing and/or benefiting from services for socially disadvantaged families, many of whom will be grappling with multiple challenges and complexities. These can be exacerbated when social disadvantage intersects with minority group status, including seeking and receiving support, navigating services, supplementing state with private services and advocacy.

Evidence informing early preventative interventions

This section describes the components and characteristics of a public health approach to child language. This approach meets the challenge of early intervention and addresses the complexities of inequity in access to support. It takes account of the prevalence of needs, and the volatility of language trajectories. Public health interventions aim to alter the course or outcome of a condition, prevent harm or improve functioning (McKean, Mensah and Reilly, 2022) through coordinated action across agencies such as health, education, social services and local government. Prevention can be enacted at three levels: primary, secondary and tertiary prevention (Figure 9.3, Table 9.3).

A mosaic of prevention

For a child language public health approach to work, action at all levels of prevention is required, it must be sustained over the early years, and it must change over development (Figure 9.4). This whole system approach creates a 'mosaic' of connected activity distributed

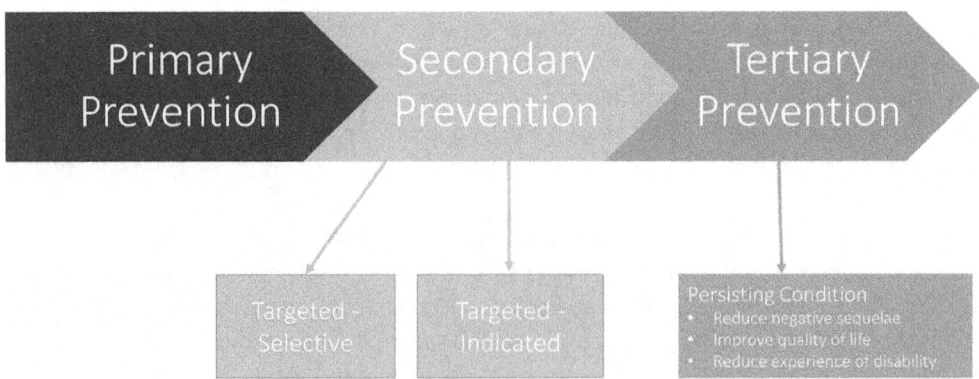

Figure 9.3 A public health framework: components

Level of prevention	Definition
Primary prevention	Acts at a whole-population, universal level and aims to reduce the incidence of a condition and to prevent its later development
Secondary prevention	Targeted at subgroups of the population. It aims to prevent a given condition from emerging or to act early to slow down or reverse its course once it has begun. This targeting can be either selective or indicated.
Targeted selective	Approaches delivered to groups most at risk of developing a condition
Targeted indicated	Approaches used when early signs and/or risks of a condition are present in the individual
Tertiary prevention	Interventions for an individual with a persisting condition. Here the focus is on reducing negative consequences, improving quality of life, and reducing an individual's experience of disability.

Table 9.3 Levels of prevention and their definitions

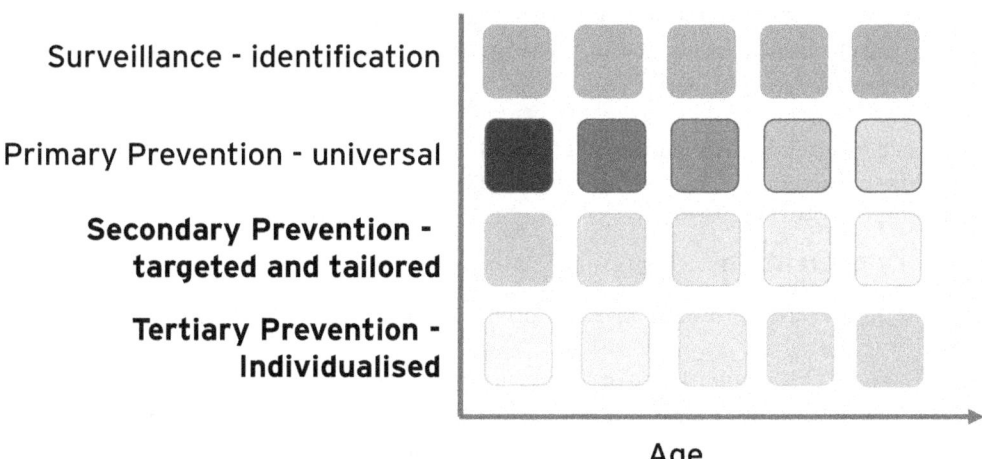

Figure 9.4 A mosaic of intervention across levels of prevention and surveillance and over time

across delivery platforms and practitioner groups, using different assessment tools, indicators of risk and interventions over time. Ideally, such a mosaic would be underpinned by connected data, allowing children's trajectories, profiles of risk and response to intervention to inform action to be assessed. The mosaic approach includes the following factors:

- A whole system approach leveraging and developing capacity across the children's workforce.
- Language as a priority outcome across children's services.
- A focus on equity of outcome not equity of provision – proportionate and tailored responses.
- Co-produced local delivery.
- Stacking interventions across development and at multiple levels of support.
- Continuous sustainable improvement and sustained investment, not short-term fixes.

This mosaic of prevention is necessary if all children in the early years are to receive the right support for optimal language outcomes. Each level of prevention *on its own* will not address children's language needs equitably or comprehensively.

- *Primary prevention*, if used in isolation, risks widening inequalities as those with most resources are more able to act upon messages regarding the provision of language enriching environments.
- *Targeted selective* interventions risk over-serving and under-serving, as not all children living in socially disadvantaged circumstances will have language problems and conversely, some children living in socially advantaged families will have language difficulties.
- *Targeted indicated* interventions again risk both over-serving and underserving children with, or at risk of, low language, due to the instability in early language development; with some children growing out of their language difficulties but also some growing into them.
- *Tertiary preventive* interventions, offered to those with a diagnosis of (D)LD, given the limited and inequitable access to services described previously, risk substantially underserving children and, crucially, miss the opportunity to tackle upstream determinants of low language early in life.

The public health framework must be provided as a whole-system approach and include all the following components (see Table 9.3 for definitions of the levels of prevention).

Primary prevention

Universal intervention provided for all children in the early years and to promote:

- awareness of the importance of language development;
- the role of parents/caregivers and the wider family in supporting children's development;
- ways to support language development as part of daily routines;
- avenues and triggers for seeking support if necessary.

Intervention delivery through multiple systems to enable equitable and sustained reach, for example:

- broadcast and social media campaigns;
- midwifery and public health nurse contacts with families;
- early years education and care providers.

Language surveillance to ensure all children's language and communication development is monitored at key points in their development and/or at educational transitions (e.g., 11-12 months; 2-2.5 years, 3 years, 4 years) (Gilroy et al., 2022).

Secondary prevention: targeted selective

The subgroup of the population most at risk of poor language development is children living with social disadvantage (Reilly et al., 2014; McKean et al., 2018; McKean, Mensah and

Reilly, 2022). There are several key actions for early years education, health, social care and voluntary sector organisations supporting families in more disadvantaged areas and those who fund and commission services.

- Prioritise the promotion of children's language development.
- Ensure teams receive training so they have the knowledge and the skills to support families and, for early education and care providers, to provide language-enriching environments (Gascoigne, 2021).
- Ensure services have the capacity to provide this support.
- Use local data with reference to knowledge of subgroups with clustering of risks to enable precise deployment of resources. For example, communities could receive additional resources where there are high levels of families experiencing several known risks: social disadvantage, large family size, maternal mental health needs, unemployment, low language at 2 years, and so on (Taylor et al., 2020; Eadie et al., 2022).
- Use universal collection and linkage of data regarding children's early language development to identify geographical areas and population subgroups where language development appears, at a group level, to be less robust than the wider population. Services should concentrate resources and efforts to address those needs.

In addition to these more localised strategies, social policy more broadly must tackle the upstream determinants of low language which cluster in families, such as overcrowding, housing instability, parental stress and more limited parental resources in terms of time and money (Taylor et al., 2020; Eadie et al., 2022; Taylor, Christensen and Zubrick, 2022).

Secondary prevention: targeted indicated

Given the volatility in early language trajectories, targeting interventions based *solely* on children's language ability before 4 years cannot be recommended. However, given that not all children with (D)LD are from socially disadvantaged families, some form of targeted indicated intervention as a component of a public health model is indicated. The recent evidence regarding the clustering and accumulation of risks and their ability to predict language outcomes suggests it may be possible to integrate child and environmental factors to create clinical 'risk models' (McKean et al., 2016; Taylor, Zubrick and Christensen, 2019; Taylor et al., 2020; Eadie et al., 2022) especially if it is possible to look at these risks over time through a surveillance model. However, further research is needed to fully evaluate such approaches when used at the individual child level and in practice. There are some promising tools and approaches available. Here are some examples:

- The Early Language Identification Measure and Intervention (ELIM-I) integrates child language abilities with other risks and has proven feasibility and acceptability for use at 2-2.5 years by health visiting teams (Law et al., 2020; Law et al., 2023).
- The Parental Responsiveness Rating Scale (PaRRIS) measures the key environmental risk of caregiver responsiveness and contingent talk (Hudson et al., 2015; Levickis et al., 2019).

Tertiary prevention

This level of support will be provided by speech and language therapists (SLTs) and other professionals with the advice and support of an SLT. The provision of primary and secondary interventions must never slow down referrals for tertiary prevention where parental concern is high, difficulties are severe or where indicators of other disabilities are present. Clear referral criteria and pathways to specialist assessment and intervention must be in place, all members of the children's workforce must be aware of them, and specialist services must be adequately resourced to meet the level of need. Key secondary consequences to low language in the early years which should be considered for tertiary prevention are socio-emotional and behavioural difficulties, social relationships and pre-literacy skills such as phonological awareness. There is currently limited evidence regarding interventions addressing these outcomes specifically in children with or at risk of (D)LD. However, it is recommended that for this group of children:

- parents should have access to advice about strategies to tackle frustration and reduce withdrawal and/or conduct difficulties as relevant to the individual child (Hutchings et al., 2007; Landry et al., 2008);
- early childhood education and care settings must have the relevant skills and knowledge in order to promote peer relationships (Fujiki and Brinton, 2017) and modify learning environments. These measures will reduce stress, improve access to learning (Dockrell, Ricketts and Lindsay, 2012) and develop key pre-literacy skills such as phonological awareness (Gillon, 2000).

Essential qualities of the mosaic of prevention

The previous section described the *components* of the public health framework that is recommended. Here the *qualities* of those components needed for its successful implementation are outlined: developmental and sustained, probabilistic, proportionate, and co-designed.

Approaches to both surveillance and intervention must differ according to the child's age and should not be seen as one-off events but as parts of pathways over time.

Surveillance

Obviously, when assessing whether children's language is developing as expected, the behaviours and skills assessed must change; but they must also differ in terms of the certainty with which a 'low' score is interpreted. As children develop, we become more certain that a low score is likely to represent a persisting difficulty and so the response should differ accordingly. For example, low scores for children with no other developmental concerns might suggest the actions listed below:

- at 11-12 months: signposting to universal resources regarding parent-child interaction and access to a parent-toddler support group

- at 2–2.5 years: two or three visits from the Health Visitor team to support a family to increase their use of responsive contingent interaction
- at 3 years: inclusion in a language-enrichment group in nursery, plus advice and monitoring of progress by the SLT
- at 4 years: elicit a referral to SLT to begin a diagnostic pathway and to receive an individualised treatment programme.

This does not mean children under the age of 4 years should not be referred for SLT or other specialist support. Certainty that a child has a persisting difficulty and would benefit from earlier SLT referral can be increased for younger children by the consideration of the additional risks discussed previously (Eadie et al., 2022; Taylor, Christensen and Zubrick, 2022; Reilly and McKean, 2023). Furthermore, a dynamic assessment approach should be adopted after each intervention to determine whether expected progress is made or not. Additional risks, lack of progress over time and/or significant parental concern should trigger earlier access to specialist support than a low language score alone.

In addition to being developmentally informed, surveillance must be sustained over time:

- to address the volatility in early language development;
- to allow earlier language scores to inform judgements regarding the accumulation of later risks (Eadie et al., 2022);
- to allow response to intervention to be considered.

Interventions

Interventions must be developmental with respect to the child language and communication skills addressed. Also, recent evidence highlights the changing nature of the qualities of adult-child interaction which maximise progress as children develop, and so parent/caregiver and early educator interventions must also be developmental in their design (Rowe and Snow, 2020).

Intervention efforts must be sustained. Single, isolated early interventions, although effective are not a 'silver bullet' and there is no clear evidence that they accelerate future progress. Also gains from a single intervention may 'wash out' if support is not sustained (e.g. McGillion et al., 2017). Molloy et al. (2021) suggest that 'stacking' of interventions is required both over time and across services and to amplify the effect of individual interventions (Heckman, 2006). Further research is required to test whether stacking interventions sequentially and/or simultaneously does indeed accumulate or at least sustain intervention effects.

Probabilistic: playing the odds to meet every child's needs

The public health framework proposed here is not deterministic and diagnosis-based but rather achieves population coverage through the four levels of the framework and over the first 4 years of a child's life. As for other areas of public health, individual interventions will inevitably overserve and underserve to a degree and this needs to be accepted and accommodated in the model. To implement this probabilistic quality, systems need to take certain actions:

- Link surveillance and intervention over time and across levels of prevention so that repeated contacts and primary preventative interventions act as 'safety nets' to ensure all children receive some level of support.
- Use research findings described above regarding clustering and accumulating risks to support practitioners to 'tip the balance' towards action for those at higher risk.
- Track children over time, allowing those receiving too low a level of intervention to be identified and support 'stepped up' as soon as possible and for accumulating risks and persisting trajectories to be identified.
- Use available local data to target geographical areas and/or subgroups of the population, using knowledge of the key factors described above which make children more likely to be vulnerable to poor language outcomes.
- Ensure interventions do not cause harm to children who receive support but do not ultimately need it, in terms of increased anxiety or stigmatisation.

More research is needed to identify the optimal configurations and content of the 'mosaic' of prevention to ensure interventions do not raise anxiety unnecessarily in those whose difficulties will resolve; and to ensure the costs of overserving are outweighed by the benefits of ensuring that all children who require support receive it.

Proportionate: tailoring for equitable benefit

For all individuals to benefit equally from interventions, differing amounts and type of support are needed, depending on individual circumstances. Professor Michael Marmot coined the term 'proportionate universalism' to refer to the universal provision of services, where the "scale and intensity . . . [are] proportionate to the level of disadvantage" (Marmot et al., 2010, p. 16). To ensure interventions achieve equitable outcomes, work is needed to understand and address the effects of an individual's circumstances on the accessibility, acceptability and effectiveness of interventions. Where family-level interventions are delivered, they must be proportionate and tailored with due regard to families' assets and adversities to ensure equity of access and benefit (McKean et al., 2022). These must also be paired with social policy that tackles inequalities in order that all families have the necessary resources to provide an optimal home learning environment in the fundamental early years. We must challenge policy that places all the responsibility on individual families to make changes in the way that they parent without tackling broader inequalities (Molloy et al., 2021).

Co-designed: tailoring to fit families and local services

Current evidence suggests that interventions and their implementation need to be adapted to fit local families' specific assets and challenges, the constraints and configuration of local services and the skills and capacity of the children's workforce (Greenwood et al., 2020).

For example, Mol et al. (2008) found that promoting parent-child interactive book-sharing is effective in socially advantaged but not socially disadvantaged families. Although the underlying intervention active ingredients of responsive contingent interactions within book-sharing contexts are therefore effective, other barriers such as time, confidence and physical resources in socially disadvantaged families make this specific approach unfeasible or unacceptable. Co-design approaches can support us to understand and address such barriers. McKean et al. (2022) report that some parents found book-reading interventions patronising, while others felt they set them up to fail as they did not engage their children's attention, leading to disruption in parent-child relationships. In both such scenarios, the barrier to engagement was not a lack of knowledge or motivation but the need to find more individualised contexts within which to promote responsive interaction which work for those specific families.

'Scaling up' interventions found to be effective in research studies for delivery by educators in the 'real world' is also challenging (Snowling et al., 2022). Barriers include competing priorities and staff turn-over; plus, a lack of the following: knowledge, skills, access to training, available time, and support (Mol, Bus and de Jong, 2009; Bleses et al., 2018). Addressing such barriers requires collaborative work to adapt current best evidence to ensure interventions can be delivered sustainably, and through accessible and acceptable methods.

Examples

BBC Tiny Happy People (now known as Cbeebies Parenting)

In 2020, the BBC launched a set of universally accessible, attractive and motivating resources to support families to provide language-enriching opportunities from before birth to school entry. This primary prevention intervention involves web resources, social media campaigns and a wealth of resources for parents/caregivers and professionals. In partnership with professionals and researchers it uses current evidence about the science of children's learning and development to motivate and inform parents/caregivers and provide practical tips and advice to integrate these into daily life. https://www.bbc.co.uk/tiny-happy-people

Stoke Speaks Out

Stoke Speaks Out was a pioneering initiative in using a 'place-based' approach to support child language development. It began in 2004 first in Stoke-on-Trent, and now across all of Staffordshire and Stoke-on-Trent. It takes a whole-system approach to ensure everyone in children's lives sees children's communication development as 'their business' and has the relevant skills and knowledge to support them.

The impetus for the initiative was local data in the area identifying that many children were starting nursery with poor language skills; by 2004, this was 64%. Stoke Speaks Out was set up to make sure everyone knows how to support children's language, and where to seek help if children are struggling. Over time, it has developed and delivered training for the whole children's workforce, enabled the development and use of identification tools and targeted interventions. Stoke Speaks Out therefore enables primary, secondary and tertiary levels of prevention, is co-designed with locally embedded practitioners, and aims to provide sustained support over the early years. https://www.stokespeaks.org/about

The Early Language Identification Measure and Intervention – ELIM-I

The Early Language Identification Measure and Intervention is used universally by Health Visiting (HV) Teams at the child's 2-2.5 year review (Law et al., 2020; McKean et al., 2022; Law et al., 2023). It aims to implement some of the key features of a public health framework including consideration of the accumulation of risks, and a proportionate and co-designed response. The ELIM-I measure draws on research regarding key risks for vulnerable language trajectories to combine both language assessment and other factors to identify children who may benefit from support. The research team also designed an accompanying intervention. They found that for an intervention to be equitable, it must be proportionate, with higher 'intensity' for higher levels of disadvantage, and also tailored, offering differing approaches depending upon the specific barriers and enablers, assets, and challenges in each family. In this approach HVs choose goals together with the family that suit the family's individual circumstances and offer different types and level of support depending upon the barriers and supports in place for that family. These can be self-directed or involve different levels of coaching and support. Research has shown the approach to be acceptable and feasible for practitioners and services (McKean et al., 2022) and co-designed training, video and print resources created in partnership with BBC Tiny Happy People (now rebranded as Cbeebies Parenting) are available to support its use. https://research.ncl.ac.uk/elim-i/elim-i/elim-itrain ingandhandbooks/. Further work is needed to test empirically whether such tailoring does deliver equitable benefits.

Summary

This chapter explores key public health concepts and summarises an important and recent body of research regarding key influences in the early years, noting that exposure to some may be time-sensitive, influences cluster together and can accumulate over time.

It demonstrates that risk profiles were associated with and characterised low language trajectories, and considered how this information could be integrated into a concept that moves beyond screening at single time points in the early years (Reilly and McKean, 2023).

Evidence was synthesised with intervention research and implementation frameworks to inform an early language public health framework of surveillance and intervention. The essential components and qualities of that framework were detailed.

References

Becker, B. (2011) 'Social disparities in children's vocabulary in early childhood. Does pre-school education help to close the gap?', *The British Journal of Sociology*, 62(1), 69-88. http://dx.doi.org/doi:10.1111/j.1468-4446.2010.01345.x.

Bleses, D., Højen, A., Dale, P.S., Justice, L.M., Dybdal, L., Piasta, S., Markussen-Brown, J., Kjærbæk, L. and Haghish, E.F. (2018) 'Effective language and literacy instruction: Evaluating the importance of scripting and group size components', *Early Childhood Research Quarterly*, 42, 256-269. http://dx.doi.org/10.1016/j.ecresq.2017.10.002.

Bronfenbrenner, U. (2005) *Making Human Beings Human: Bioecological Perspectives on Human Development*. Thousand Oaks, CA: SAGE.

Christensen, D., Taylor, C.L. and Zubrick, S.R. (2017) 'Patterns of multiple risk exposures for low receptive vocabulary growth 4-8 years in the longitudinal study of Australian children', *PLoS One*, 12(1), e0168804. http://dx.doi.org/10.1371/journal.pone.0168804.

Dean, H. (2007) 'Poor parents? The realities of work-life balance in a low-income neighbourhood', *Benefits: A Journal of Poverty and Social Justice*, 15(3), 271-282. http://dx.doi.org/10.51952/ylfa8554.

Di Sante, M. and Potvin, L. (2022) 'We need to talk about social inequalities in language development', *American Journal of Speech and Language Pathology*, 31(4), 1894-1897. http://dx.doi.org/10.1044/2022_ajslp-21-00326.

Dubois, P., St-Pierre, M.C., Desmarais, C. and Guay, F. (2020) 'Young adults with developmental language disorder: A systematic review of education, employment, and independent living outcomes', *Journal of Speech, Language, and Hearing Research*, 63(11), 3786-3800. http://dx.doi.org/10.1044/2020_JSLHR-20-00127.

Eadie, P., Levickis, P., McKean, C., Westrupp, E., Bavin, E.L., Ware, R.S., Gerner, B. and Reilly, S. (2022) 'Developing preschool language surveillance models - cumulative and clustering patterns of early life factors in the early language in Victoria Study Cohort', *Frontiers in Pediatrics*, 10. http://dx.doi.org/10.3389/fped.2022.826817.

Fujiki, M. and Brinton, B. (2017) 'Social communication intervention for children with language impairment'. In R. McCauley, M.F. Fey and R. Gillam (eds), *Treatment of Language Disorders*, 2nd edn. Baltimore, MD: Brookes Publishing, pp. 421-449.

Gascoigne, M. (2021) 'Equity for all: Children's speech and language therapy services in Scotland'. Better Communication CIC and Scottish Government. Available at: https://www.bettercommunication.org.uk/downloads/2022%20Equity%20for%20All%20Final%20for%20Publication.pdf

Gillon, G. (2000) 'The efficacy of phonological awareness intervention for children with spoken language impairment', *Language Speech and Hearing Services in Schools*, 31, 126-141.

Gilroy, V., Jackson, V., Stephen, R., Charlton, J. and McKean, C. (2022) *Campaigning for more responsive parenting: Lessons learned from the NSPCC's Look, Say, Sing, Play Campaign*. London: NSPCC.

Greenwood, C.R., Schnitz, A.G., Carta, J.J., Wallisch, A. and Irvin, D.W. (2020) 'A systematic review of language intervention research with low-income families: A word gap prevention perspective', *Early Childhood Research Quarterly*, 50, 230-245. http://dx.doi.org/10.1016/j.ecresq.2019.04.001.

Heckman, J.J. (2006) 'Skill formation and the economics of investing in disadvantaged children', *Science*, 312(5782), 1900-1902.

Hudson, S., Levickis, P., Down, K., Nicholls, R. and Wake, M. (2015) 'Maternal responsiveness predicts child language at ages 3 and 4 in a community-based sample of slow-to-talk toddlers', *International Journal of Language and Communication Disorders*, 50(1), 136-142. http://dx.doi.org/10.1111/1460-6984.12129.

Hutchings, J., Bywater, T., Daley, D., Gardner, F., Whitaker, C., Jones, K., Eames, C. and Edwards, R (2007) 'Parenting intervention in Sure Start services for children at risk of developing conduct disorder: pragmatic randomised controlled trial', *British Medical Journal*, 334(7595), 678-682.

Landry, S.H., Smith, K.E., Swank, P.R. and Guttentag, C.L. (2008) 'Responsive parenting: The optimal timing of an intervention across early childhood', *Developmental Psychology*, 44(5), 1335-1353.

Law, J., Charlton, J. and Asmussen, K. (2017) *Language as a Child Wellbeing Indicator*. London: Early Intervention Foundation.

Law, J. and Charlton, J. (2022) 'Interventions to promote language development in typical and atypical populations'. In J. Law,. S. Reilly, and C. McKean (eds), *Language Development: Individual Differences in a Social Context*. Cambridge: Cambridge University Press, pp. 470-494.

Law, J., Charlton, J., McKean, C., Watson, R., Roulstone, S., Holme, C., Gilroy, V., Wilson, P. and Rush, R. (2020) *Identifying and Supporting Children's Early Language Needs*. Newcastle upon Tyne: Newcastle University

Law, J., Charlton, J., Wilson, P., Rush, R., Gilroy, V. and McKean, C. (2023) 'The development and productivity of a measure for identifying low language abilities in children aged 24-36 months', *BMC Pediatrics*, 23(1), 495. http://dx.doi.org/10.1186/s12887-023-04079-x.

Law, J., Clegg, J., Rush, R., Roulstone, S. and Peters, T.J (2019) 'Association of proximal elements of social disadvantage with children's language development at 2 years: An analysis of data from the Children in Focus (CiF) sample from the ALSPAC birth cohort', *International Journal of Language and Communication Disorders*, 54(3), 362-376. http://dx.doi.org/10.1111/1460-6984.12442.

Levickis, P., McKean, C., Walls, E. and Law, J. (2019) 'Training community health nurses to measure parent-child interaction: a mixed-methods study', *European Journal of Public Health*. http://dx.doi.org/10.1093/eurpub/ckz155.

Levickis, P., Patel, P., McKean, C., Smith, J., Hackworth, N., Law, J. and Reilly, S. (2022) 'A review of interventions to promote language development in early childhood'. In J. Law, S. Reilly, and C. McKean (eds), *Language Development: Individual Differences in a Social Context*. Cambridge: Cambridge University Press, pp. 443–469.

Määttä, S., Laakso, M.L., Tolvanen, A., Ahonen, T. and Aro, T. (2012) 'Developmental trajectories of early communication skills', *Journal of Speech, Language, and Hearing Research*, 55, 1083–1096.

Marmot, M., Atkinson, A., Bell, J., Black, C., Broadfoot, P., Cumberlege, J., Diamond, I., Gilmore, I., Ham, C., Meacher, M. and Mulgan, G. (2010) *Strategic Review of Health Inequalities in England Post-2010: Fair Society Healthy Lives: The Marmot Review*. London: Institute of Health Equity.

McGillion, M., Pine, J.M., Herbert, J.S. and Matthews, D. (2017) 'A randomised controlled trial to test the effect of promoting caregiver contingent talk on language development in infants from diverse socioeconomic status backgrounds', *Journal of Child Psychology and Psychiatry and Allied Disciplines*, 58(10), 1122–1131. http://dx.doi.org/10.1111/jcpp.12725.

McKean, C., Law, J., Mensah, F., Cini, E., Eadie, P., Frazer, K. and Reilly, S. (2016) 'Predicting meaningful differences in school-entry language skills from child and family factors measured at 12 months of age', *International Journal of Early Childhood*, 48(3), 329–351. http://dx.doi.org/10.1007/s13158-016-0174-0.

McKean, C., Law, J., Morgan, A. and Reilly, S. (2018) 'Developmental language disorder'. In S. Rueschemeyer and G.M. Gaskell (eds), *Oxford Handbook of Psycholinguistics*. Oxford: Oxford University Press.

McKean, C., Mensah, F.K., Eadie, P., Bavin, E.L., Bretherton, L., Cini, E. and Reilly, S. (2015) 'Levers for language growth: Characteristics and predictors of language trajectories between 4 and 7 years', *PLoS ONE*, 10(8). http://dx.doi.org/10.1371/journal.pone.0134251.

McKean, C., Mensah, F. and Reilly, S. (2022) 'Language trajectories in childhood: The nature and drivers of individual differences and their implications for intervention', In J. Law, S. Reilly, and C. McKean (eds), *Language Development: Individual Differences in a Social Context*. Cambridge: Cambridge University Press, pp. 259–280.

McKean, C. and Reilly, S. (2023) 'Creating the conditions for robust early language development for all: Part two: Evidence informed public health framework for child language in the early years', *International Journal of Language and Communication Disorders*, 58(6), 2242-2264. http://dx.doi.org/ https://doi.org/10.1111/1460-6984.12927

McKean, C., Watson, R., Charlton, J., Roulstone, S., Homle, C., Gilroy, V. and Law, J. (2022) '"Making the most of together time": Development of a Health Visitor-led intervention to support children's early language and communication development at the 2-2(1/2)-year-old review', *Pilot Feasibility Stud*, 8(1), 35. http://dx.doi.org/10.1186/s40814-022-00978-5.

McKean, C, Wraith, D., Eadie, P., Cook, F., Mensah, F. and Reilly, S. (2017) 'Subgroups in language trajectory from 4 to 11 years: The nature and predictors of stable, improving and declining language trajectory groups', *Journal of Child Psychology and Psychiatry*, 58(10), 1081-1091. http://dx.doi.org/10.1111/jcpp.12790.

Mol, S.E., Bus, A.G. and de Jong, M.T. (2009) 'Interactive book reading in early education: A tool to stimulate print knowledge as well as oral language', *Review of Educational Research*, 79(2), 979–1007. http://dx.doi.org/10.3102/0034654309332561.

Mol, S.E. Bus, A.G., de Jong, M.T. and Smeets, D.J.H. (2008) 'Added value of dialogic parent-child book readings: A meta-analysis', *Early Education and Development*, 19(1), 7-26. http://dx.doi.org/10.1080/10409280701838603.

Molloy, C., Moore, T., O'Connor, M., Villanueva, K., West, S. and Goldfeld, S. (2021) 'A novel 3-part approach to tackle the problem of health inequities in early childhood', *Academic Pediatrics*, 21(2), 236-243. http://dx.doi.org/10.1016/j.acap.2020.12.005.

Morgan, P.L., Hammer, C.S., Farkas, G., Hillemeier, M.M., Maczuga, S., Cook, M. and Morano, S. (2016) 'Who receives speech/language pathology services by 5 years of age in the United States?', *American Journal of Speech-Language Pathology*, 25, 183-199.

Mountford, H.S., Braden, R., Newbury, D.F, and Morgan, A.T. (2022) 'The genetic and molecular basis of developmental language disorder: A review', *Children*, (5), 586. https://www.mdpi.com/2227-9067/9/5/586.

Norbury, C.F., Gooch, D., Wray, C., Baird, G., Charman, T., Simonoff, E., Vamvakas, G. and Pickles, A. (2016) 'The impact of nonverbal ability on prevalence and clinical presentation of language disorder: Evidence from a population study', *Journal of Child Psychology and Psychiatry*, 57(11), 1247-1257.

Reilly, S., Cook, F., Bavin, E.L., Bretherton, L., Cahir, P., Eadie, P., Gold, L., Mensah, F., Papadopoullos, S. and Wake, M. (2018) 'Cohort profile: The early language in Victoria Study (ELVS)', *International Journal of Epidemiology*, 47(1), 11-20. http://dx.doi.org/10.1093/ije/dyx079.

Reilly, S. and McKean, C. (2023) 'Creating the conditions for robust early language development for all: Part 1: Evidence informed child language surveillance in the early years', *International Journal of Langauge and Communication Disorders*, http://dx.doi.org/https://doi.org/10.1111/1460-6984.12929.

Reilly, S., Tomblin, B., Law, J., McKean, C., Mensah, F.K., Morgan, A., Goldfeld, S., Nicholson, J.M. and Wake, M. (2014) 'Specific language impairment: A convenient label for whom?', *International Journal of Language and Communication Disorders*, 49(4), 416-451. http://dx.doi.org/10.1111/1460-6984.12102.

Rowe, M.L. and Snow, C.E. (2020) 'Analyzing input quality along three dimensions: interactive, linguistic, and conceptual', *Journal of Child Language*, 47(1), 5-21. http://dx.doi.org/10.1017/S0305000919000655.

Skeat, J. Wake, M., Ukoumunne, O.C., Eadie, P., Bretherton, L. and Reilly, S. (2014) 'Who gets help for preschool communication problems? Data from a prospective community study', *Child: Care, Health and Development*, 40(2), 215-222. http://dx.doi.org/10.1111/cch.12032.

Snowling, M.J., Duff, F.J., Nash, H.M. and Hulme, C. (2016) 'Language profiles and literacy outcomes of children with resolving, emerging, or persisting language impairments', *Journal of Child Psychology and Psychiatry*, 57, 1360-1369.

Snowling, M.J. West, G., Fricke, S., Bowyer-Crane, C., Dilnot, J., Cripps, D., Nash, M. and Hulme, C. (2022) 'Delivering language intervention at scale: Promises and pitfalls', *Journal of Research in Reading*, 45(3), 342-366. http://dx.doi.org/https://doi.org/10.1111/1467-9817.12391.

Taylor, C.L. Christensen, D., Lawrence, D., Mitrou, F. and Zubrick, S.R. (2013) 'Risk factors for children's receptive vocabulary development from four to eight years in the longitudinal study of Australian children', *PLOS one*, 8(9), e73046. http://dx.doi.org/10.1371/journal.pone.0073046.

Taylor, C.L. Christensen, D., Stafford, J., Venn, A., Preen, D. and Zubrick, S.R. (2020) 'Associations between clusters of early life risk factors and developmental vulnerability at age 5: A retrospective cohort study using population-wide linkage of administrative data in Tasmania, Australia', *BMJ Open*, 10(4), e033795.

Taylor, C.L., Christensen, D. and Zubrick, S.R. (2022) 'Creating equitable opportunities for language and literacy development in childhood and adolescence'. In J. Law, S. Reilly and C. McKean (eds), *Language Development: Individual Differences in a Social Context*. Cambridge: Cambridge University Press, pp. 231-256.

Taylor, C.L., Zubrick, S.R. and Christensen, D. (2019) 'Multiple risk exposures for reading achievement in childhood and adolescence', *Journal of Epidemiology and Community Health*, 73(5), 427-434.

Taylor, M. and Edwards, B. (2012) 'Housing and children's wellbeing and development: evidence from a national longitudinal study', *Family Matters*, 91, 47-61.

Ukoumunne, O. C., Wake, M., Carlin, J., Bavin, E. L., Lum, J., Skeat, J., Williams, J., Conway, L., Cini, E., & Reilly, S. (2012) 'Profiles of language development in pre-school children: a longitudinal latent class analysis of data from the Early Language in Victoria Study', *Child: care, health and development*, 38(3), 341-349. https://doi.org/10.1111/j.1365-2214.2011.01234.x.

US Preventive Services Task Force (2024) 'Screening for Speech and Language Delay and Disorders in Children: US Preventive Services Task Force Recommendation Statement', *JAMA*, 331(4), 329-334. http://dx.doi.org/10.1001/jama.2023.26952.

Zambrana, I.M., Pons, F., Eadie, P. and Ystrom, E. (2014) 'Trajectories of language delay from age 3 to 5: Persistence, recovery and late onset.' *International Journal of Language and Communication Disorders*, 49, 304-316.

Zubrick, S.R., Taylor, C.L. and Christensen, D. (2015) 'Patterns and predictors of language and literacy abilities 4-10 years in the Longitudinal Study of Australian Children', *PLoS ONE*, 10, e0135612.

10 Developmental Language Disorder (DLD)

Courtenay Norbury and Susan Ebbels

What you'll learn in this chapter

- How to describe the core features of developmental language disorder (DLD)
- How to discuss changes in terminology to describe children's language-learning deficits
- An understanding of the diagnostic issues that surround DLD, particularly the role of non-verbal cognitive ability
- How to interpret assessment results and formulate a diagnostic statement
- How to summarise the current evidence base for interventions targeting oral language at the universal, targeted, and specialist levels in a multi-tiered system of support, including the speech-language therapist's role at each level.

Key information about DLD

Developmental Language Disorder (DLD) is a lifelong form of neurodiversity that may be diagnosed when a child is struggling to learn his or her own language (Bishop et al., 2016). Prevalence estimates vary depending on the definitions and assessments used to measure language; however, recent international studies converge on a prevalence of 6-8% of school-aged children with language skills that are significantly below age expectations and result in functional impacts, e.g. Australia, 6.4%: (Calder et al., 2022); England, 7.5%: (Norbury et al., 2016); China, 8.6%: (Wu et al., 2023). DLD is more common in areas of socio-economic deprivation, with prevalence rates as high as 13% in the most disadvantaged neighbourhoods (Norbury et al., 2021). DLD is also more common in highly vulnerable groups, for example, 60% of children in care (Clegg et al., 2021) and 71% of children sentenced in the youth justice system between April 2019 and March 2020 met criteria for language disorder (Youth Justice Board, Ministry of Justice, 2021). In addition, children diagnosed with mental health conditions are significantly more likely to have language needs than peers (NHS Digital, 2018).

Definition

International diagnostic frameworks including DSM-5-TR (American Psychiatric Association, 2022) and ICD-11 (World Health Organization, 2019) include the following characteristics in the definition of language disorder:

DOI: 10.4324/9781003671626-14

- persistent difficulties in understanding and/or producing language across modalities (i.e. spoken, written, sign language);
- language abilities below chronological age expectations;
- differences in language leading to functional impacts in communication, social participation, academic achievement, and/or occupational performance;
- language difficulties are evident early in development and are not the consequence of an acquired pathology (e.g. traumatic brain injury, stroke, tumour);
- difficulties with language are not attributable to sensory impairment, motor difficulties, or another medical or neurological condition, and are not better explained by intellectual disability;
- language differences may occur in any area of language (phonology, semantics, morphology, pragmatics), either in isolation or in combination.

Terminology

Unlike other neurodevelopmental conditions, such as autism, dyslexia, and ADHD, there has been a lack of consistency in the terms used to describe language differences, resulting in numerous challenges to public awareness, research funding, and service provision (McGregor, 2020). For instance, Bishop (2010) found that 130 different terms for language difficulties had been used at least once in a research publication, and 33 distinct forms (e.g. specific language impairment, language delay, language disability, language disorder, or developmental language disorder) had been used 600 times or more.

To address this inconsistency, the international CATALISE consortium invited key stakeholders (families, speech-language therapists, researchers, teachers, etc.) to review evidence and agree on terminology and diagnostic criteria (Bishop et al., 2017). CATALISE recommended the term, 'Developmental Language Disorder' (DLD) for a condition in which language is not developing as expected, but no other associated biomedical condition is present.

DLD supersedes the term 'specific language impairment' (SLI), previously used in research. DLD is a more inclusive term – all children with SLI would meet criteria for DLD, but DLD also includes children with lower non-verbal cognitive ability scores (an exclusion criterion for SLI). DLD is distinguished from 'Language Disorder associated with X', the term used when language difficulties are associated with other neurodevelopmental conditions such as autism or intellectual disability.

More recently, there has been increased sensitivity around the use of the term 'disorder'. Here, we suggest that a difference may become a disorder when it disadvantages the individual in their society (Tomblin, 2006). There is substantial evidence that limited language skills prevent individuals from fully participating in society, compromise well-being, and limit self-advocacy (Snow, 2021). Thus, both strengths and challenges associated with language disorder should be acknowledged and addressed to maximise future opportunities. Furthermore, the use of 'disorder' underscores the need for services and support (Bishop, 2017). In addition, adults with lived experience have described the positive impacts that a diagnosis and a consistent label can have for raising awareness and promoting self-advocacy (Wilmot et al., 2024).

Indicators of complexity/challenge/co-occurrence

Language disorder very rarely occurs in isolation; children presenting with language as a primary concern are very likely to experience co-occurring symptoms, such as behavior problems (Yew and O'Kearney, 2013), motor/coordination deficits (Flapper and Schoemaker, 2013), and reading disorders (Snowling et al., 2020). In addition, other conditions may mask underlying language deficits. For example, approximately 60% of young people presenting to child and adolescent mental health clinics have language disorders, often undiagnosed (Cohen et al., 2013). Thus, children with language disorder and co-occurring developmental concerns will form a substantial proportion of the average clinician's caseload.

Differentiating conditions are biomedical conditions in which language disorder occurs as part of a more complex developmental condition, which may have a specific diagnostic/intervention pathway. CATALISE recommended the term 'Language disorder associated with X', where X is a differentiating condition, such as brain injury, autism, acquired epileptic aphasia, cerebral palsy, genetic conditions associated with intellectual disability and oral language limitations associated with sensorineural hearing loss (Bishop et al., 2017).

For differentiating conditions, the child will likely require specific support for language and communication needs, but intervention pathways may be focused on distinctive features of the biomedical condition. We often assume that language interventions should be diagnosis-specific, however, there is no published research directly comparing language intervention approaches across neurodevelopmental conditions (Donolato et al., 2023). Instead, interventions that focus on language tend to use similar methods and have common approaches to increasing and structuring language input to facilitate learning (Donolato et al. 2023).

Causes of DLD

Clinicians and researchers have known for some time that DLD tends to run in families, and twin studies have established that DLD arises from a combination of genetic and environmental risk factors (Mountford et al., 2022). A common myth is that language disorders arise because parents don't spend enough time talking to their children. Understanding genetic influences on DLD reminds us that many parents and siblings may also have language challenges, and this may affect talk within the home. Genetic influences can affect a child's environmental experience. For example, children with language disorders may select more solitary activities that make fewer demands on verbal skills but also offer fewer opportunities to learn or use language in social contexts.

Genetic influences are thought to affect the way the brain develops. Unlike cases of adult stroke, there are no gross lesions of neurological structures in the left hemisphere for children with DLD. Instead, current hypotheses are focused on disruptions to connections between brain regions that may impede learning language from the usual input (Ullman et al., 2024). The implication for intervention is that these children with DLD have a biological difference that makes language learning harder. They therefore require more language input and/or input that is structured in such a way that it is easier to learn, for example by using visual cues to make the rules of grammar explicit.

Important points about SLT practice in DLD

To improve early identification and timely treatment, many have called for universal screening (Adlof and Hogan, 2019). However, for under-5s, universal screening is not recommended given the low levels of screen accuracy, high rates of spontaneous recovery, and lack of evidence indicating positive benefits of screening on later language outcomes (see Chapter 9 of this book and Bishop et al., 2017 for discussion). For school-aged children, language skills tend to become more stable and screening followed by intervention can yield at least small, short-term positive benefits for children with low language proficiency (West et al., 2021). A review of screening tools is provided by Bao et al. (2024). Many screens have high false-positive rates, meaning that most individuals who screen positive will not have language disorder on further assessment. It is therefore important for services to articulate how children and families with positive screening results will be managed. It is unclear whether screening reduces prevalence or incidence of DLD; the possibility remains that it is better to focus intervention efforts on those for whom there are language concerns (cf. Bishop et al., 2017).

Diagnosis is a key role for the SLT

CATALISE (Bishop et al., 2016; Bishop et al., 2017) provided clinicians with agreed criteria and terminology to facilitate consistency in diagnosis, yet SLTs still report a number of barriers to providing a DLD diagnosis, including case complexities, worries about giving a 'wrong' diagnosis, lack of confidence or knowledge about diagnostic criteria, concerns about stigma for individuals with a diagnosis, and service-level issues, including not having enough clinical time for assessment and diagnosis, and/or services withholding diagnoses if there is no intervention pathway available (Harvey, 2023). Some of these barriers may be addressed through further training and mentorship. Others appear to be in violation of the Health and Care Professionals Council (HCPC) Standards of Proficiency for Speech and Language Therapists. For instance, section 2.5 asks us to 'respect and uphold the rights, dignity, values and autonomy of service users, including their role in the assessment, diagnostic, treatment and/or therapeutic process'. Families and individuals with lived experience include 'we are diagnosed early' as one of their five key visions for people with DLD to have a better future (https://www.afasic.org.uk/a-vision-for-dld-for-the-uk/). In addition, adults report that a diagnosis can be life-changing and is key to raising awareness and advocating for their own needs (Wilmot et al., 2024). Thus, where appropriate, a diagnosis of DLD should be made and discussed, and a summary of strategies and reasonable adjustments provided, even if no further treatment option is available.

Early intervention is important, but later intervention is also necessary

It almost goes without saying that early intervention is critical to children and their families, and this is reflected in government policies that prioritise funding for early intervention. These policies tend to be predicated on the assumption that intervening early will attenuate the need for services later. However, there is growing evidence that (1) after school entry, language is a stable trait, much like height or weight (Bornstein et al., 2018), and (2) the positive benefits of short-term interventions tend to fade out over time (Bailey et al., 2020). In addition, families and adults with lived experience of DLD report that the transition to secondary school was a challenging period in which language difficulties adversely affected learning, social relationships, and well-being (Wilmot et al., 2024). This is not surprising given that the language demands of school and society become increasingly sophisticated as young people get older and transition to adult life. Together, these two factors suggest that a 'cure' may not be a realistic goal of interventions. Instead, services should be planning support and intervention across the life span, with the goal of upskilling individuals and attenuating the negative impacts of DLD on quality of life.

Understanding children's needs in DLD

In a multi-cultural society, diagnosis requires integration of information from various sources, including family and teacher reports, a sample of expressive language, and observation of classroom learning (Castilla-Earls et al., 2020). Formal assessment is also recommended, using culturally-fair, process-oriented tasks such as non-sense word repetition (which taps the phonological memory and encoding skills thought to underlie word learning), sentence repetition, dynamic assessment and/or fast mapping (in which children are taught and asked to retain new word labels or word meanings), or rapid automatic naming (such as saying all the days of the week in rapid sequence).

Common approaches to assessment

Case history

Possible 'red flags' for language disorder include parent concern, a positive family history of language, literacy, or learning difficulties, poor understanding of what others say, and functional impact at home or at school. Additional red flags that warrant onward referral to other professionals include prematurity, language regression, broader health or developmental concerns (motor, cognition, sensory), lack of social engagement, and/or adverse childhood experiences.

Clinical observations

Informal observation during the assessment session can be an invaluable way to establish how the child currently communicates and uses compensatory strategies. The clinician should note whether the child produces single words or phrases or sentences, accuracy of speech sounds or other vocalisations, responds to his or her name or follows simple verbal instructions, uses gesture or pointing, or shows, points, or talks about new things in the environment with caregivers. Informal conversation samples, in which the child and SLT converse, can provide more detail about the level and quality of the child's expressive language, including speech production, utterance length and complexity, fluency, and vocal quality.

In general, children with DLD say less, use simple grammar, may take longer to respond to what has been said or to express themselves, may seem to forget what has been said or only follow part of an instruction, may need more repetition, may use more general vocabulary ('doing the scissors' instead of 'cutting') and may leave out key pieces of information in recounting an event. They may also rely more on non-verbal strategies to communicate, including use of gestures or pictures/symbols.

Standardised assessment of comprehension and expression

While an estimate of expressive language is possible from informal assessment, it can be more challenging to accurately gauge a child's level of understanding. Standardised assessments carried out by SLTs can provide important information about the child's comprehension and expressive language skills in each language domain relative to peers of the same age and from the same language community.

There remains limited consensus as to precise cut-offs that are associated with language disorder (Bishop et al., 2016). The most used cut-off for research diagnosis is -1.25SD below the normative mean (bottom 10th centile), while a cut-off of -1.5SD (bottom 7th centile) on a composite language score was most closely aligned with functional impact on early academic attainment (Norbury et al., 2016).

Rating scales

Standardised tests provide an estimate of language abilities in optimal speaking and listening conditions. However, we are often more interested in how children use language in everyday contexts and rely on parent and teacher rating scales to inform us. The *Children's Communication Checklist-2* (CCC-2; (Bishop, 2003) provides an overview of structural (speech, syntax, vocabulary) and pragmatic (coherence, initiation, non-verbal communication, use of context) language skills, with two additional sub-scales tapping potential autism characteristics related to social relationships and specific interests. Low scores on the pragmatic sub-scales of the CCC-2 are associated with both academic underachievement and increased rates of social, emotional, and behavioral concerns in a population sample. However, pragmatic challenges usually co-occur with language difficulties and/or an increase in autism behaviors (Saul et al., 2023). The CCC-2 can usefully signpost the clinician to areas that require further evaluation.

For all behaviourally defined conditions (e.g. autism, dyslexia), the diagnostic label is our best hypothesis, based on available evidence, and should not be set in stone. Clinicians can convey this by: (1) outlining family concerns and reasons for referral; (2) assessing child strengths and challenges; (3) using evidence that supports the proposed diagnosis; and (4) making a statement such as, 'this diagnosis is based on information available at the point of testing. It may change if new information comes to light, or the picture may change as the child develops.' It is also possible to convey uncertainty and request that the child returns for assessment in 6-12 months to establish persistence (or otherwise) of language challenges. Finally, it may be that more information is required from other professionals to make a differential diagnosis. Making time to talk to families some time after giving the diagnosis is important as they may not be able to take in all the information at the time of the assessment and may have further questions.

Supporting children's needs in DLD

Support and intervention services for children are often conceptualised as being split into tiers or levels (e.g. Fuchs and Fuchs, 2006; Ebbels et al., 2019). Education distinguishes between *Tiers 1, 2* and *3*, alongside which SLTs provide *universal*, *targeted* and *specialist* services. As far as language and, in particular, DLD are concerned, Tier 1 focuses on universal prevention of language difficulties by providing language-rich, inclusive communication environments and high-quality teaching within educational settings for all children. Parallel to Tier 1, SLTs provide universal services, which typically focus on continuing professional development sessions aimed at raising awareness of DLD, helping staff to identify DLD and promote accommodations which will support children with DLD to participate fully. Tier 2 focuses on short-term catch-up using manualised interventions or programmes for children who are performing just below age expectations, often delivered to small groups of children by education staff and without direct SLT involvement. SLTs may provide targeted services to support Tier 2 by sign-posting schools to evidence-based programmes with a good training and support system. A potentially very important role for SLTs at Tier 2 however, is to liaise with schools about the next steps for children who still have language difficulties after completion of these interventions. Tier 3 focuses on individual children with identified language difficulties, including DLD, who require individualised interventions. SLTs may provide specialist assessment services within Tier 3, establishing the individual profile of each child and planning, devising and monitoring the child's progress with an individualised intervention programme. The SLT may provide specialist intervention directly, or they may train and support a non-specialist to deliver indirect Tier 3 intervention (most often a parent, a speech and language therapy assistant or a teaching assistant). This latter situation is a hybrid between specialist and targeted as the assessment, planning and monitoring is specialist, but intervention delivery is not. See Chapter 2 of this book for in-depth discussion of the whole-systems approach.

Tier 1 /universal

Large-scale randomised control trials have shown that Tier 1 whole-class teaching using language programmes can improve aspects of language, especially vocabulary, in preschool and primary-aged children (Hagen et al., 2017; Jiang et al., 2019; Petersen Douglas et al., 2022; West et al., 2024). However, the effect sizes are usually small and there is no evidence that these programmes help children with DLD. In fact, West et al. (2024) reported that effect sizes were considerably smaller for children with identified language concerns relative to their peers in the classroom. This raises the possibility that Tier 1 programmes may inadvertently widen the gap between children with and without language difficulties. Other studies (Bleses et al., 2018) showed no effect of Tier 1 intervention on children's language skills. In addition, a meta-analysis (Markussen-Brown et al., 2017) showed that professional development for education staff had little or no effect on child outcomes. Similarly, a recent large randomised-controlled trial of an intensive professional development programme demonstrated significant improvements in teacher knowledge about child language and literacy development and instruction (Goldfeld et al., 2021), but no impact on teacher talk within the classroom (Eadie et al., 2022) nor child language and literacy outcomes (Goldfeld et al., 2022).

SLTs are typically not involved in the Tier 1 studies mentioned above. In terms of universal services delivered by SLTs, we know of no robust trials or meta-analyses demonstrating that these are effective (cf. Smith et al., 2017). However, we recognise that raising awareness and promoting inclusive practices are a vital part of an SLT's role and therefore call for urgent research on the most effective ways to do this. We also caution against exclusive delivery of SLT via universal services, given the lack of robust data concerning the effectiveness of such services and the potential widening of the gap between children with and without language difficulties.

Tier 2/targeted

Several manualised intervention programmes focused on language are now available for schools to use at Tier 2. Many of these programmes are supported by randomised control trials demonstrating that they can improve the expressive language, narrative and vocabulary of school-aged children with low language proficiency (Hagen et al., 2017; Joffe et al., 2019; West et al., 2021; Gillam et al., 2022; Petersen Douglas et al., 2022) when delivered with fidelity by well-trained and regularly supported education staff, and especially when language outcomes are explicitly taught within the intervention (Rogde et al., 2019). However, the programmes with the most robust evidence require significant commitment from school staff. For example, the Nuffield Early Language Intervention (NELI) programme requires 30 intervention hours in small groups and 10 individual sessions per child. Many schools struggle to comply with these levels of input, offering <50% of intended therapy sessions (Dimova et al., 2020; Disley, 2024). Increased compliance leads to better language outcomes (Dimova et al., 2020) while low levels of provision were not effective (Smith et al., 2023). Very few of the above studies involved SLTs or discuss what happens to children when they have completed the NELI.

Tier 3/specialist

Tier 3 interventions are for children with identified language and communication needs, including DLD, and are individually tailored to those needs. This requires a detailed, specialist assessment process that identifies individual intervention targets, and regular monitoring of a child's progress so that the programme may be adapted as the child's needs change. An SLT intervention programme would ideally focus on all of the following: (1) improving the child's language skills, (2) helping the child to develop strategies to support their learning, participation and self-advocacy, and (3) working with others in the child's environment to increase their own use of strategies and accommodations that maximise the child's communication success.

We know of no trials investigating the effectiveness of teaching individualised strategies to children with DLD, or to communication partners in their environment. However, teachers, allied health professionals and parents/carers report that strategies such as providing extra time and visual support do help children with DLD (Ziegenfusz et al., 2025). While we know these accommodations are important, people with lived experience of DLD report that others struggle to use accommodations consistently (Wilmot et al., 2024). Thus, trials that focus on maintaining enhanced communication behaviours of significant others are needed.

Most studies of Tier 3 interventions consider specialist intervention provided by an SLT. In general, these tend to be small-scale studies that report positive outcomes in primary and secondary-aged children, particularly so for expressive language, at the word (Steele and Mills, 2011; Lowe et al., 2018), sentence (Ebbels, 2014; Cleave et al., 2015) and narrative (Pico et al., 2021) levels. For receptive language, there are far fewer studies, and the evidence is mixed (Tarvainen et al., 2020; 2021), though generally meta-analyses reveal smaller effect sizes for receptive versus expressive language outcomes (Donolato et al., 2023). Intervention effects also tend to be larger for bespoke outcome measures that are closely aligned with treatment content, for example, taught vocabulary, and smaller for more distal measures such as standardised tests (Donolato et al., 2023).

The vast majority of studies of Tier 3 SLT intervention involved specialist intervention delivered by an SLT. However, in clinical practice, SLTs often use a consultative model (Ebbels et al., 2019) where they train and support other non-specialists (often parents or teaching assistants) to provide indirect Tier 3 intervention. Intervention provided by a parent who has received training from an SLT can lead to improved expressive language in pre-school children (DeVeney et al., 2017; Roberts et al., 2019), especially when parents have received a high level of coaching from an SLT (Tosh et al., 2017). Very few studies have investigated the effectiveness of teaching assistants delivering intervention under the supervision of an SLT. Those that have found positive effects when intervention is delivered by an assistant employed by a research team (Boyle et al., 2009) or specialist language support service (Mecrow et al., 2010), but not when delivered by school staff (McCartney et al., 2010). Implementation quality and dosage are likely factors; fewer than expected intervention sessions were provided and staff had very little training and support during the study (McCartney et al., 2010). Similarly, Rogde et al. (2019) found interventions delivered by school staff were less effective than interventions delivered by external agents (clinicians, researchers). Implementation quality also moderated treatment effects – school staff are often under-resourced to provide traditional methods of intervention. For indirect Tier 3 intervention to be effective, the intervention provider needs to receive sufficient coaching, support, and monitoring to ensure that intervention is provided with fidelity and at the required dosage.

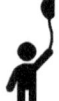

Max's story

Max is a 12-year-old boy with DLD. His speech is clear, but he speaks slowly, and it takes a long time to find the words he wants to say. He avoids situations where he might have to talk. For example, he loves swimming, but didn't go for a week when he cut his leg because he was worried about people asking him questions about it. He often doesn't understand what other people are saying but just smiles and nods so they don't know he doesn't understand. He is keen to make friends but can't keep up with conversations. When they tell jokes, he assumes they are laughing at him and storms away in anger. He says it is like 'experiencing everything on catch-up' – by the time he has figured out what they are talking about, they've moved on. School is even worse – reading is a struggle and most lessons involve complex vocabulary and sentences. Lots of information he is expected to know isn't explicitly stated and many words and phrases mean more than one thing. Yesterday, in science, was a typical example. The topic was 'The Greenhouse Effect' and even though he was listening carefully, Max was still confused. When he asked 'Sir, where is the *green* house?', everyone laughed, and the teacher accused him of messing around. Max feels stupid and is certain other students think he's stupid. His mum is worried that he is becoming isolated and took him to see a psychologist, but she had never heard of DLD before. Max finds it particularly difficult to explain how he feels. His mum asked the school for additional help from the speech and language therapist. Together they agreed ways to support communication, for example, using visuals, not cold calling Max to answer questions in class, and summarising key lesson concepts in bullet points. A period of intervention was offered that focused on developing understanding of figurative expressions for emotion and including causal connectives in short narratives ('I'm over the moon because I smashed my exam!'). The SLT included regular communication with Max's family and school staff so they could reinforce what he was learning in therapy.

Summary

Developmental language disorder (DLD) is a common and usually life-long condition that impacts every aspect of a young person's life. Speech and language therapy plays a vital role in upskilling young people in the language they need to communicate successfully with family, peers, and in formal situations, such as school or work. Diagnosis is paramount because it provides an opportunity for young people to understand and advocate for themselves. Assessment should highlight both communication strengths and challenges in order to inform a tailored and individualised approach to intervention.

Most services now operate a multi-tiered system of support, though resource limitations have shifted focus to more universal forms of provision. Universal provision is important and should enhance language skills for all children, but the current evidence base suggests that whole class instruction and explicit teacher education programmes have limited impact on the language skills of children with DLD and may in fact widen the gap between those with and without DLD.

Targeted and specialist short-term interventions can improve specific aspects of language but rarely have long-term impacts. Planning for regular periods of intervention, particularly around points of transition, can give young people the language they need for specific purposes, increase tools and strategies for self-advocacy, attenuate the potential negative impacts of DLD, and enable young people to thrive as they become adults.

Recommended resources

RADLD – Raising Awareness of Developmental Language Disorder – RADLD and RADLD - YouTube. Available at: https://www.youtube.com/RADLD

Raising Awareness of Developmental Language Disorder. Available at: https://radld.org/

References

Adlof, S.M. and Hogan, T.P., 2019. If we don't look, we won't see: measuring language development to inform literacy instruction. *Policy Insights from the Behavioral and Brain Sciences*, 6, 210-217. https://doi.org/10.1177/2372732219839075

American Psychiatric Association, 2022. *Diagnostic and Statistical Manual of Mental Disorders*, DSM-5-TR. edn. Washington, DC: American Psychiatric Association Publishing. https://doi.org/10.1176/appi.books.9780890425787

Bailey, D.H., Duncan, G.J., Cunha, F., Foorman, B.R. and Yeager, D.S., 2020. Persistence and fade-out of educational-intervention effects: mechanisms and potential solutions. *Psychological Science in the Public Interest*, 21, 55-97. https://doi.org/10.1177/1529100620915848

Bao, X., Komesidou, R. and Hogan, T.P., 2024. A review of screeners to identify risk of developmental language disorder. *American Journal of Speech-Language Pathology*, 33, 1548-1571. https://doi.org/10.1044/2023_AJSLP-23-00286

Bishop, D.V.M., 2003. *The Children's Communication Checklist*, 2nd edn. London: The Psychological Corporation,

Bishop, D.V.M., 2010. Which neurodevelopmental disorders get researched and why? *PLoS ONE* 5, e15112. https://doi.org/10.1371/journal.pone.0015112

Bishop D. V. M. (2017). Why is it so hard to reach agreement on terminology? The case of developmental language disorder (DLD). *International Journal of Language & Communication Disorders*, 52(6), 671-680. https://doi.org/10.1111/1460-6984.12335

Bishop, D.V.M., Snowling, M.J., Thompson, P.A. Greenhalgh, T., 2017. Phase 2 of CATALISE: A multinational and multidisciplinary Delphi consensus study of problems with language development: terminology. *Journal of Child Psychology and Psychiatry*, 58, 1068-1080. https://doi.org/10.1111/jcpp.12721

Bishop, D.V.M., Snowling, M.J., Thompson, P.A., Greenhalgh, T. and Consortium, 2016. CATALISE: A multinational and multidisciplinary Delphi consensus study: Identifying language impairments in children. *PLoS ONE* 11, e0158753. https://doi.org/10.1371/journal.pone.0158753

Bleses, D., Højen, A., Justice, L.M., Dale, P.S., Dybdal, L., Piasta, S.B., Markussen-Brown, J., Clausen, M. and Haghish, E.F., 2018. The effectiveness of a large-scale language and preliteracy intervention: The spell randomized controlled trial in Denmark. *Child Development*, 89, e342-e363. https://doi.org/10.1111/cdev.12859

Bornstein, M.H., Hahn, C.-S., Putnick, D.L. and Pearson, R.M., 2018. Stability of core language skill from infancy to adolescence in typical and atypical development. *Science Advances*, 4, eaat7422. https://doi.org/10.1126/sciadv.aat7422

Boyle, J.M., McCartney, E., O'Hare, A. and Forbes, J., 2009. Direct versus indirect and individual versus group modes of language therapy for children with primary language impairment: principal outcomes from a randomized controlled trial and economic evaluation. *International Journal of Language and Communication Disorders*, 44, 826-846. https://doi.org/10.1080/13682820802371848

Calder, S.D., Brennan-Jones, C.G., Robinson, M., Whitehouse, A. and Hill, E., 2022. The prevalence of and potential risk factors for Developmental Language Disorder at 10 years in the Raine Study. *Journal of Paediatrics and Child Health*, 58, 2044-2050. https://doi.org/10.1111/jpc.16149

Castilla-Earls, A., Bedore, L., Rojas, R., Fabiano-Smith, L., Pruitt-Lord, S., Restrepo, M. A. and Peña, E. 2020. Beyond scores: Using converging evidence to determine speech and language services eligibility for dual language learners. *American Journal of Speech-Language Pathology*, 29, 1116-1132. https://doi.org/10.1044/2020_AJSLP-19-00179

Cleave, P.L., Becker, S.D., Curran, M.K., Van Horne, A.J.O. and Fey, M.E., 2015. The efficacy of recasts in language intervention: A systematic review and meta-analysis. *American Journal of Speech-Language Pathology*, 24, 237-255. https://doi.org/10.1044/2015_AJSLP-14-0105

Clegg, J., Crawford, E., Spencer, S. and Matthews, D., 2021. Developmental Language Disorder (DLD) in young people leaving care in England: A study profiling the language, literacy and communication abilities of young people transitioning from care to independence. *International Journal of Environmental Research and Public Health*, 18, 4107. https://doi.org/10.3390/ijerph18084107

Cohen, N.J., Farnia, F. and Im-Bolter, N., 2013. Higher order language competence and adolescent mental health. *Journal of Child Psychology and Psychiatry*, 54, 733-744. https://doi.org/10.1111/jcpp.12060

DeVeney, S.L., Hagaman, J.L. and Bjornsen, A.L., 2017. Parent-implemented versus clinician-directed interventions for late-talking toddlers: A systematic review of the literature. *Communication Disorders Quarterly*. 39, 293-302. https://doi.org/10.1177/1525740117705116

Dimova, S., Ilie, S., Brown, E.R., Broeks, M., Culora, A. and Sutherland, A., 2020. *The Nuffield Early Language Intervention: Evaluation Report*. London: Education Endowment Foundation.

Disley, E., 2024. *The Nuffield Early Language Intervention Scale-Up*. London: Education Endowment Foundation.

Donolato, E., Toffalini, E., Rogde, K., Nordahl-Hansen, A., Lervåg, A., Norbury, C. and Melby-Lervåg, M., 2023. Oral language interventions can improve language outcomes in children with neurodevelopmental disorders: A systematic review and meta-analysis. *Campbell Systematic Reviews*, 19, e1368. https://doi.org/10.1002/cl2.1368

Eadie, P., Stark, H., Snow, P., Gold, L., Watts, A., Shingles, B., Orsini, F., Connell, J. and Goldfeld, S., 2022. Teacher talk in early years classrooms following an oral language and literacy professional learning program. *Journal of Research on Educational Effectiveness*, 15, 302–329. https://doi.org/10.1080/19345747.2021.1998938

Ebbels, S., 2014. Effectiveness of intervention for grammar in school-aged children with primary language impairments: A review of the evidence. *Child Language Teaching and Therapy*, 30, 7–40. https://doi.org/10.1177/0265659013512321

Ebbels, S.H., McCartney, E., Slonims, V., Dockrell, J.E., Norbury, C.F., 2019. Evidence-based pathways to intervention for children with language disorders. *International Journal of Language and Communication Disorders*, 54, 3–19. https://doi.org/10.1111/1460-6984.12387

Flapper, B.C.T. and Schoemaker, M.M., 2013. Developmental Coordination Disorder in children with specific language impairment: Co-morbidity and impact on quality of life. *Research in Developmental Disabilities*, 34, 756–763. https://doi.org/10.1016/j.ridd.2012.10.014

Fuchs, D. and Fuchs, L.M., 2006. Introduction to response to intervention: what, why, and how valid is it? *Reading Research Quarterly*, 41, 93–99.

Gillam, S.L., Vaughn, S., Roberts, G., Capin, P., Fall, A.-M., Israelsen-Augenstein, M., Holbrook, S., Wada, R., Hancock, A., Fox, C., Dille, J., Magimairaj, B.M. and Gillam, R.B., 2022. Improving oral and written narration and reading comprehension of children at-risk for language and literacy difficulties: Results of a randomized clinical trial. *Journal of Educational Psychology*, https://doi.org/10.1037/edu0000766

Goldfeld, S., Snow, P., Eadie, P., Munro, J., Gold, L., Le, H.N.D., Orsini, F., Shingles, B., Connell, J., Watts, A. and Barnett, T., 2022. Classroom promotion of oral language: outcomes from a randomized controlled trial of a whole-of-classroom intervention to improve children's reading achievement. *AERA Open*, 8, 23328584221131530. https://doi.org/10.1177/23328584221131530

Goldfeld, S., Snow, P., Eadie, P., Munro, J., Gold, L., Orsini, F., Connell, J., Stark, H., Watts, A. and Shingles, B., 2021. Teacher knowledge of oral language and literacy constructs: results of a randomized controlled trial evaluating the effectiveness of a professional learning intervention. *Scientific Studies of Reading*, 25, 1–30. https://doi.org/10.1080/10888438.2020.1714629

Hagen, Å.M., Melby-Lervåg, M. and Lervåg, A., 2017. Improving language comprehension in preschool children with language difficulties: A cluster randomized trial. *Journal of Child Psychology and Psychiatry*, 58, 1132–1140. https://doi.org/10.1111/jcpp.12762

Harvey, H., 2023. Diagnostic procedures of paediatric speech and language therapists in the UK: Enabling and obstructive factors. *International Journal of Language and Communication Disorders*, 58, 1454–1467. https://doi.org/10.1111/1460-6984.12871

Jiang, H., Logan, J., and Language and Reading Research Consortium (LARRC), 2019. Improving reading comprehension in the primary grades: mediated effects of a language-focused classroom intervention. *Journal of Speech, Language and Hearing Research*, 62, 2812–2828. https://doi.org/10.1044/2019_JSLHR-L-19-0015

Joffe, V.L., Rixon, L. and Hulme, C., 2019. Improving storytelling and vocabulary in secondary school students with language disorder: A randomized controlled trial. *International Journal of Language and Communication Disorders*, 54, 656–672. https://doi.org/10.1111/1460-6984.12471

Lowe, H., Henry, L., Müller, L. and Joffe, V.L., 2018. Vocabulary intervention for adolescents with language disorder: A systematic review. *International Journal of Language and Communication Disorders*, 53, 199–217. https://doi.org/10.1111/1460-6984.12355

Markussen-Brown, J., Juhl, C.B., Piasta, S.B., Bleses, D., Højen, A. and Justice, L.M., 2017. The effects of language- and literacy-focused professional development on early educators and children: A best-evidence meta-analysis. *Early Child Research Quarterly*, 38, 97–115. https://doi.org/10.1016/j.ecresq.2016.07.002

McCartney, E., Boyle, J., Ellis, S., Bannatyne, S. and Turnbull, M., 2010. Indirect language therapy for children with persistent language impairment in mainstream primary schools: outcomes from a cohort intervention. *International Journal of Language and Communication Disorders*, 100824014249025. https://doi.org/10.3109/13682820903560302

McGregor, K.K., 2020. How we fail children with developmental language disorder. *Language, Speech and Hearing Services in Schools*, 51, 981–992. https://doi.org/10.1044/2020_LSHSS-20-00003

Mecrow, C., Beckwith, J. and Klee, T., 2010. An exploratory trial of the effectiveness of an enhanced consultative approach to delivering speech and language intervention in schools. *International Journal of Language and Communication Disorders*, 45, 354–367. https://doi.org/10.3109/13682820903040268

Mountford, H.S., Braden, R., Newbury, D.F. and Morgan, A.T., 2022. The genetic and molecular basis of developmental language disorder: A review. *Children*, 9, 586. https://doi.org/10.3390/children9050586

NHS Digital, 2018. *Mental Health of Children and Young People in England, 2017*. Available at: https://digital.nhs.uk/data-and-information/publications/statistical/mental-health-of-children-and-young-people-in-england/2017/2017

Norbury, C., Gooch, D., Wray, C., Baird, G., Charman, T., Simonoff, E., Vamvakas, G. and Pickles, A., 2016. The impact of nonverbal ability on prevalence and clinical presentation of language disorder: evidence from a population study. *Journal of Child Psychology and Psychiatry*, 57, 1247–1257. https://doi.org/10.1111/jcpp.12573

Norbury, C., Griffiths, S., Vamvakas, G., Baird, G., Charman, T., Simonoff, E. and Pickles, A., 2021. Socioeconomic disadvantage is associated with prevalence of developmental language disorders, but not rate of language or literacy growth in children from 4 to 11 years: Evidence from the Surrey Communication and Language in Education Study (SCALES). Available at SSRN: https://ssrn.com/abstract=3814832 or http://dx.doi.org/10.2139/ssrn.3814832

Petersen Douglas, B., Staskowski, M., Spencer, T.D., Foster, M.E. and Brough, M.P. 2022. The effects of a multitiered system of language support on kindergarten oral and written language: a large-scale randomized controlled trial. *Language, Speech and Hearing Services in Schools*, 53, 44–68. https://doi.org/10.1044/2021_LSHSS-20-00162

Pico, D.L., Hessling Prahl, A., Biel, C.H., Peterson, A.K., Biel, E.J., Woods, C. and Contesse, V.A., 2021. Interventions designed to improve narrative language in school-age children: a systematic review with meta-analyses. *Language, Speech and Hearing Services in Schools*, 52, 1109–1126. https://doi.org/10.1044/2021_LSHSS-20-00160

Roberts, M.Y., Curtis, P.R., Sone, B.J. and Hampton, L.H., 2019. Association of parent training with child language development: a systematic review and meta-analysis. *JAMA Pediatrics*, 173, 671. https://doi.org/10.1001/jamapediatrics.2019.1197

Rogde, K., Hagen, Å.M., Melby-Lervåg, M. and Lervåg, A., 2019. The effect of linguistic comprehension instruction on generalized language and reading comprehension skills: A systematic review. *Campbell Systematic Reviews*, 15, e1059. https://doi.org/10.1002/cl2.1059

Saul, J., Griffiths, S. and Norbury, C.F., 2023. Prevalence and functional impact of social (pragmatic) communication disorders. *Journal of Child Psychology and Psychiatry*, 64, 376–387. https://doi.org/10.1111/jcpp.13705

Smith, A., Staunton, R., Sahasranaman, A. and Worth, J., 2023. *Impact Evaluation of Nuffield Early Language Intervention (NELI) Wave Two*. Education Endowment Foundation, London.

Smith, C., Williams, E. and Bryan, K., 2017. A systematic scoping review of speech and language therapists' public health practice for early language development: Systematic scoping review of SLT public health. *International Journal of Language and Communication Disorders*, 52, 407–425. https://doi.org/10.1111/1460-6984.12299

Snow, P.C., 2021. SOLAR: The science of language and reading. *Child Language Teaching and Therapy*, 37, 222–233. https://doi.org/10.1177/0265659020947817

Snowling, M.J., Hayiou-Thomas, M.E., Nash, H.M. and Hulme, C., 2020. Dyslexia and Developmental Language Disorder: comorbid disorders with distinct effects on reading comprehension. *Journal of Child Psychology and Psychiatry*, 61, 672–680. https://doi.org/10.1111/jcpp.13140

Steele, S.C. and Mills, M.T., 2011. Vocabulary intervention for school-age children with language impairment: A review of evidence and good practice. *Child Language Teaching and Therapy*, 27, 354–370. https://doi.org/10.1177/0265659011412247

Tarvainen, S., Launonen, K. and Stolt, S., 2021. Oral language comprehension interventions in school-age children and adolescents with developmental language disorder: A systematic scoping review. *Autism and Developmental Language Impairments*, 6, 23969415211010423. https://doi.org/10.1177/23969415211010423

Tarvainen, S., Stolt, S. and Launonen, K., 2020. Oral language comprehension interventions in 1–8-year-old children with language disorders or difficulties: A systematic scoping review. *Autism and Developmental Language Impairments*, 5, 2396941520946999. https://doi.org/10.1177/2396941520946999

Tomblin, J.B., 2006. A normativist account of language-based learning disability1,2. Learning *Disabilities Research & Practice*, 21, 8–18. https://doi.org/10.1111/j.1540-5826.2006.00203.x

Tosh, R., Arnott, W. and Scarinci, N., 2017. Parent-implemented home therapy programmes for speech and language: a systematic review: Home programmes for speech and language: a review. *International Journal of Language and Communication Disorders*, 52, 253–269. https://doi.org/10.1111/1460-6984.12280

Ullman, M.T., Clark, G.M., Pullman, M.Y., Lovelett, J.T., Pierpont, E.I., Jiang, X. and Turkeltaub, P.E., 2024. The neuroanatomy of developmental language disorder: a systematic review and meta-analysis. *Nature: Human Behaviour*, 8, 962–975. https://doi.org/10.1038/s41562-024-01843-6

West, G., Lervåg, A., Birchenough, J.M.H., Korell, C., Rios Diaz, M., Duta, M., Cripps, D., Gardner, R., Fairhurst, C. and Hulme, C., 2024. Oral language enrichment in preschool improves children's language skills: A cluster randomised controlled trial. *Journal of Child Psychology and Psychiatry*, 65, 1087–1097. https://doi.org/10.1111/jcpp.13947

West, G., Snowling, M.J., Lervåg, A., Buchanan-Worster, E., Duta, M., Hall, A., McLachlan, H. and Hulme, C., 2021. Early language screening and intervention can be delivered successfully at scale: Evidence from a cluster randomized controlled trial. *Journal of Child Psychology and Psychiatry*, 62, 1425–1434. https://doi.org/10.1111/jcpp.13415

Wilmot, A., Boyes, M., Sievers, R., Leitão, S. and Norbury, C., 2024. Impact of developmental language disorders on mental health and well-being across the lifespan: A qualitative study including the perspectives of UK adults with DLD and Australian speech-language therapists. *BMJ Open*, 14, e087532. https://doi.org/10.1136/bmjopen-2024-087532

World Health Organization, 2019. *International Statistical Classification of Diseases and Related Health Problems*, 11th edn. Geneva: WHO.

Wu, S., Zhao, J., De Villiers, J., Liu, X.L., Rolfhus, E., Sun, X., Li, X., Pan, H., Wang, H., Zhu, Q., Dong, Y., Zhang, Y. and Jiang, F., 2023. Prevalence, co-occurring difficulties, and risk factors of developmental language disorder: first evidence for Mandarin-speaking children in a population-based study. *Lancet Regional Health - Western Pacific*, 34, 100713. https://doi.org/10.1016/j.lanwpc.2023.100713

Yew, S.G.K. and O'Kearney, R., 2013. Emotional and behavioural outcomes later in childhood and adolescence for children with specific language impairments: meta-analyses of controlled prospective studies: SLI and emotional and behavioural disorders. *Journal of Child Psychology and Psychiatry*, 54, 516–524. https://doi.org/10.1111/jcpp.12009

Youth Justice Board, Ministry of Justice, 2021. Assessing the needs of sentenced children in the youth justice system 2019/20. Available at: https://assets.publishing.service.gov.uk/media/604a3ee28fa8f540179c6ab7/experimental-statistics-assessing-needs-sentenced-children-youth-justice-system-2019-20.pdf

Ziegenfusz, S., Westerveld, M.F., Fluckiger, B. and Paynter, J., 2025. Stakeholder perspectives on educational needs and supports for students with developmental language disorder. *International Journal of Language and Communication Disorders*, 60, e13134. https://doi.org/10.1111/1460-6984.13134

PART IV

Communication

11 Severe and profound learning disabilities
A school-based approach

Rachel Sawford and Ann Miles

What you'll learn in this chapter

- The meaning of the diagnostic terms Severe Learning Disabilities (SLD) and Profound and Multiple Learning Disabilities (PMLD)
- How to best support children with the primary diagnosis of SLD and PMLD through the Communication at the Heart of the School (CATHS) approach
- The importance of attunement
- True partnership
- How CATHS works in practice.

Key information about severe and profound learning disabilities

This chapter discusses working with children who have a primary diagnosis of SLD and PMLD. We will discuss the challenges with supporting this particular client group. These challenges will be addressed through the CATHS approach. CATHS provides an assessment and guidance on interventions as well as suggesting an effective service delivery model.

Children with SLD and PMLD have significant cognitive impairments. They are likely to have difficulties with short-term memory, creating a mental picture, imagination, curiosity and the ability to generalise and transfer skills. Many children may also have one or more additional barriers to learning such as attachment disorders, trauma disorders, autism, sensory impairments and physical disabilities. The majority will have lifelong communication needs. This makes for a complex picture.

According to the most recent government figures (Department for Health and Social Care, 2020), the prevalence of children in England aged between 5 and 15 years with learning disabilities is:

- 29,492 children identified as having Severe Learning Difficulties
- 10,032 children identified as having Profound and Multiple Learning Difficulties.

The same government figures also show that 12% of children with a primary Special Educational Need (SEN) of SLD and 15% of children with a primary SEN need of PMLD are educated in a mainstream school. Most children will be in special educational settings. Some

DOI: 10.4324/9781003671626-16

may be educated at home or have significant medical needs which take priority. Speech and Language Therapists (SLTs) need to be prepared to support children in a variety of different environments.

Terminology

Using the term 'developmental age' can help everyone to understand the level at which the child is engaging with the world. For example, a child can be described as at the '18-month level'. However, there are difficulties in using this terminology: children with significant cognitive impairment and additional barriers to learning may be communicating and playing in the same way as a neurotypical 18-month-old but they are not learning in the same way. For example, they tend not to explore new things or try out new ideas. CATHS uses the term 'developmental age' as a quick and easy way of recognising the level of language and engagement of children while acknowledging this is not a true description of the child's functioning. The CATHS approach is for children with a developmental age of between birth and 4-5 years.

The CATHS approach: principles, structure and underpinning framework

The main principles of CATHS are:

- Language is intertwined with cognitive development.
- Language is used for different purposes or functions.
- We recognise the value of communication for the sake of social interaction, where meaning is less important. Sometimes called small talk, phatic communication establishes a social bond and is, perhaps, the most important form of communication, especially for those with language difficulties.

CATHS is a complete approach to working with children with SLD and PMLD. It is inclusive of other language programmes and gives guidance when other programmes will add value. CATHS consists of:

- the Communication and Cognitive Framework;
- an assessment leading to a Future Plan;
- a Service Delivery Model: Pathway and Intervention Packages;
- guidance for communication-rich classrooms.

The Communication and Cognitive Framework

The Communication and Cognitive Framework underpins CATHS and provides a common language and approach for both education staff and SLTs to work in partnership (Figure 11.1). In the framework, communication and cognitive development is broken down into six broad categories across four developmental bands, spanning from 0 months to 4½ years.

Communication functions

Communication functions refer to the jobs that we want our communications to do for us. As children develop, the demands placed on their communication become more complex. For example, at an early developmental level, children *share information* by showing something important to them, e.g., a stone they have found, but as they develop understanding and language, children want to *describe* in lots of detail something important to them, e.g., a favourite TV programme. The key communicative functions at each band are listed on the framework and this is the foundation of the CATHS Communication Assessment.

Mode

The Mode refers to the way children communicate. At the earliest developmental levels, the mode is informal, making use of body language, vocalisations, gestures and facial expression. As the child develops, their mode becomes more formal, using speech and the written word.

Communication Functions	Mode of Communication	Cognitive Learning (How children learn)	Classroom Interventions	Good Practice
BAND 1 PRE-INTENTIONAL (Birth–3 months)				
UNDERSTANDING Turn towards a soothing tone of voice.	Communication partners assign meaning to behaviours such as crying, stilling, increasing activity.	Engagement is through sensory experiences.	Intensive Interaction. Affective Communication Assessment.	Ensure the child is at the centre of the social environment. Regular undivided interaction from an adult.
BAND 1 EMERGING INTENTIONAL (3–5 months)				
UNDERSTANDING Show recognition of familiar people or activities. EXPRESSION Communication partners interpret the child's behaviours. *Likes, Dislikes, Wants, Rejects, Distinguishes between the familiar and the unfamiliar.*	Communication partners assign meaning to behaviours such as crying, stilling, increasing activity, smiling and vocalising.	Most engagement is through sensory experiences. Offer one stimulus at a time (person or object or activity).	Intensive interaction. Environmental support to develop consistent sensory cues including songs and movement cues. Affective Communication Assessment.	Regular individual interaction from an adult. Observe and interpret patterns of responses. Sensory cues to important events or activities.
BAND 1 INTENTIONAL (5–9 months)				
UNDERSTANDING Understands signifiers such as objects of reference, songs or familiar routines. EXPRESSION *Draws attention, Requests, Greetings, Protests and rejects, Gives information, Responds (Leading to Yes and No).*	Children may express themselves through vocalising, looking, facial expression, reaching and other gestures.	People and object play is integrated (see explanation of columns). Causal understanding (cause and effect) develops. People and object permanence develops.	Intensive interaction. Early signing. Objects of reference. Affective Communication Assessment.	Regular individual interaction from an adult. Communication partners respond to all attempts to communicate. Develop routines where consistent language is used and offer consistent cues such as songs to key activities.

Figure 11.1 The Communication and Cognitive Framework
Source: Sawford and Miles (2021).

BAND 2 (9–18 months)				
UNDERSTANDING Understands signifiers such as objects of reference, signs and key words. EXPRESSION Greets, Existence/Shared Attention, Disappearance, Recurrence, Possession, Rejection, Non-Existence, Location, Action, Agent, Object, Attribute.	Expression frequently consists of a combination of methods such as gesture, reaching, leading, vocalising and using objects, signing and/or words.	Learning takes place through the child's own physical activity. Combines objects in play. Sorts objects in play using their own criteria. Simple one element pretend play.	Intensive Interaction. Signing. Photos leading to concrete symbols presented in a variety of ways.	Create an environment to facilitate independent play where the adult can join the child in their choice of activity. Create situations where the child is motivated to use language to activate. Look for opportunities to model the first words (sign and spoken word).
BAND 3 (18 months–3 years)				
UNDERSTANDING 1–3 key words in each phrase. EXPRESSION Conversation skills, Requests, Gives information, Directs, Describes Questions, Repairs misunderstandings. (persists with communication intent)	Uses words, signs and symbols in short sentences and phrases, e.g.: 'Mummy go work' May continue to use several modes of expression in the same phrase.	Relates only to the present (very little concept of the past or future). Sequences ideas in play. Develops understanding of basic concepts of size, colour, numbers and position.	Intensive Interaction. Signing. Special Time. Symbols presented in a variety of ways, e.g. through communication books and/or Voice Output Communication Aids (VOCA).	Provide a variety of play environments, real life experiences and books to extend vocabulary. Model language one step ahead of the child. Model how to ask questions.
BAND 4 (3 + years)				
UNDERSTANDING Understands abstract ideas and language out of context e.g. past and future. EXPRESSION Gives and Shares Information, Describes, Questions, Reasons and Predicts, Plans and Evaluates.	Uses complex sentences containing joining words such as 'and', 'because'.	Language is used for learning e.g. to plan and evaluate activities, negotiate, predict what may happen, question to find out information. Begins to use early number and reading skills.	Signing. Special Time. Access to both high and low tech Augmentative and Alternative Communication which should be aiming to use written words. Access to early literacy schemes.	The role of the communication partner is as an active listener who shares ideas, clarifies meanings and explains. Asks cognitively challenging questions.

Figure 11.1 (Continued)

This is a typical developmental pattern. This column also includes advice when alternative, augmentative modes may be appropriately introduced. Modes such as sign, symbols or voice output devices have been found to be essential for children who find it hard to use speech (see Chapter 4).

Cognition

Children use language to express ideas they already understand, so in simple terms, the child needs to experience and understand the concept of 'big' before they can give the concept the word label.

Severe and profound learning disabilities 157

Progression in learning cannot happen without sufficient language skills to ask questions, to check misunderstandings, or to use abstract words. Concepts such as the past and future cannot be discussed without knowledge of words such as 'tomorrow'. For example, in the classroom, many children cannot progress in maths once they are beyond the initial stages of practical activities because their language skills do not include the words to understand and use abstract ideas, such as multiplication.

An understanding of cognitive development informs us about learning at different developmental levels. For example, at the earliest levels children can focus on either an object or a person; they cannot integrate the two things. Knowing how children learn means communication learning experiences can be pitched at the correct level.

Cognitive and communication skills can develop at different paces. While it is not unusual among children with SLD and PMLD that communication skills appear at a lower level than practical abilities, an extreme gap between them would require extra assessment. There are two common reasons for this mismatch:

- A child's physical disabilities may mean the child is unable to access speech. The child may be able to understand significantly more than they can express. In this case, alternative means of communication need to be considered.
- Some children show splinter skills in practical activities, such as reciting the alphabet, however, without a firm foundation of language development, including abstract concepts, further learning is impacted.

Classroom interventions

This column in Figure 11.1 lists compatible approaches and interventions that are needed to create communication-rich classrooms. These are the most appropriate and effective additional interventions for each developmental level. SLTs can ensure classroom staff have the correct skills to support the children in their class.

Good practice

This column in Figure 11.1 provides a quick checklist of essential strategies to be used by classroom staff.

Understanding children's needs in CATHS

CATHS assessment

Good practice starts with a good quality assessment. Children diagnosed with SLD and PMLD with complexities do not fit easily into many standard assessments. Therefore, the assessment must be flexible, and as individual as the children themselves.

The CATHS assessment is *narrative*; the assessor is asked to observe the child's behaviours and then categorise that information under the language functions at the appropriate developmental band (see Figure 11.2). It assesses understanding, language functions and cognitive development. The assessment is formative and leads to a plan of where to go next.

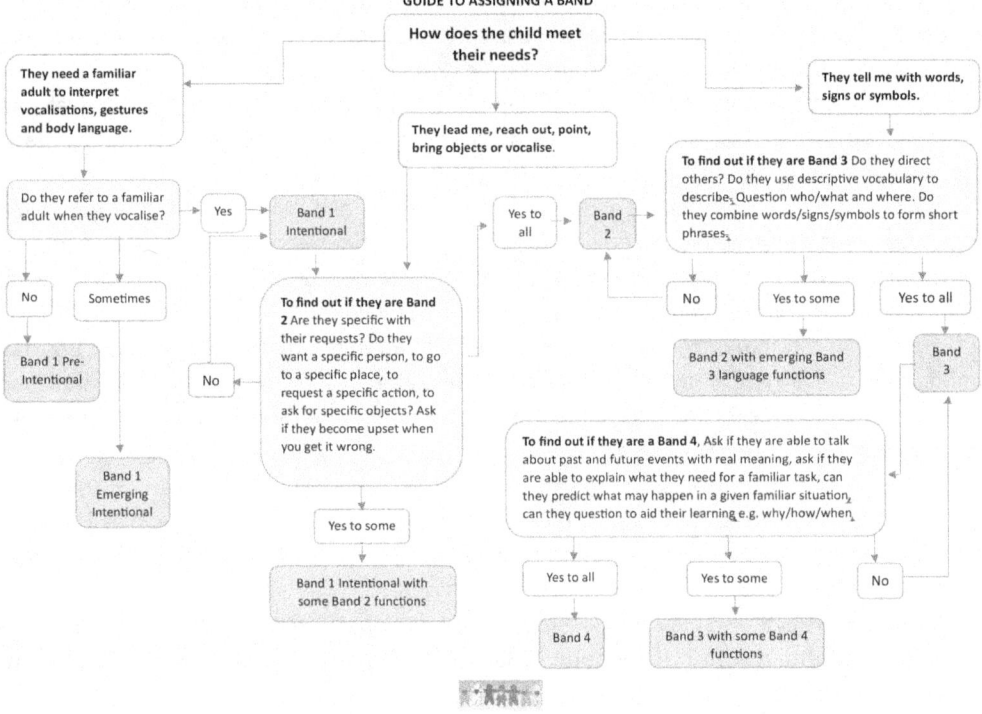

Figure 11.2 Guide to assigning a band

The Future Plan

The Future Plan contains everything which is necessary to support the child's communication. It includes:

- 'What Works Well'
- Approaches to Communication Development
- Moving Forward
- Education, Health and Care Plan objective
- Speech and Language Therapy Provision.

This is the document which guides classroom practice and therapy input. It is shared as a report.

The complexity of the learning disabilities means that communication skills can take a long time to develop. Initially, the child may use the new skill on one or two occasions with familiar adults. As they become more confident, the skill appears in more situations and with a greater range of people. Only then can it be said that it is truly established. In the early stages, this fragile skill can be lost if the circumstances change or if the child no longer has a use for it. Continuing successful strategies will give the child more opportunities to consolidate their successful communications: 'If it works, keep doing it.' This is recorded in the 'What Works Well' section of the Future Plan.

SLTs are often required to identify 'targets' for children to achieve within a time limit. This is challenging with a group of children whose learning needs are complex, significant and unpredictable. Their progress is dependent on numerous factors including health, attunement and environment. However, we can identify a general direction of what would be progress for a particular child. This may mean looking at gaps in the assessment profile or where skills are newly acquired. Other targets may mean looking at consolidating newly learnt skills. These goals focus on lateral progress.

Sawford and Miles (2021, p. 16) describe lateral progress in several ways:

- Increasing the frequency with which the skill is used.
- Extending the range of situations and people in which they can use the skill.
- A tendency to be more spontaneous in the use of the skill.
- A feeling of increased competence and maturity that those who know the child well will be able to describe. To validate these subjective 'feelings', it is important to be objective through moderation, discussions with others and careful observations of the child in a range of contexts.

Supporting children's needs with CATHS

Service delivery model

The most common SLT service delivery model is a care package which involves an initial assessment from which an intervention plan is created. This is usually a set number of sessions (6-8) where the therapist works directly with the child, focusing on a specific skill. The package is completed by a review or discharge.

CATHS recognises that this group of children needs an approach to Speech and Language Therapy that is at odds with this time-limited medical model of care packages. The complex nature of children with co-existing conditions alongside their cognitive impairment means they will have lifelong communication needs.

A service delivery model that supports children with lifelong learning needs is about enhancing the communication environment, so the children learn and practise the skills needed in daily life, all day, every day. This involves empowering others to be able to offer continuing support.

Working in partnership

SLTs cannot work in isolation; many children with SLD and PMLD will have contact with a range of professionals. These may include:

- education staff
- Allied Health Professionals (AHPs)
- specialist advisory teachers
- educational psychologists
- medical practitioners
- social care professionals, and
- Child and Adolescent Mental Health Services (CAMHS).

Communication at the earliest level involves attunement; being able to recognise, interpret and respond to the child's behaviours and communications. Sometimes a child's communication can be very subtle and only those who know the child well notice. Attunement comes from frequently engaging with the child. The work of the Intensive Interaction Institute provides guidance in the development of attunement skills for staff (Nind and Hewett, 2006).

Family members and school staff are the people who can develop attuned relationships with the child. It is with these groups that the SLT must work most closely.

Working with families

Families are a crucial part of the assessment process. They will be forming and adapting communication strategies continually at home, whether they are doing this consciously or not. The lead assessor's job is to tease out and identify what these strategies are and why they work.

Families contribute to the CATHS assessment in the following ways:

- Taking part in the assessment meeting, through contributing examples of their child's communication in the home.
- Helping to formulate the Future Plan.
- Informing the professionals about what is reasonable and practical at home.
- Engaging with the process through regular sharing of information from a home perspective (Sawford and Miles, 2021).

It is typical for children to present differently in different environments. Understanding this means a higher quality plan can be put in place. For example, if a child is communicating a function at home that they are not in school, this can guide the school's work with the child.

Working within the education system

Children need to learn communication skills in the environment in which they will use them. School is where children spend much of their day and it plays an important part in their social life. It is also the place where the teachers and support staff know the child well and have frequently built attuned relationships.

A communication-rich classroom is one where children are interested and engaged. Understanding the child's cognitive level and individual learning preferences can guide activity planning which both appeals and can be used to extend learning. When children are engaged, they are learning in many different ways, including reinforcing previous knowledge, exploring new ideas and extending previously learnt skills. SLTs and education staff use the Communication and Cognitive Framework to develop a communication-rich classroom.

The first step in developing a partnership is to carry out joint assessments of the children. The classroom staff contribute examples to the assessment which becomes a shared document. Creating the Future Planning page together means that both parties will be invested in its success and will work to create a communication rich environment. It is important that communication goals, strategies and interventions are functional for the child and are embedded into the child's environment. This means the SLT working directly in the classroom.

Severe and profound learning disabilities 161

These are the roles of the therapist when working alongside school staff in the classroom:

- Getting to know the children's learning preferences and interests.
- Trialling new strategies and sharing the results with class staff.
- Modelling successful strategies.
- Working with staff to make changes which enhance the communication opportunities in the classroom.
- Noting any staff training needs.
- Making written observations of children's communications and sharing these with class staff.

Communication-rich classrooms

The CATHS model of service delivery recommends creating communication-rich classrooms through embedding best communication practice within the environment. By doing this, the SLTs are:

- supporting all the children in the classroom;
- ensuring goals, interventions and strategies are more meaningful and realistic;
- ensuring opportunities for rehearsal are frequent and purposeful;
- ensuring strategies are more easily generalised to everyday life;
- working with those who know the child best;
- upskilling staff to support numerous children; and
- identifying those who need more targeted/specialist therapeutic work.

Asad's story

I (Rachel, SLT) first had contact with Asad when he was 8 years old. He had recently moved to the area with his family. Before he started the school, I made a scheduled telephone call where I explained several points.

- I work in partnership with my education colleagues.
- I will work in Asad's classroom, supporting Asad and his peers alongside his teachers; children are rarely withdrawn from class.
- The goal of therapy is to support children to effectively communicate their message.
- In the classroom I model best practice and set up opportunities for the children to practise and develop their communication skills.

I asked about Asad's interaction skills at home and started his initial communication assessment. The 'How to Assign a Band' flow diagram (Figure 11.2) helped to place Asad into a communication band. From the information Asad's mum gave me, I felt his communication was at a band 2 level.

Asad started school and I visited him in his classroom on a few occasions and made some observations. After about six weeks, when Asad had settled and built relationships with the staff, I completed his communication assessment with his teacher and his mother (Figure 11.3). Together, we made a Future Plan considering Asad's communication at

BAND TWO

NAME:	Asad
DOB:	
DATE:	
COMPLETED BY:	Ann Miles - Class Teacher Rachel Sawford - Speech and Language Therapist Asad's mother

BACKGROUND
Medical information
Learning disability. Vision corrected by glasses.

SUMMARY
Asad communicates for a range of purposes including to request a person, an action, to go to a place, to indicate he would like more of something and to indicate something that belongs to him. He uses means such as gestures, vocalisations, facial expression and is starting to use some signs and single spoken words. Asad understands familiar phrases spoken in context. He enjoys interacting with others and has formed positive relationships with familiar adults. Examples from home have been reported by Asad's mother. This is a working document that grows as Asad's communication develops.

ASSESSMENT OF COMMUNICATION SKILLS
UNDERSTANDING
Understanding of signifiers such as objects, signs and key words.
Asad is understanding language in everyday contexts and in routine. For example: • His mother said "time to put on your shoes" as his school bus arrived, Asad looked for them but returned screaming and pointing to his feet. Asad's mother found that his shoes had been left in a different place and he couldn't find them. This is also an example of non-existence. • His teacher said "sit down" while holding his wellingtons, he sat and held out his feet.
EXPRESSION
GREETS *How do they communicate "hello" and "goodbye"?*
• Asad greets his LSA with a big smile when coming off the bus. • Asad gets very excited when his Grandad visits, he shouts and leaps into his arms.
EXISTENCE/SHARED ATTENTION *How do they acknowledge an object or event exists?*
Asad demonstrates shared attention through nonverbal means.

Figure 11.3 Asad's communication assessment

	• Asad approached Mr G. excitedly looking down at his new shoes, jumping and kicking out his feet. Mr G. pointed and said "nice shoes". Asad was pleased and moved on to Mrs K. but this time he pointed to his feet.
DISAPPEARANCE *What do they do when an object or person disappears?*	
Asad has not demonstrated disappearance in school.	
RECURRENCE *How do they request more?*	
Asad indicates more by repeating the action. Occasionally he has said and signed "more". • Asad laughed as the balloon deflated, flying around the room. When it landed, he collected it bringing it back saying "more". • When we finished singing "Baby Shark", he repeated the last action. I said, "Do you want more?" He repeated "more" and signed. • When the swing stopped, Asad shook the ropes and looked at Mr G. Mr G. didn't notice so Asad yelled "more". When Mr G. turned round, Asad signed more.	
POSSESSION *Can they indicate that something belongs to them?*	
Asad indicates possession through vocalising and pulling items towards him. • During snack Asad screamed as another pupil went to take his biscuit. He frowned and snatched it back angrily vocalising. • When Asad's brother took his spiderman toy, he pulled it back and shouted, clearly complaining.	
REJECTION *How do they refuse an object or activity?*	
When Asad has been asked to finish something enjoyable, he communicates through body language, vocalisation and more recently shouting "stop" and "no." • When Mrs S encouraged Asad to join relaxation time, he swiped her hands away shouting "no". • Asad put out his hand and said "stop" loudly when L touched his cars.	
NON-EXISTENCE *How do they communicate that something is missing?*	
Asad knows where his favourite items are stored. When they are misplaced he will seek assistance from adults leading them to where he last saw them or where he believes they should be. • Asad was searching for something. He took Mrs K's hand, leading her to the cupboard. He pushed her hand onto the handle. When she opened the door he pushed her hand to the empty top shelf and angrily vocalised. • Mum said "put on your shoes", Asad looked for them, and returned shouting. Mum realised his shoes had been left outside and he couldn't find them.	
LOCATION *How do they indicate the position of people or objects?*	
Asad will indicate location through gestures.	

Figure 11.3 (Continued)

	• Asad took Grandad's hand and sat him on the chair next to him. • Asad gave Mrs K the Soft Play photo asking to go there.
ACTION *How do they comment on/request an action?*	
Asad indicates that he would like a specific action through gesture, vocalisations and signing. • The SALT joined Asad playing with the toy cars, she modelled "go" when he held a car at the top of the ramp. After a few times, Asad imitated her and said "g" before he let the car go. • Asad struggled with the little wind up toys. He shook it and shouted at me. I said/signed, "help?" He gave it to me and copied the "help" sign. • We were stomping in puddles. When I paused, he touched my legs and jumped, telling me to bounce.	
AGENT *How do they indicate a person?*	
Asad has formed relationships with familiar members of staff and indicates who he would like to engage with through vocalisations and body language. • Asad wanted to be in Mr G.'s group today. He pointed to Mr. G. and said "Gu Gu" • Asad pushed the supply member of staff away when she held out her hand to take him to Forest School. He then ran up to his teacher and took her hand. • Asad had said "Gan gan", meaning grandma for the first time.	
OBJECT *How do they label objects?*	
Asad does not label objects in school, however, at home Asad has said "bider" referring to his spiderman toy. • At his grandparents' house Asad asks to lie in their hammock by standing at their back door making a swinging motion.	
ATTRIBUTE *How do they comment on/request the property of an object?*	
Asad indicates attribute through facial expression and body language. • When a spikey leaf pricked his finger, Asad showed his finger to the adult and frowned. • When Asad got tomato puree on his hands, he wiped them on the adult next to him, frowning, showing her his hands.	
INTERACTION SKILLS *This should be based on the Fundamentals of Communication.*	
Asad enjoys interacting with familiar adults. He is aware of people and initiates interacting with others.	

Figure 11.3 (Continued)

| COGNITIVE SKILLS ||
From *Mary Sheridan's Birth to Five Years* (Sharma & Cockerill, 2014)	
Looks for fallen or hidden (in sight) objects.	Achieved
Shows causal understanding (cause and effect).	Achieved
Plays social games (e.g. peek a boo or pat a cake).	Achieved
Initiates joint attention.	Achieved
Functional use of toys (e.g. pushes cars, pretends to drink).	Asad found a plastic toy hairdryer, he put it to his head. When the adult joined in with him, he lost interest and moved on.
Early symbolic play: use of toys or dolls/others.	Asad puts spiderman on the table next to a plate at snack time.
Acts out familiar actions in play or imitating day to day activities.	Asad moved the chairs in the room, he was trying to create the Circle Time set-up.
Other examples of cognitive development skills.	

Figure 11.3 (Continued)

166 *Supporting Children's Speech, Language and Communication Needs*

FUTURE PLANNING AND STRATEGIES

NAME: Asad   **D.O.B:**   **DATE OF PLAN:**

WHAT WORKS WELL?
Maintaining skills
Lots of opportunities for active play. Familiar adults who can play, join in with his games and respond to his communications. A play environment where he can choose to engage in active play, outdoor learning environment, toys with a function such as cars and toys representing real objects. A responsive environment with opportunities for spontaneous communication.
APPROACH TO COMMUNICATION DEVELOPMENT
<ul><li>Use signing and key words to help develop understanding.</li><li>Access to photographs, signing, simple speech.</li><li>Clear language with little ambiguity, repeating the vocabulary.</li><li>Accept all communication attempts and respond appropriately.</li><li>Model key signs as you speak, e.g., "it's time to play outside", sign 'play' and 'outside'.</li><li>Model one step ahead.</li><li>Familiar items stored in the same place.</li><li>Repeat activities so they become predictable before changing them or extending them.</li><li>Consistent expectations.</li><li>Provide items that can be combined e.g. spoon and cup, bricks, train engine and carriages, etc.</li><li>Provide real objects, e.g., telephones, cups, etc.</li></ul>
MOVING FORWARD
Any further considerations, assessment or support *Should a short-term outcome be required.*
<ul><li>Opportunities to practise and refine a range of words and signs which can be used to indicate the language functions, e.g., object labels, people's names, gone, here/there (name of places - trampoline), mine, look.</li><li>Provide toys that encourage symbolic play.</li><li>Further observations and assessment of Asad's cognitive abilities.</li><li>When Asad requests the hammock at his grandparents' house, they will model the word "hammock" and wait for him to respond.</li></ul>
EDUCATION HEALTH AND CARE PLAN OBJECTIVE
E1: To spontaneously communicate all band 2 language functions in a manner that is understood by familiar and unfamiliar communication partners.
SPEECH AND LANGUAGE THERAPY
Asad attends a specialist provision where the following is offered:

Figure 11.3 (Continued)

> - A specialist environment offered by the school.
> - Teachers with specialist training.
> - The availability of Communication Assistants.
> - A curriculum modified to meet the needs of a child with a learning disability.
> - The Speech and Language Therapist liaises directly with the child's teacher on request to set up communication objectives and agree implementation.
>
> This forms the classroom-based environmental package.

Figure 11.3 (Continued)

home and school. As Asad was not assessed at band 3 or 4, there was no need to withdraw him for formal assessments.

I was timetabled to spend six sessions in Asad's class. He was interacting frequently and comfortably with his class staff, and he was happy when I joined in with his games. There were specific strategies that worked well:

- Burst pause, e.g., each time the spinning top fell over, the adult pauses with an expectant facial expression, inviting Asad to communicate.
- One step ahead, e.g., when he makes a sound such as 'g' for go, staff model 'go'.
- Signing alongside single words and phrases in context.
- Access to photos on the outside of cupboards indicating what is inside, and photos of places around the school on a transition board.

CATHS has an integrated practice model, and I have an embedded working context, so while in Asad's class I spent time with a couple of children who needed greater levels of support. Enhancing the communication environment for any one child supports the communication and education of all the children in the classroom. For example, Beatrice doesn't respond to the general Intensive Interaction style of the classroom and initiates interactions through hair pulling. I recommended using Intensive Interaction as a focused individual intervention. I liaised with the Intensive Interaction coordinator in school, and she did further training with class staff.

Caleb is in a wheelchair and has a visual impairment. Caleb communicates through repetitive learnt phrases (scripts) and loves staff singing to him. Our Future Plan had involved extending his scripts and presenting them in a lyrical fashion. I noticed staff purely responding to his demands by singing the song he has initiated without trying to extend. I modelled using song to communicate transitions and comment on classroom events, e.g. 'I heard the door close'. These wider examples show how I worked in an integrated way to support communication for all children within the classroom.

Summary

The complexity of children with a diagnosis of PMLD and SLD means professionals must never forget that their learning needs will be lifelong. The nature of the children's barriers to learning means learning new skills is difficult. It is therefore imperative that we ensure we are teaching skills for life.

The goal is for children to be effective and efficient communicators in all situations. It is not about giving the child a system which is only effective when working with the SLT. It is about working in the environment with those who know the child best and starting from the child; looking at what it is they want to communicate and giving opportunities to extend their desire to communicate for new purposes. Alongside this, we need to ensure the child has means of communication that work for them. Their engagement in this process is pivotal; engagement means the child sees a purpose in the activity and is motivated to learn.

The CATHS approach is all about the child, not the system. It starts with assessing the child's successful interactions and the Future Plan focuses on exploring how their current skills can be refined and extended. A key factor is the environment around the child, which can be strengthened to both support and further develop skills.

References

Department for Health and Social Care (2020) *Education and Children's Social Care*. Available at: https://www.gov.uk/government/publications/people-with-learning-disabilities-in-england/chapter-1-education-and-childrens-social-care-updates (accessed November 2024).

Nind, M. and Hewett, D. (2006) *Access to Communication*. 2nd edn. London: David Fulton Publishers.

Sawford, R. and Miles, A. (2021) *Communication at the Heart of the School*. London: Routledge.

Sharma, A. and Cockerill, H. (2014) *Mary Sheridan's Birth to Five Years: Children's Developmental Progress*. 4th edn. Abingdon: Routledge.

12 Stammering

Ben Bolton-Grant

What you'll learn in this chapter

- What stammering is, including its visible (overt) and hidden (covert) features
- The impact of the environment on the stammering experience
- The multifactorial nature of stammering
- Key differences between transient and persistent stammering
- Approaches to information-gathering
- Approaches to supporting children who stammer
- The importance of creating a supportive environment
- Promoting acceptance and confidence in individuals who stammer.

Key information about stammering

Stammering, or stuttering, is a neuro-developmental difference affecting the flow and rhythm of speech. While some features of stammering are visible, much of the experience remains hidden. The 'iceberg' analogy (Figure 12.1) illustrates this: the visible tip represents overt features, while the submerged section symbolises covert features, which are deeply felt but unseen. Additionally, the water surrounding the iceberg reflects the environment, shaping how stammering is experienced and evolves over time (Sheehan, 1970).

Overt features of stammering

'Overt' means open and visible. It refers to the parts of stammering that can be heard and seen by other people. These relate to speech and non-speech characteristics.

Speech characteristics

- *Repetitions*: Sounds and single syllables are repeated. For example, 'm-m-m-my name is Ben', 'my-my-my name is Ben', 'my name is B-B-B-Ben'.
- *Prolongations*: The articulators freeze but the airstream and phonation (if producing a voiced sound) continue. For example, 'mmmmmy name is Ben', 'my name issssss Ben', 'my naaaaaaame is Ben'.
- *Blocks*: The articulators, airstream and phonation all stop, meaning there is a complete stoppage to the forward flow of speech. For example, '. . . my name is Ben', 'my . . . name is Ben', 'my name is . . . Ben' (Wingate, 1964).

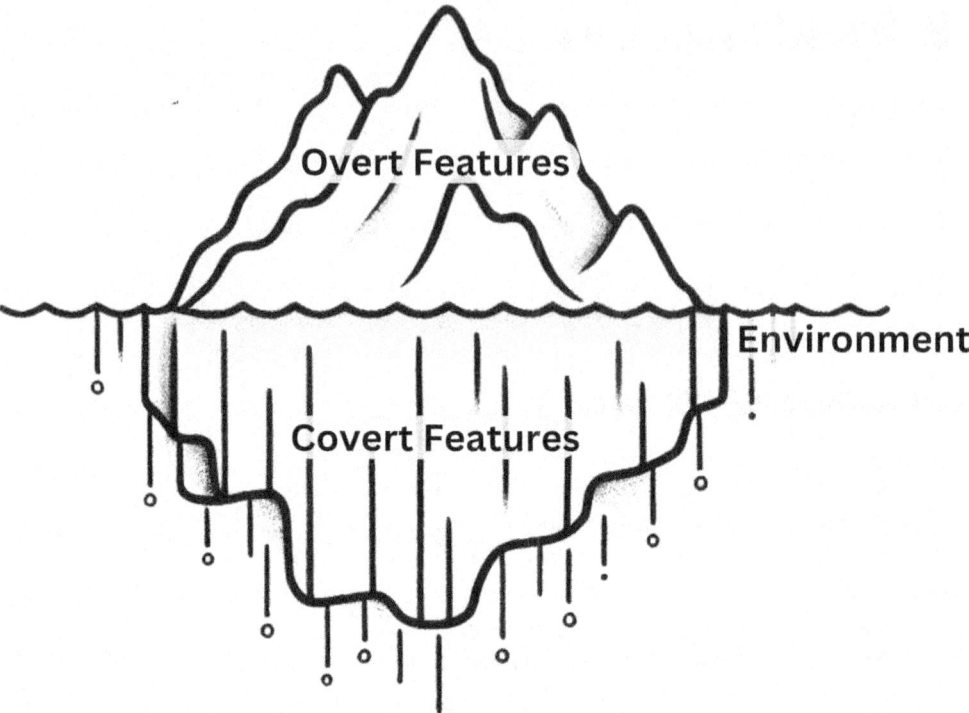

Figure 12.1 Iceberg showing overt stammering features above the waterline and covert features below

These can also be referred to as 'primary features' (Guitar, 2024) because they are the first part of stammering to emerge.

Non-speech characteristics

All of the speech characteristics described above may be accompanied by varying levels of physical tension and struggle, which lead to overt non-speech characteristics. For example, someone may grimace when stammering, show tension in the face, jaw, neck or other parts of their body. Tension in the vocal folds may lead to unusual changes in voice quality or pitch during moments of stammering. These non-speech characteristics are sometimes referred to as 'secondary features' (Guitar, 2024) as they develop after, and as a result of the speech (or primary) characteristics as the speaker tries to stop the stammering from happening.

Covert features of stammering

'Covert' means hidden and refers to the parts of stammering that an observer may be unaware of. These are the thoughts, feelings and behaviours that the person experiences as a result of stammering. These develop over time through an interplay between the person's overt stammering and their environment (Guitar, 2024).

Thoughts

Over time, the way in which a child thinks about themselves and about stammering will change as their awareness increases. This can impact on their self-identity (Daniels and Gabel, 2004) and self-esteem (Yovetich, Leschied and Flicht, 2000; Blood and Blood, 2004; Cook and Howell, 2014; Adriaensens, Beyers and Struyf, 2015). This includes both a fear of negative evaluation from other people, for example, peers, teachers, family members and strangers (Langevin et al., 2009; Blood and Blood, 2016) as well as negative evaluation of one's self (Miers et al., 2009; Eggers, Millard and Kelman, 2021). Thoughts about moments of stammering can be pervasive, with older children and teenagers experiencing attentional bias which means they are more likely to notice moments of difficulty associated with stammering compared to neutral or positive moments (Harley, 2018; Rodgers, Lau and Zebrowski, 2020; Eggers, Millard and Kelman, 2021). They are also likely to anticipate moments of stammering (Tichenor and Yaruss, 2019), which can lead to increased levels of fear and anxiety in speaking situations.

Feelings

As children grow more aware of their stammer, negative and difficult emotions are likely to develop. People who stammer have reported feelings of shame, guilt, worry, embarrassment, emotional pain and exhaustion, hopelessness, and fear (Tichenor and Yaruss, 2019), and are more likely to experience anxiety or be diagnosed with an anxiety disorder (Iverach and Rapee, 2014). This anxiety appears to build from childhood and begins to go beyond typical levels of anxiety by adolescence (Smith et al., 2014).

Behaviours

Behavioural features of stammering often develop as a way for the speaker to try to avoid or escape from the unpleasant physical experiences, and the thoughts and feelings associated with stammering. For example, choosing not to speak, removing themselves from a situation, substituting feared sounds or words, or using other methods to avoid detection by conversation partners (Tichenor and Yaruss, 2019).

The environment

A child's environment significantly influences their experience of stammering. Societal stigma often portrays stammering negatively compared to fluent speech (Boyle, 2018), affecting how children perceive themselves. Subtle reactions, such as well-meaning advice trying to help the child speak fluently, and incorrect stereotypes such as believing children who stammer to be self-conscious or shy (Craig et al., 2003), can harmfully impact children. Overt stigma, including teasing, bullying, and exclusion, can start as early as preschool and often persists through school and beyond (Langevin, Packman and Onslow, 2009; Blood et al., 2011).

Incidence and prevalence

Most stammering is developmental, beginning in early childhood as communication develops, typically between ages 2 and 5 (Yairi and Ambrose, 2005). Incidence in early childhood is 5–9% (Mansson, 2000; Yairi and Ambrose, 2005; Reilly et al., 2009), decreasing to a 1% prevalence in adults (Cavenagh et al., 2015; Gattie, Lieven and Kluk, 2024).

Transient versus persistent stammering

Around 74% of young children who start to stammer will experience transient stammering, which resolves over time, while 26% develop persistent stammering (Yairi and Ambrose, 1999). This suggests not all children who stammer will require speech and language therapy. Although predicting persistence is challenging, certain indicators can help guide decisions about who may or may not require support (see Table 12.1).

Aetiology

Stammering usually starts in early childhood and is influenced by genetic, motor, linguistic, and emotional factors (Smith and Weber, 2017):

- *Genetic factors*: Stammering often runs in families (Ward, 2008; Kraft and Yairi, 2011), suggesting a genetic predisposition.
- *Motor factors*: Children who stammer may have less stable speech-motor systems (Smith and Weber, 2017), which become more unstable with complex linguistic tasks (Kleinow and Smith, 2000).
- *Linguistic factors*: Children who stammer often have subtle differences in language processing and production (Ntourou, Conture and Lipsey, 2011; Reilly et al., 2013; Millager et al., 2014), with many also having phonological disorders (LaSalle and Wolk, 2011).
- *Emotional factors*: Children who stammer show greater negative affect (Eggers, Millard and Kelman, 2021) and reactivity (Ntourou, Conture and Walden, 2013) compared with children who don't stammer, which can increase struggle and secondary behaviours (Eggers, Luc and Van den Bergh, 2013).

Indicator for transience	*Indicator for persistence*
Being female	Being male
No family history of persistent stammering	Family history of persistent stammering
Earlier onset	Later onset
Lower frequency of overt stammering	Higher frequency of overt stammering
Good phonological skills	Poor phonological skills
Good language skills	Poor language skills

Table 12.1 Indicators of transient versus persistent stammering
Source: Singer et al. (2020).

Term	Definition
Stammering	Stammering is the term typically used in the UK. It is used as a neutral and objective way in general use and in more formal ways such as research.
Stuttering	Stuttering and stammering mean the same thing and can be used interchangeably, but stuttering is more typically used in North America and Australia
Dysfluency	Dysfluency has traditionally been used to describe stammering, with 'dys' implying disorder. As stammering is increasingly seen as a difference rather than a defect (Simpson, Campbell and Constantino, 2021), this term has been criticised for reinforcing stigma. However, some parts of the stammering community are reclaiming it as a positive identity marker (e.g., dysfluent.org).
Disfluency	Disfluency can be used to describe non-fluent elements of speech that occur in everyone's speech, whether they stammer or not. This includes interjections, revisions, hesitations.
Normal non-fluency	Normal non-fluency can be used to refer to an increase in disfluencies associated with early language development that reduces as the child's language system matures
Fluency	Fluency has been used as the opposite to stammering and has often been seen as a desirable outcome. A focus on fluency risks stigmatising stammering.

Table 12.2 Terminology used in stammering

Important points about SLT practice in stammering

Terminology and context

As you read more about stammering, you will find a range of terminology being used. It's important to understand what these mean and the role that language plays in either adding to or reducing the stigma around stammering (see Table 12.2).

Stammering-affirming practice

Stammering-affirming practice validates the experiences of people who stammer, fostering acceptance and promoting positive identities. It emphasises empowerment and self-advocacy, and recognises stammering as a valid communication style rather than a disorder (Constantino, 2023). Early interactions with speech and language therapy shape how children perceive stammering as they grow. Therapists must use neutral language, avoiding terms like 'good day' for fluent speech and 'bad day' for stammering, as this reinforces stigma. The goal is to support natural and easy communication, whether or not stammering occurs.

Understanding children's needs in stammering

Given the multifactorial nature of stammering, our information gathering must be similarly multifactorial to help us fully understand our client and their context.

History and underlying factors

Our goal is to understand the child and their family's experience with stammering, identify indicators of persistence, and explore factors contributing to its development. Using the multifactorial nature of stammering, we can build a client profile by gathering relevant information:

- age of the child at the onset of stammering
- time since onset
- gender
- family history of stammering
- details about the onset and development of the stammer
- child and/or parents' impressions of stammering
- cultural views of stammering
- parents' description of the child's temperament
- language development
- phonological development.

We use various tools to gather information, starting with a referral or pre-appointment questionnaire to collect background details. A detailed conversation with the child and/or family follows to explore their experiences, concerns, and hopes. Depending on the child's age and family preferences, this discussion may occur without the child, allowing open communication. If needed, formal or informal assessments of the child's language and phonological skills may be conducted based on initial findings.

Overt features

Traditional SLT practice often used a medical model which focused on reducing or eliminating stammering, starting with a detailed analysis of overt features, such as syllables stammered and the duration of stammering. While some clients and families may expect this, excessive focus on overt features can increase stigma and negatively impact how clients view themselves and therapy (Sisskin, 2023). A stammering-affirming approach instead prioritises helping clients speak comfortably and confidently, regardless of stammering.

However, understanding overt stammering features remains important. Observing interactions with the child and family can reveal core features, secondary behaviours, and signs of tension. Since stammering varies by situation, the therapy setting may not reflect the full range of the child's stammering. Therefore, discussions with the child and family about how stammering sounds, looks, and feels are vital to gaining a comprehensive understanding.

Covert features

Covert features develop over time, but even young children can show awareness in the moment of stammering. Visible tension and struggle often indicate underlying covert features driving these behaviours. Finding out about these elements requires careful consideration of the child's age, level of awareness of stammering and family dynamics. You will likely use a range of information-gathering tools, working with both the child and their family.

Working with the family

Case history

Including an exploration of insights the family have about what the child thinks and feels about stammering is essential, particularly for younger children or those who do not have the awareness or language skills needed to engage in the discussion themselves, but it should be included with all families. We need to identify two key aspects:

1. covert features observed in the child
2. family members' reactions to stammering.

By comparing the child's and the family's reactions, we can determine if they align or differ, guiding our next steps in supporting both the child and their family.

Formal measures

The use of formal assessment tools to gather the views of family members can be helpful. One such tool is the Palin Parent Rating Scale (Millard and Davis, 2016) which is completed by parents or guardians of children who stammer to assess:

- the impact of stammering on the child
- the severity of stammering and its impact on the parent
- the parent's knowledge and confidence in managing stammering.

Working with the child

If a child has an awareness of stammering and is able to enter into a conversation about it, then we may work directly with them to explore the covert aspects of their stammer.

Drawing

We may ask the child to draw emotions, thoughts and situations related to stammering, using this as the basis for a discussion in which the child can explain their drawing can help elicit further information.

We can also use the iceberg analogy to support exploring stammering by drawing an iceberg and asking the client to add details of their stammer. Throughout this process, we should ask open questions, paraphrase, clarify, and gently probe to help the child explore stammering and feel understood.

Scaling

The use of scaling questions is well established with older children and adults and can be a useful way to explore all aspects of stammering. Scaling questions can be as broad or as specific as needed, and make use of numeric and descriptive scales. They can also be phrased to either focus on the area of perceived difficulty or the intended outcome. Here are two examples of scaling.

How bothered are you about stammering?

1_____10
(not at all)_____(extremely)

Or

How happy do you feel about talking?				
Very sad	Sad	OK	Happy	Very happy

Some formal assessment tools make use of scaling questions, but using them in an informal and flexible way, with the clinician asking questions specific to the client can lead to a rich and holistic understanding.

Formal measures

There is a range of formal assessment tools available to help explore a client's experiences of stammering. It is not always essential to make use of formal tools, and it is up to individuals to select which, if any, are appropriate for their situation. Indicators that formal assessment might be useful are:

- the child has awareness of their stammer
- the child would benefit from structured questions to respond to.

The following are some common formal assessments used with children who stammer:

- A-19 Scale for children who stammer (Andre and Guitar, 1979).
- Behavior Assessment Battery for School-Age Children Who Stutter (BAB) (Brutten and Vanryckeghem, 2007).
- KiddyCAT (Communication Attitude Test for Preschool and Kindergarten Children Who Stutter) (Vanryckeghem and Brutten, 2007).
- Wright and Ayre Stuttering Self-Rating Profile (WASSP) (Wright and Ayre, 2000).
- Overall Assessment of the Speaker's Experience of Stuttering (OASES) (Yaruss and Quesal, 2006).

✍ Supporting children's needs in stammering

Supporting children who stammer and their families requires a flexible and tailored approach based on the profile that you have built and the client and family preferences. We must keep stammering-affirming practice in mind throughout this, supporting our clients and their families to move to a place in which communication is viewed as easy, enjoyable and authentic. To do this, we need to draw on a range of indirect approaches in which we work with the people around the child to change their communication environment, and direct approaches in which we work with the child to change aspects of their overt and/or covert features of stammering.

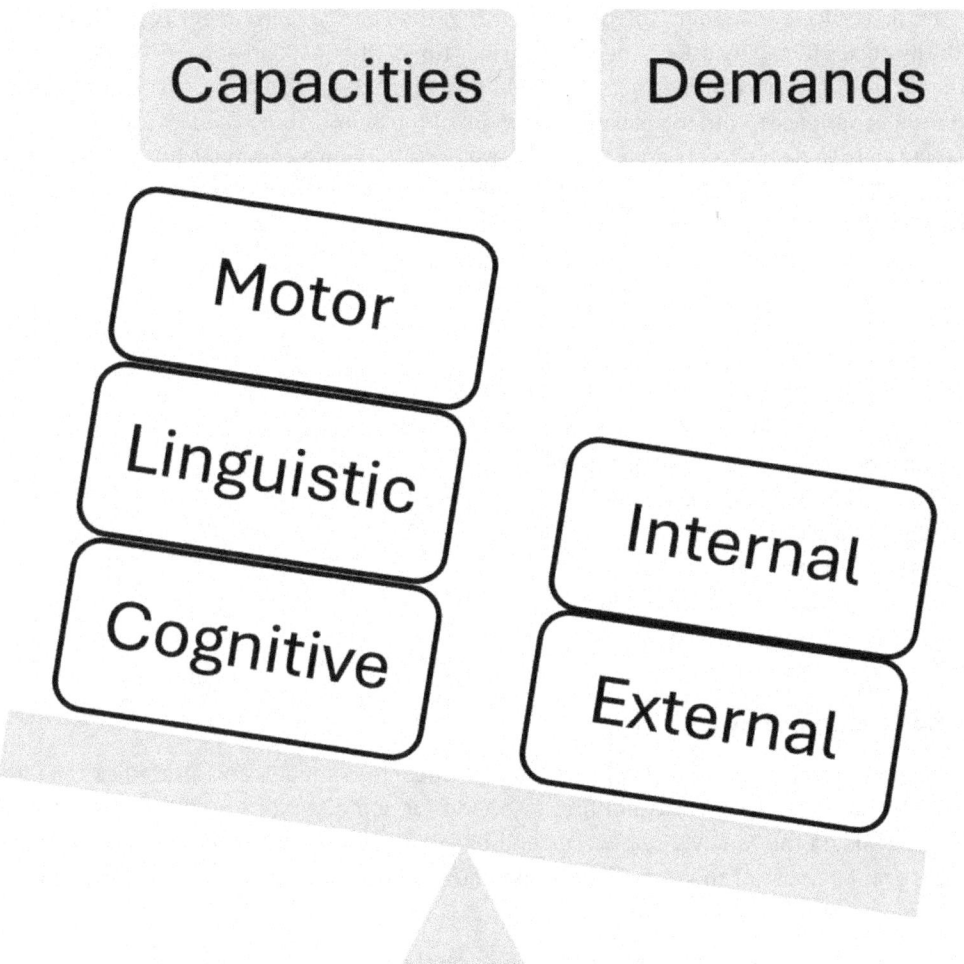

Figure 12.2 The Demands and Capacities model

Environmental and indirect approaches

The demands and capacities model (Starkweather and Gottwald, 1990) is a useful conceptual framework when considering how to support children who stammer. The model suggests that when the demands placed on the child's communication system outweigh their capacity to communicate, stammering increases. As this continues, the child's awareness of stammering is likely to increase, leading to the development of secondary features and struggle. It can be helpful to picture this as a set of balance scales, with demand on one side and capacity on the other (see Figure 12.2).

Demands can be internal (anxiety, self-expectations) or external (situational pressures). Capacities include language skills, coping strategies, and support systems. Balancing demands and capacities is key, aiming to reduce communication demands and enhance capacity.

The first step to managing the demands within the child's environment is to explore this with the child's family by asking them to consider times when talking appears easier or more difficult. From this, we can then consider what it is about these situations that leads to these different experiences, with the aim of doing more of the helpful things and less of the unhelpful. We can then help parents adjust their interactions to reduce communication demands on their child. Parent interactions are key to helping children who stammer communicate more easily and naturally.

Strategies to reduce demands during interactions:

- following child's lead in play
- letting child solve problems
- commenting rather than questioning
- language at child's level
- language related to the child's focus
- time to initiate, respond and finish
- slowed rate of talking
- use of pausing
- using eye contact, position, touch, humour
- praise and encouragement.

Advice and information

Providing information about the Demands and Capacities model, and strategies for families to try out at home, is a useful first step, and for some families is all the support they will need. Using the family's own words and observations will help them to engage in this process and be part of the decision-making about what will happen next. For example, we might say:

> You say that he stammers more when he's on the spot or answering questions. You are right, being less on the spot can help talking feel easier. Can you think of ways that we can help him feel less on the spot?

Having information to refer back to and share with other important people in the child's life is also crucial. We should provide the family with written information to take away with them in the form of leaflets that have been developed in-house, published materials, websites, and social media, etc. We should be mindful of both the quality and content of the information we give and be specific about what information we are suggesting to families to safeguard against them finding unhelpful information.

Special Time

Setting up 'Special Time' is a more structured way to address changes in the child's communication environment. Changing the way that you interact with your child can be difficult for parents to implement throughout the day with all the demands of a busy family life. Special Time is intended to be a protected time each day in which parents can focus on any strategies that they are using. Families are asked to spend 5 minutes giving the child their undivided attention in an activity chosen by the child, focusing on one or two helpful strategies.

Parent-Child Interaction Therapy (PCI)

Parent-Child Interaction Therapy (PCIT) is a structured indirect approach to supporting children who stammer by creating a supportive communication environment through the use of parent-interaction strategies, such as the ones listed above. 'Palin-PCI' (Kelman and Nicholas, 2020) is well established, widely used, and well supported by research. It involves several elements:

- Parents using interaction strategies during daily special time sessions.
- Six weeks of weekly sessions with an SLT in which these are reviewed, followed by a 6-week consolidation period.
- Videoing to support feedback and coaching to help parents enhance their use of communication strategies.
- Family strategies to manage the home communication environment.

Palin PCI has been found to reduce stammering and increase confidence in communicating in children aged between 3 and 7 years old. It has also been found to reduce parental anxiety about stammering and increase parental confidence in supporting a child who stammers (Millard, Nicholas and Cook, 2008; Millard, Edwards and Cook, 2009; Millard and Cook, 2010; Millard, Zebrowski and Kelman, 2018). This research has used multiple case studies, which means that, while it provides positive outcomes that give us confidence that it is an effective support approach, it does not have a comparison or control group, and so findings must be applied with some caution.

Awareness-raising

Awareness-raising is an increasingly large part of the speech and language therapy role when working with people who stammer. Through this work we can change our client's environment, leading to fewer stigmatising and unhelpful reactions to stammering, which in turn allows our clients to communicate comfortably and authentically. This awareness-raising may happen in specific environments, particularly in homes and schools for children who stammer. However, considering the larger environment and society as a whole is also important. Speech and language therapists should be involved in public awareness-raising and campaigning as part of their allyship to the stammering community. Key elements in successful awareness-raising which leads to a change in public attitudes are:

- education
- protest
- contact with people who stammer (Boyle, Dioguardi and Pate, 2016).

Working with schools

Working with schools may involve school visits during which the speech and language therapist can observe the child in school to consider the demands in different parts of that environment. Information should then be shared with school staff, including the child's teacher, teaching assistants, SENCO, lunchtime supervisors and all the staff the child may interact with daily. This may include providing written or recorded information or providing direct training with one or more members of staff.

As well as working with the staff in a school to create a supportive environment SLTs also should consider working with a child's peer group, engaging the child who stammers in the decision-making around what information is shared with their classmates and how this is done. It may be that the child wants to give the information directly to the class themselves, in which case, the SLT's role is to support them to plan and deliver a presentation about stammering. Alternatively, they might wish their class to know about stammering but not want to give the information themselves, in which case the speech and language therapist can deliver the presentation on the child's behalf. They may or may not choose to be part of the group when this happens and we should support them to be as involved as they feel they want to be.

Direct approaches

The Lidcombe Programme

The Lidcombe Programme (Onslow, Packman and Harrison, 2003) is a structured approach where speech and language therapists train parents to conduct daily sessions, providing positive reinforcement for fluent speech. This method aims to increase fluency and reduce stammering. While it may be criticised for potentially stigmatising stammering, it has strong evidence from randomised control trials showing its effectiveness in young children, especially those under 7 (Jones et al., 2005; Packman and Onslow, 2012; O'Brian et al., 2013; O'Brian, Smith and Onslow, 2014). At this age, children's brains are more adaptable, allowing them to develop neural pathways for fluent speech. However, its effectiveness decreases in older children.

Stammering modification

Stammering modification is a direct speech approach used with older children who stammer, as it requires awareness and insight. It aims to reduce the struggle and tension experienced during stammering and replace it with an easier, more relaxed version of stammering.

Cognitive behavioural therapy (CBT)

It is unlikely that solely focusing on overt features of stammering will lead to a successful change in a child's attitudes towards speaking. Support should be planned to address the underlying thoughts, feelings and reactions to stammering (covert features). Cognitive behavioural therapy uses a range of techniques, including cognitive restructuring, relaxation techniques, and exposure therapy to help reduce negative thoughts, feelings and reactions, leading to a positive and accepting attitude towards stammering (Kelman and Wheeler, 2015; Obiweluozo et al., 2021).

An integrated approach

Due to the dynamic and individual nature of stammering our clients are likely to require an individualised and dynamic approach to supporting them. This means adopting an integrated approach in which speech and language therapists draw on a range of approaches to address the overt, covert and environmental features of their clients' experience of stammering.

Group therapy

Due to the social nature of the experience of stammering, addressing this through a social structure such as a group seems to be a natural choice. Groups can be used in order to work on a range of different therapy approaches, including addressing speech directly, working on thoughts and feelings, creating a supportive environment and helping our clients consider how they can change their communication environment at home and in school. Outside of the therapist-planned activities within the group, spending time with other people who stammer can have a transformative effect on our clients' experiences. Being in a situation with other people who stammer, who are in the same boat and understand their experiences creates an environment in which clients are free to experiment with thinking about stammering in a different way (Liddle, James and Hardman, 2011).

Jacob's story

Jacob began stammering at the age of 3. His parents, noticing this and aware that his uncle also stammers, sought speech and language therapy to address their concerns before Jacob started school. They were particularly worried about how the stammer might affect his confidence and communication.

In therapy, the focus was on supporting the family rather than 'fixing' Jacob's stammer. The speech and language therapist helped them explore the communication environment, teaching strategies like slowing down their speech, reducing time pressure, and maintaining positive interactions with Jacob. These changes aimed to build his confidence and create a supportive environment at home. Jacob's parents also learned about the importance of accepting his stammer, which helped them feel more equipped to support him.

Fast forward to when Jacob was 10, his stammer began to bother him more. He started withdrawing from speaking situations, avoiding raising his hand in class, and feeling increasingly anxious. Some of his friends had made comments about his stammer, which led to teasing and affected his confidence. His parents noticed he was speaking with more tension and struggle.

Jacob returned to speech and language therapy, where the focus shifted to addressing his thoughts and feelings about stammering. Using cognitive behavioural therapy (CBT), Jacob explored his reactions to stammering and learned how to reframe negative thoughts. Stammering modification techniques helped reduce the physical tension in his speech. Additionally, Jacob joined a therapy group for children who stammer, where he found a community of peers who understood his experiences.

Through therapy and the support of his 'tribe', Jacob became more confident and accepting of his stammer. This newfound self-assurance empowered him to take a speaking role in his school production, a moment that highlighted his resilience and growth.

Summary

Stammering is multifactorial in nature due to the interplay between genetic, motor, linguistic, and emotional factors. These are influenced by the environment and society and lead to overt and covert features. Speech and language therapy should adopt a stammering-affirming approach that promotes acceptance, empowerment, and positive self-identity by combining direct and indirect approaches and addressing both the visible and hidden aspects of stammering. Addressing the client's environment is crucial, leading to a supportive environment that fosters authentic and confident communication.

Recommended resources

Action for Stammering Children (ASC) is a UK-based charity focused on supporting children and young people who stammer, along with their families. Its mission is to ensure that every child and young person who stammers has access to effective support and feels empowered to reach their full potential. Available at: https://actionforstammeringchildren.org/

Stamma is the public-facing name of the British Stammering Association (BSA), a UK-based charity dedicated to supporting people who stammer. Its mission is to create a society that understands, accepts, and values stammering as a valid form of communication, free from stigma and discrimination. Their website is full of information and resources for people who stammer, families, teachers, employers and speech and language therapists. Available at: https://stamma.org/

References

Adriaensens, S., Beyers, W. and Struyf, E. (2015) 'Impact of stuttering severity on adolescents' domain-specific and general self-esteem through cognitive and emotional mediating processes', *Journal of Communication Disorders*, 58, 43–57. https://doi.org/10.1016/j.jcomdis.2015.10.003.

Andre, S. and Guitar, B. (1979) *A-19 Scale for Children Who Stammer.* Burlington, VT: University of Vermont.

Blood, G.W. and Blood, I.M. (2004) 'Bullying in adolescents who stutter: Communicative competence and self-esteem', *Contemporary Issues in Communication Science and Disorders*, 31(Spring), 69–79. https://pubs.asha.org/doi/pdf/10.1044/cicsd_31_S_69.

Blood, G.W. and Blood, I.M. (2016) 'Long-term consequences of childhood bullying in adults who stutter: Social anxiety, fear of negative evaluation, self-esteem, and satisfaction with life', *Journal of Fluency Disorders*, 50, 72–84. https://doi.org/10.1016/j.jfludis.2016.10.002.

Blood, G.W., Blood, I.M., Tramontana, G.M., Sylvia, A.J., Boyle, M.P. and Motzko, G.R. (2011) 'Self-reported experience of bullying of students who stutter: Relations with life satisfaction, life orientation, and self-esteem', *Perceptual and Motor Skills*, 113(2), 353–364. https://doi.org/10.2466/07.10.15.17.PMS.113.5.353-364.

Boyle, M.P. (2018) 'Enacted stigma and felt stigma experienced by adults who stutter', *Journal of Communication Disorders*, 73, 50–61. https://doi.org/10.1016/j.jcomdis.2018.03.004.

Boyle, M.P., Dioguardi, L. and Pate, J.E. (2016) 'A comparison of three strategies for reducing the public stigma associated with stuttering', *Journal of Fluency Disorders*, 50, 44–58. http://dx.doi.org/10.1016/j.jfludis.2016.09.004.

Brutten, G.J. and Vanryckeghem, M. (2007) *Behavior Assessment Battery for School-Age Children Who Stutter (BAB).* San Diego, CA: Plural Publishing Inc.

Cavenagh, P., Costelloe, S., Davis, S. and Howell, P. (2015) 'Characteristics of young children close to the onset of stuttering', *Communication Disorders Quarterly*, 36(3), 162–171. http://dx.doi.org/10.1177/1525740114549955.

Constantino, C. (2023) 'Fostering positive stuttering identities using stutter-affirming therapy', *Language, Speech, and Hearing Services in Schools*, 54(1), 42-62. https://doi.org/10.1044/2022_LSHSS-22-00038.

Cook, S. and Howell, P. (2014) 'Bullying in children and teenagers who stutter and the relation to self-esteem, social acceptance, and anxiety', *Perspectives on Fluency and Fluency Disorders*, 24(2), 46-57. https://doi.org/10.1044/ffd24.2.46.

Craig, A., Hancock, K., Tran, Y. and Craig, M. (2003) 'Anxiety levels in people who stutter', *Journal of Speech, Language, and Hearing Research*, 46, 1197-1206 https://doi.org/10.1044/1092-4388(2003/093).

Daniels, D.E. and Gabel, R.M. (2004) 'The impact of stuttering on identity construction', *Topics in Language Disorders*, 24(3), 200-215. http://www.csun.edu/~ainslab/readings/Rimsky/Craig_2003_Anxiety%20levels%20in%20people%20who%20stutter.pdf.

Eggers, K., Luc, F. and Van den Bergh, B.R. (2013) 'Inhibitory control in childhood stuttering', *Journal of Fluency Disorders*, 38(1), 1-13. https://doi.org/10.1016/j.jfludis.2012.10.001.

Eggers, K., Millard, S. and Kelman, E. (2021) 'Temperament and the impact of stuttering in children aged 8-14 years', *Journal of Speech, Language, and Hearing Research*, 64(2), 417-432. https://doi.org/10.1044/2020_JSLHR-20-00095.

Gattie, M., Lieven, E. and Kluk, K. (2024) 'Adult Stuttering Prevalence II: Recalculation, subgrouping and estimate of stuttering community engagement', *Journal of Fluency Disorders*, 1-15. https://doi.org/10.1016/j.jfludis.2024.106086.

Guitar, B. (2024) *Stuttering: An Integrated Approach to Its Nature and Treatment*. 6th edn. Philadelphia, PA: Lippincott Williams & Wilkins.

Harley, J. (2018) 'The role of attention in therapy for children and adolescents who stutter: Cognitive behavioral therapy and mindfulness-based interventions', *American Journal of Speech-Language Pathology*, 27(3S), 1139-1151. https://doi.org/10.1044/2018_AJSLP-ODC11-17-0196.

Iverach, L. and Rapee, R.M. (2014) 'Social anxiety disorder and stuttering: Current status and future directions', *Journal of Fluency Disorders*, 40, 69-82. http://dx.doi.org/10.1016/j.jfludis.2013.08.003.

Jones, M., Onslow, M., Packman, A., Williams, S., Ormond, T., Schwarz, I. and Gebski, V. (2005) 'Randomised controlled trial of the Lidcombe programme of early stuttering intervention', *British Medical Journal*, 331(7518), 659-661. http://dx.doi.org/10.1136/bmj.38520.451840.E0.

Kelman, E. and Nicholas, A. (2020) *Palin Parent-Child Interaction Therapy For Early Childhood Stammering*. New York: Routledge.

Kelman, E. and Wheeler, S. (2015) 'Cognitive behaviour therapy with children who stutter', *Procedia-Social and Behavioral Sciences*, 193, 165-174. https://doi.org/10.1016/j.sbspro.2015.03.256.

Kleinow, J. and Smith, A. (2000) 'Influences of length and syntactic complexity on the speech motor stability of the fluent speech of adults who stutter', *Journal of Speech, Language, and Hearing Research*, 43(2), 548-559. https://pubs.asha.org/doi/abs/10.1044/jslhr.4302.548.

Kraft, S.J. and Yairi, E. (2011) 'Genetic bases of stuttering: The state of the art, 2011', *Folia Phoniatrica Et Logopaedica*, 64(1), 34-47. http://dx.doi.org/10.1159/000331073.

Langevin, M., Kleitman, S., Packman, A. and Onslow, M. (2009) 'The Peer Attitudes Toward Children who Stutter (PATCS) scale: An evaluation of validity, reliability and the negativity of attitudes', *International Journal of Language & Communication Disorders*, 44(3), 352-368. https://doi.org/10.1016/j.jfludis.2009.05.001.

Langevin, M., Packman, A. and Onslow, M. (2009) 'Peer responses to stuttering in the preschool setting', 18(23), 264-276. https://doi.org/10.1044/1058-0360(2009/07-0087).

LaSalle, L.R. and Wolk, L. (2011) 'Stuttering, cluttering, and phonological complexity: Case studies', *Journal of Fluency Disorders*, 36(4), 285-289. https://doi.org/10.1016/j.jfludis.2011.04.003.

Liddle, H., James, S. and Hardman, M. (2011) 'Group therapy for school-aged children who stutter: A survey of current practices', *Journal of Fluency Disorders*, 36(4), 274-279. https://doi.org/10.1016/j.jfludis.2011.02.004.

Mansson, H. (2000) 'Childhood stuttering: incidence and development', *Journal of Fluency Disorders*, 25, 47-57. https://doi.org/10.1016/S0094-730X(99)00023-6.

Miers, A.C., Blöte, A.W., Bokhorst, C.L. and Westenberg, P.M. (2009) 'Negative self-evaluations and the relation to performance level in socially anxious children and adolescents', *Behaviour Research and Therapy*, 47(12), 1043-1049. https://doi.org/10.1016/j.brat.2009.07.017.

Millager, R.A., Conture, E.G., Walden, T.A. and Kelly, E.M. (2014) 'Expressive language intratest scatter of preschool-age children who stutter', *Contemporary Issues in Communication Science and Disorders*, 41(Spring), 110-119. https://pubs.asha.org/doi/pdf/10.1044/cicsd_41_S_110.

Millard, S.K. and Cook, F.M. (2010) 'Working with young children who stutter: Raising our game', *Seminars in Speech and Language*, 31(4), 250-261. http://dx.doi.org/10.1055/s-0030-1265758.

Millard, S.K. and Davis, S. (2016) 'The Palin Parent Rating Scales: Parents' perspectives of childhood stuttering and its impact', *Journal of Speech, Language, and Hearing Research*, 59(5), 950-963. https://pubs.asha.org/doi/abs/10.1044/2016_JSLHR-S-14-0137.

Millard, S.K., Edwards, S. and Cook, F.M. (2009) 'Parent-child interaction therapy: Adding to the evidence', *International Journal of Speech-Language Pathology*, 11(1), 61-76. http://dx.doi.org/10.1080/17549500802603895.

Millard, S.K., Nicholas, A. and Cook, F.M. (2008) 'Is parent-child interaction therapy effective in reducing stuttering?', *Journal of Speech, Language, and Hearing Research*, 51(3), 636-650. http://dx.doi.org/10.1044/1092-4388(2008/046).

Millard, S.K., Zebrowski, P. and Kelman, E. (2018) 'Palin Parent–Child Interaction Therapy: The bigger picture', *American Journal of Speech-Language Pathology*, 27(3S), 1211-1223. https://pubs.asha.org/doi/abs/10.1044/2018_AJSLP-ODC11-17-0199.

Ntourou, K., Conture, E.G. and Lipsey, M.W. (2011) 'Language abilities of children who stutter: A meta-analytical review', *American Journal of Speech-Language Pathology*, 20(3), 163-179. https://doi.org/10.1044/1058-0360(2011/09-0102).

Ntourou, K., Conture, E.G. and Walden, T.A. (2013) 'Emotional reactivity and regulation in preschool-age children who stutter', *Journal of Fluency Disorders*, 38(3), 260-274. https://doi.org/10.1016/j.jfludis.2013.06.002.

Obiweluozo, P.E., Ede, M.O., Onwurah, C.N., Uzodinma, U.E., Dike, I.C. and Ejiofor, J.N. (2021) 'Impact of cognitive behavioural play therapy on social anxiety among school children with stuttering deficit: A cluster randomised trial with three months follow-up', *Medicine*, 100(19), e24350. https://pmc.ncbi.nlm.nih.gov/articles/PMC8133212/pdf/medi-100-e24350.pdf.

O'Brian, S., Iverach, L., Jones, M., Onslow, M., Packman, A. and Menzies, R. (2013) 'Effectiveness of the Lidcombe Program for early stuttering in Australian community clinics', *International Journal of Speech-Language Pathology*, 15(6), 593-603. http://dx.doi.org/10.3109/17549507.2013.783112.

O'Brian, S., Smith, K. and Onslow, M. (2014) 'Webcam delivery of the lidcombe program for early stuttering: A phase I clinical trial', *Journal of Speech, Language, and Hearing Research*, 57(3), 825-830. http://dx.doi.org/10.1044/2014_JSLHR-S-13-0094.

Onslow, M., Packman, A. and Harrison, E. (2003) *The Lidcombe Program of Early Stuttering Intervention: A Clinician's Guide*. Austin, TX: Pro-Ed.

Packman, A. and Onslow, M. (2012) 'Investigating optimal intervention intensity with the Lidcombe Program of early stuttering intervention', *International Journal of Speech-Language Pathology*, 14(5), 467-470. http://dx.doi.org/10.3109/17549507.2012.689861.

Reilly, S., Onslow, M., Packman, A., Cini, E., Conway, L., Ukoumunne, O.C., Bavin, E.L., Prior, M., Eadie, P., Block, S., and Wake, M. (2013) 'Natural history of stuttering to 4 years of age: A prospective community-based study', *Pediatrics*, 132(3), 460-467. https://doi.org/10.1542/peds.2012-3067.

Reilly, S., Onslow, M., Packman, A., Wake, M., Bavin, E.L., Prior, M., Eadie, P., Cini, E., Bolzonello, C., and Ukoumunne, O.C. (2009) 'Predicting stuttering onset by the age of 3 years: A prospective, community cohort study', *Pediatrics*, 123, 271-277. https://doi.org/10.1542/peds.2007-3219.

Rodgers, N.H., Lau, J.Y. and Zebrowski, P.M. (2020) 'Attentional bias among adolescents who stutter: Evidence for a vigilance-avoidance effect', *Journal of Speech, Language, and Hearing Research*, 63(10), 3349-3363. https://doi.org/10.1044/2020_JSLHR-20-00090.

Sheehan, J.G. (1970) *Stuttering: Research and Therapy*. New York: Harper and Row.

Simpson, S., Campbell, P. and Constantino, C. (2021) 'Stammering: Difference not defect'. Available at: https://www.redefiningstammering.co.uk/wp-content/uploads/2021/04/Stammering-Difference-Not-Defect.pdf.

Singer, C.M., Hessling, A., Kelly, E.M., Singer, L. and Jones, R.M. (2020) 'Clinical characteristics associated with stuttering persistence: A meta-analysis', *Journal of Speech, Language, and Hearing Research*, 63(9), 2995-3018. https://doi.org/10.1044/2020_JSLHR-20-00096.

Sisskin, V. (2023) 'Disfluency-affirming therapy for young people who stutter: Unpacking ableism in the therapy room', *Language, Speech, and Hearing Services in Schools*, 54(1), 114-119. https://doi.org/10.1044/2022_LSHSS-22-00015.

Smith, A. and Weber, C. (2017) 'How stuttering develops: The multifactorial dynamic pathways theory', *Journal of Speech, Language, and Hearing Research*, 60(9), 2483-2505. https://doi.org/10.1044/2017_JSLHR-S-16-0343.

Smith, K.A., Iverach, L., O'Brian, S., Kefalianos, E. and Reilly, S. (2014) 'Anxiety of children and adolescents who stutter: A review', *Journal of Fluency Disorders*, 40, 22-34. https://doi.org/10.1016/j.jfludis.2014.01.003.

Starkweather, C.W. and Gottwald, S.R. (1990) 'The demands and capacities model II: Clinical applications', *Journal of Fluency Disorders*, 15(3), 143-157. https://doi.org/10.1016/0094-730X(90)90015-K.

Tichenor, S.E. and Yaruss, J.S. (2019) 'Stuttering as defined by adults who stutter', *Journal of Speech, Language, and Hearing Research*, 62(12), 4356-4369. http://dx.doi.org/10.1044/2019_JSLHR-19-00137.

Vanryckeghem, M. and Brutten, G.J. (2007) *KiddyCAT Communication Attitude Test for Preschool and Kindergarten Children Who Stutter.* San Diego, CA: Plural Publishing Inc.

Ward, D. (2008) 'The aetiology and treatment of developmental stammering in childhood', *Archives of Disease in Childhood*, 93(1), 68-71. http://dx.doi.org/10.1136/adc.2006.109942.

Wingate, M.E. (1964) 'A standard definition of stuttering', *Journal of Speech and Hearing Disorders*, 29(4), 484-489. https://doi.org/10.1044/jshd.2904.484.

Wright, L. and Ayre, A. (2000) *Wright & Ayre Stuttering Self-Rating Profile.* Bicester: Winslow.

Yairi, E. and Ambrose, N.G. (1999) 'Early childhood stuttering I: Persistency and recovery rates', *Journal of Speech, Language, and Hearing Research,* 42(5), 1097-1112. https://doi.org/10.1044/jslhr.4205.1097.

Yairi, E. and Ambrose, N.G. (2005) *Early Childhood Stuttering: For Clinicians by Clinicians.* Austin, TX: Pro-ed.

Yaruss, J.S. and Quesal, R.W. (2006) 'Overall Assessment of the Speaker's Experience of Stuttering (OASES): Documenting multiple outcomes in stuttering treatment', *Journal of Fluency Disorders*, 31(2), 90-115. http://dx.doi.org/10.1016/j.jfludis.2006.02.002.

Yovetich, W.S., Leschied, A.W. and Flicht, J. (2000) 'Self-esteem of school-age children who stutter', *Journal of Fluency Disorders*, 25(2), 143-153. https://doi.org/10.1016/S0094-730X(00)00031-0.

13 Neurodivergent children
A neuro-affirming lens on autism, ADHD and beyond

Lynne Bremner and Marion Rutherford

What you'll learn in this chapter

- The important role of Speech and Language Therapists in identifying and planning to meet the needs of neurodivergent children and young people and their families
- Definitions, diagnostic criteria and prevalence for neurodevelopmental conditions
- The importance of the neurodiversity paradigm and a neurodevelopmental approach
- How the *Communication Assessment in an ICF Framework* can guide assessment and interventions relevant to neurodivergent people
- Key principles of a neuro-affirming approach.

Key information about neurodivergence

Neurodevelopment is the complex process by which the nervous system, particularly the brain, develops from the prenatal period into adulthood. This process involves the growth, differentiation, and maturation of neurons (nerve cells) and their connections, allowing for the development of sensory, motor, cognitive, emotional, communication and social functions. Neural circuits in the brain are shaped by interactions between the brain and the environment in early development. This process can be affected by heredity, biology and the environment (for example exposure to alcohol in utero, prematurity, quality of interactions with caregivers) leading to different neurodevelopmental trajectories. Some ways of developing reflect the experiences of most people and are seen as neurotypical; others might follow a trajectory more like a minority of people and could be described as neurodivergent or neurominority. The accepted terminology continues to evolve.

Different neurodevelopmental trajectories are common. This chapter will introduce essential knowledge and understanding about neurodivergent people, to support you to be an accessible and affirming speech and language therapy (SLT) practitioner and colleague.

Being neurodivergent is not necessarily problematic for an individual but difficulties and support needs can arise throughout life, depending on a range of factors. Physical and mental health inequalities and reduced participation in employment, education and other key areas of life are commonly experienced by neurodivergent people. Intersectionality and belonging to more than one group with protected characteristics increase the risk of exclusion or negative life outcomes (Equality Act, 2010), for example, being neurodivergent and

Diagnosis	Prevalence in children (%)	Selected references
Autism	2.8-3.9	Maciver, Rutherford, Johnston and Roy, 2023; Centers for Disease Control and Prevention, 2023
Attention Deficit Hyperactivity Disorder (ADHD)	3-5	Sayal et al., 2018
Fetal Alcohol Spectrum Disorder (FASD)	3-5	Scottish Intercollegiate Guidelines Network (SIGN), 2019
Intellectual Disability	2.5	Mencap, 2020
Developmental Language Disorder (DLD)	7.5	Norbury et al., 2016
Developmental Coordination Disorder (DCD)	5	Blank et al., 2019
Specific learning difficulty (dyslexia, dyscalculia)	3-10	Francés et al., 2022

Table 13.1 Neurodevelopmental diagnoses and prevalence

Co-occurrence

Data reported about the co-occurrence of neurodevelopmental conditions are to some extent limited by the nature of diagnostic services which tend to have a single condition lens. If clinicians look for autism, they see autism and this diagnosis is given, but if the same child attends for ADHD assessment, this might be their diagnosis. In single condition pathways, individuals may be told only that they 'do not have x condition' but are not necessarily assessed with a neurodevelopmental lens to fully understand their profile. This approach is being challenged and over time we are likely to see changes in service delivery which in turn will change what we know about co-occurrence (see Table 13.2). Neurodevelopmental pathways are designed to better identify co-occurring conditions (Male et al., 2020; Rutherford and Johnston 2022).

There is also high co-occurrence of diagnosed neurodevelopmental conditions in stammerers (Briley et al., 2018), people with situational mutism (Keville et al., 2023), avoidant/restrictive food intake disorder (Nyholmer et al., 2024), eating disorders (Christiansen et al., 2024) and other groups with communication support needs.

Diagnoses	Co-occurrence
Autism in people with ADHD	14.4% of USA children (3-17 years) with ADHD had co-occurring autism (Danielson et al., 2024)
ADHD in autistic people	A systematic review found wide variation in prevalence of ADHD in young autistic people from 0-86% (Bougeard et al., 2021). Pooled estimate of lifetime prevalence of ADHD in autistic people was 40.2% (Rong et al., 2021).
Intellectual disability (ID) in autistic people	37.9% of US autistic children aged 8 have ID (Maenner et al., 2023)
Autism in people with intellectual disability	1.2% of US children had ID, of whom 39% are autistic (Patrick, 2021) 21.7% of people with ID in Scotland in 2011 were also autistic (Dunn et al., 2020)

Table 13.2 Co-occurrence of neurodevelopmental diagnoses

female, being from a black or minority ethnic background, having also experienced childhood trauma or living in poverty. Early or timely recognition and support for needs arising at different life stages are recommended in government policy across the four nations of the UK (Scottish Government, 2004; 2017; Department for Education and Department of Health, 2015; Department of Education Northern Ireland, 2020; Morgan, 2020; Welsh Government, 2021).

Definitions, diagnostic criteria and prevalence

For SLTs in training, research and clinical practice, diagnostic categories provide a framework to support decision-making, understanding needs in context and planning to meet individual needs. Understanding broad diagnostic descriptions is a starting point, but individuals with the same diagnosis may present differently based on age, developmental stage, gender, physical and social environment, how well support needs are met, and masking to fit in rather than being their authentic self. A deeper understanding comes from a non-judgmental approach, engaging with neurodivergent individuals, and learning from their experiences.

Some key information to know and critically consider includes:

- *Neurodevelopmental disorders* are defined and diagnosed using international diagnostic criteria, with DSM 5 (American Psychiatric Association, 2013) and ICD 11 (World Health Organization (WHO, 2019) being the current reference manuals.
- The International Classification of Functioning – Children and Young People (ICF-CY) is a biopsychosocial model, used to consider how a range of in-person and environment factors interact to support or challenge participation or involvement in all areas of daily life (WHO, 2007).
- The language and positionality of diagnostic manuals do not reflect the neurodiversity paradigm or neurodivergent community preferences (Keating et al., 2023).
- The use of neuro-affirming mindsets and language is evolving (Rutherford and Johnston, 2022).
- Around 10–15% of people are neurodivergent (Gillberg, 2021) and co-occurrence is to be expected. It is rare to only experience one neurodevelopmental condition, although services are not yet as effective as they could be in identifying co-occurrence (Lang et al., 2024).
- In Scottish schools, 2.6% of primary school children were autistic (Maciver, Rutherford, Johnston and Roy, 2023); and 3.9% in secondary. In the USA, 4% of children were diagnosed as autistic (Yan et al., 2024). Prevalence rates for common neurodevelopmental conditions are given in Table 13.1.
- In some populations, the prevalence of neurodevelopmental conditions is higher, for example, in those who experience involvement with crime (Day et al., 2024), substance misuse, mental illness (Pehlivanidis et al., 2020) and eating disorders (Brown et al., 2024). Autistic children and young people are significantly more likely to have suicidal thoughts, and adults are eight times more likely to die by suicide (Brown et al., 2024).

Diagnoses	Co-occurrence
Language delay or disorder in people with ADHD	14.8% of US children (3–17 years) with ADHD had co-occurring speech/language disorder (Danielson et al., 2024). Some 27% of children with DLD in China had hyperactivity or inattention (Wu et al., 2023).
Language delay or disorder in autistic people	70.4% of 8-year-old autistic children had delayed language (Etyemez et al., 2022).
Developmental coordination disorder and ADHD	21.7% of US children (3–27 years) with ADHD had co-occurring developmental co-ordination delay (Danielson et al., 2024).
Premature birth and neurodivergence	Autistic children were more likely to be born preterm (Khachadourian et al., 2023). There is a positive association between early and preterm birth and likelihood of being autistic (Xie et al., 2017; Crump et al., 2023). Preterm children are two times more likely to have DCD than full term peers (Panceri et al., 2024).

Table 13.2 (Continued)

What we might notice

There are areas across conditions where we see differences in development, processing, preferences, understanding, actions and responses:

- speech and language
- communication and social interaction
- sensory
- motor
- thinking styles
- executive function and planning
- attention
- learning
- participation

Practitioners must take a holistic approach, avoiding a narrow focus on one area of development. For instance, difficulty understanding emotion vocabulary may stem from various factors, including attention patterns, external influences, developmental stage and profile, interoception and alexithymia. Interoception refers to the body's ability to sense internal signals, such as hunger, thirst, or pain. It links physical sensations to emotions. Some neurodivergent individuals may not easily recognise or respond to these internal cues. This is linked to alexithymia, which is a difficulty in describing, identifying and expressing feelings and emotions and differentiating between emotional and physical sensations (Van Bael et al., 2024).

Important points about SLT practice with neurodivergent children

Two main topics influence contemporary SLT practice in this area: the neurodiversity paradigm and a neurodevelopmental approach.

The neurodiversity paradigm

Neurodiversity, a term introduced into popular parlance in the 1990s, refers to the natural variation in neurocognitive functioning among all individuals, encompassing neurotypical individuals and those with neurological differences (Kapp, 2020; Botha et al., 2024). Emerging in the 1990s, the neurodiversity movement evolved as an extension of the autism rights movement. It advocates recognising and celebrating diverse ways of thinking, emphasises the importance of neurodiversity for society, and calls for equality for neurominorities (Raymaker, 2020).

The neurodiversity movement has led to the paradigm shift in how SLTs understand neurodevelopmental differences (DeThorne and Searsmith, 2021; Gaddy and Crow, 2023). Advances in scientific research have also contributed to the shift. Sonuga-Barke (2020) highlights recent findings that challenge previous assumptions, suggesting neurodevelopmental conditions such as autism and ADHD are not distinct 'disorders' rooted in specific brain function differences, nor are they solely associated with impairment. Contemporary thinking within a dimensional approach recognises the continuous nature of many manifestations and an understanding that outcomes arise due to interaction between the person and their environment (Miller et al., 2019).

The paradigm shift has prompted a re-evaluation of speech and language therapy practice. Historically, many practitioners working with children with neurodevelopmental differences operated within the medical model framework, putting the child's 'impairments' at the centre and taking a deficit-based approach to intervention with a focus on treating or 'curing' to align with neurotypical expectations (Pellicano and den Houting, 2022). For example, teaching an autistic child to meet the neurotypical expectation to make eye contact with others.

More recent SLT practice has been shaped by the social model, which emphasises the significant influence of a person's physical and social environment – including societal attitudes and behaviours – on the experience and impact of neurodevelopmental differences. This has led to SLTs focusing increasingly on environmental adaptations such as supporting teachers to implement visual supports and creating predictable settings or supporting parents and carers to adapt their communication and play. Through the neurodiversity paradigm, we recognise that the outcome measures SLTs use are often historically related to neurotypical expectations. Professionals rather than neurodivergent individuals held the power to decide what is important and which outcomes should be measured.

Neuro-affirming practice is emerging in response to the broad acceptance of the neurodiversity paradigm by many neurodivergent individuals, clinicians and professional bodies. Building on the social model of disability, this practice focuses on evening out the balance of power between neurodivergent individuals and practitioners and celebrating difference. Guidance on neuro-affirming practice is emerging (Gaddy and Crow, 2023; RCSLT, 2023) and as a result SLTs are reflecting on whether their assessment and support approaches are neuro-affirming. For example, do the outcomes prioritise neurotypical norms instead of acknowledging and valuing diverse ways of being (Rutherford and Johnston, 2022)?

The neurodevelopmental approach

The work of Gillberg and other researchers has influenced a shift in the design and delivery of healthcare services for neurodivergent children and young people. Services are increasingly adopting a neurodevelopmental, transdiagnostic and multidisciplinary approach (Gillberg, 2021; Rutherford et al., 2021; Astle et al., 2022). Gillberg's approach is based on the high likelihood of co-occurrence of neurodevelopmental conditions, operating under the assumption that co-occurrence is almost always present. He also highlighted that early indicators are shared across neurodevelopmental conditions (Gillberg, 2010). This perspective has led to the development of integrated neurodevelopmental services and pathways, where practitioners consider a range of neurodevelopmental conditions as part of a multidisciplinary team. This comprehensive approach has the potential to enhance their ability to understand and address an individual's support needs (Male et al., 2020).

Understanding neurodivergent children's needs

SLTs have many shared and transferable assessment roles in identifying, observing, assessing, diagnosing and supporting neurodivergent children and their families. Assessment has a range of aims and, depending on these, SLTs will need to delve, probe, extend or summarise their approach. In this section, we will focus on aspects of assessment in which SLTs should be particularly confident.

Two key reasons for assessment are:

- differential diagnosis. Neurodivergent individuals, whether diagnosed as children or adults, feel that diagnosis is important (de Broise et al., 2022; Guilbaud et al., 2021). SLTs play a key role in differential diagnosis as part of the diagnostic team or contributing to it;
- understanding and planning to meet needs.

This chapter will focus on the latter with reference to Figure 13.1. When planning an assessment approach aligned with Figure 13.1, the importance of person + environment= outcome (Beardon, 2020) is key, with the need to consider both the child's or young person's strengths and needs together with their environment, to investigate whether there is a mismatch. Therefore, assessment should focus on an individual's characteristics (e.g., developmental stage, communication domains impacted, needs identified) and the nature of the environments in which the person is participating, including their impact on others in the environment.

In a multi-agency assessment, while bringing their expertise to the team approach, each team member must be more concerned with a holistic understanding of the child in their environment than their uni-professional perspective. A well-rounded clinician collaborates with and learns from colleagues across disciplines, ensuring a more integrated and effective approach to assessment and intervention. Nevertheless, it is key that SLTs understand developmental stage and trajectories and in particular communication stages from early development, before words or symbolic understanding to complex conversational communication.

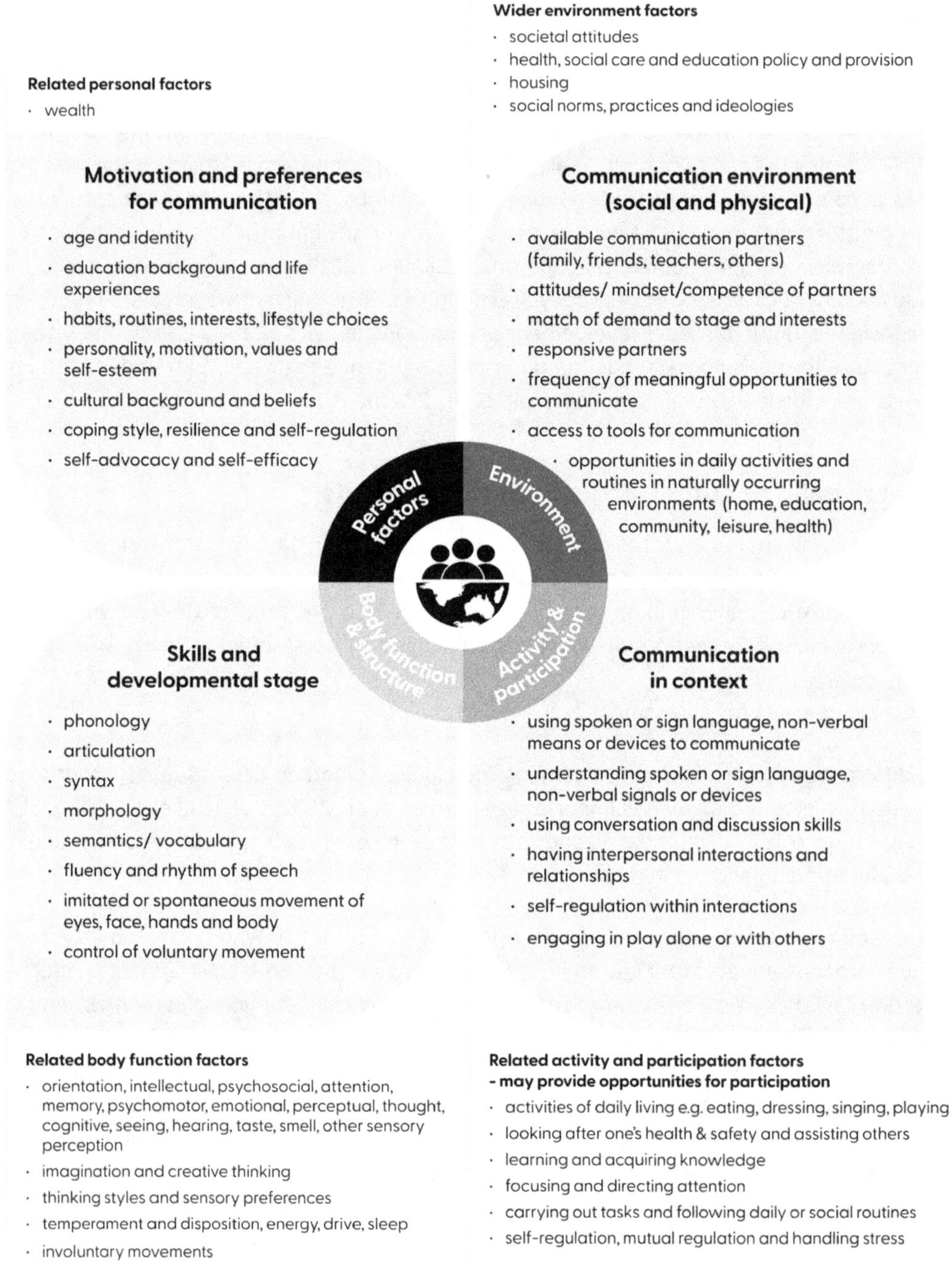

Related personal factors
· wealth

Wider environment factors
· societal attitudes
· health, social care and education policy and provision
· housing
· social norms, practices and ideologies

Motivation and preferences for communication

· age and identity
· education background and life experiences
· habits, routines, interests, lifestyle choices
· personality, motivation, values and self-esteem
· cultural background and beliefs
· coping style, resilience and self-regulation
· self-advocacy and self-efficacy

Communication environment (social and physical)

· available communication partners (family, friends, teachers, others)
· attitudes/ mindset/competence of partners
· match of demand to stage and interests
· responsive partners
· frequency of meaningful opportunities to communicate
· access to tools for communication
· opportunities in daily activities and routines in naturally occurring environments (home, education, community, leisure, health)

Skills and developmental stage

· phonology
· articulation
· syntax
· morphology
· semantics/ vocabulary
· fluency and rhythm of speech
· imitated or spontaneous movement of eyes, face, hands and body
· control of voluntary movement

Communication in context

· using spoken or sign language, non-verbal means or devices to communicate
· understanding spoken or sign language, non-verbal signals or devices
· using conversation and discussion skills
· having interpersonal interactions and relationships
· self-regulation within interactions
· engaging in play alone or with others

Related body function factors
· orientation, intellectual, psychosocial, attention, memory, psychomotor, emotional, perceptual, thought, cognitive, seeing, hearing, taste, smell, other sensory perception
· imagination and creative thinking
· thinking styles and sensory preferences
· temperament and disposition, energy, drive, sleep
· involuntary movements

Related activity and participation factors – may provide opportunities for participation
· activities of daily living e.g. eating, dressing, singing, playing
· looking after one's health & safety and assisting others
· learning and acquiring knowledge
· focusing and directing attention
· carrying out tasks and following daily or social routines
· self-regulation, mutual regulation and handling stress

Figure 13.1 Communication assessment in an ICF framework

Source: Based on the work of WHO 2001, 2007; Rutherford and Johnston 2022; Bölte et al., 2024.

Creating a neuro-affirming environment for assessment

A well-regulated child and family will make for a more effective assessment. Therefore, before embarking on an assessment, SLTs should consider the environment, e.g., minimise sensory triggers, provide clear directions, make the experience predictable by providing a clear overview of the process and use the child or young person's preferred terms (see Doherty et al., 2023, for an overview).

Digital approaches can play a role in effective and efficient assessments and can be a positive and efficient way to undertake aspects of assessment, for example, clinical history conversations with families without children being present or direct observation at home using synchronous or non-synchronous recordings. Clinicians recognise it can save travel time, avoid disruption to family routines and childcare, and reduce demand on clinical space (Charlton et al., 2024; Stroupková et al., 2024).

Undertaking assessment within an ICF framework

Effective assessment is essential for understanding a child's needs and planning support, while ongoing evaluation helps the clinician determine whether agreed goals are met. Planning effective assessment requires the exploration of three key areas (described below):

- *A clear understanding of the nature of the concern raised.* Understanding the needs and concerns of the child, their family and the referrer is crucial in creating a targeted, supportive and effective assessment environment.
- *Establishment of the child/young person's communication/developmental stage.* The child's developmental and communication stage can be estimated through initial conversations with the child, family and referrer. This allows the SLT to select further assessment methods and focus. Due to the heterogeneity of neurodevelopmental conditions, SLTs must be able to assess a wide range of areas. For instance, when assessing a young pre-verbal child, the focus would be on early communication skills, such as joint attention and communication strategies. In contrast, for a child with conversational-level language, the assessment would emphasise higher-level skills, including conversational abilities and the capacity to share emotions and interests.
- *Case history.* Typically gathered from a parent and carer and, where possible, the child, with information from the referrer, the focus of the case history is early development and current communication/presentation. This information allows the identification of factors that will influence the interpretation of communication skills. These aspects include medical and physical factors, such as deafness, vision, learning disability, medical conditions, and birth history; and family history including developmental, medical and social aspects. Tools such as developmental questionnaires and caregiver interviews provide a preliminary understanding of the child's communication skills and challenges within naturally occurring environments.

After evaluating this information, a decision can be made on whether and how to proceed with the assessment.

The model for neurodevelopmental assessment provided in Figure 13.1 outlines key areas considered in a comprehensive SLT assessment. It is influenced by the ICF-CY (WHO, 2007), ICF core sets for autism (Bölte et al., 2024) and principles of the neurodiversity paradigm. The model reflects the two domains of the bio-psycho-social ICF model (WHO, 2007): functioning and disability, and contextual factors. The functioning and disability domain includes *speech and language skills*, as well as *communication in context*, which focuses on how these skills are applied in real-life interactions. The contextual factors influencing communication are the *communication environment*, such as social and physical settings, as well as the individual's *motivations and preferences*, which drive their engagement in communication.

Although the ICF may not initially appear aligned with the neurodiversity paradigm, Bölte et al. (2021) argue that the framework can reconcile with the neurodiversity paradigm. This is based on its inclusion of environmental factors, along with their potential positive or negative impacts on an individual's participation, together with direct attention on an individual's strengths and abilities and a holistic approach to an individual's functioning and health.

Based on the initial information gathering and evaluation, SLTs identify areas from the model to prioritise for assessment. Using their clinical judgement, they choose methods to gain a holistic understanding of the child's strengths, needs, and communication environment. Practical aspects, such as expertise and time available, will be part of the decision-making process. A neuro-affirming lens on this would include consideration of strengths-based approaches, affirming language and being mindful of the risks of comparisons to neurotypical norms (Maciver et al., 2023).

The three main ways further information can be gathered are outlined below.

Asking the child/young person and those proximal to them

They are key informants about a child or young person's current abilities, motivations and preferences. There are a range of tools to gather this information in both a standardised and formal way. Examples include the Children's Communication Checklist-2 (Bishop, 2003), a standardised tool designed to measure language, and pragmatic/social interaction differences, and the SCERTS Assessment Process-Parent Interview (Prizant et al., 2006). Individuals may benefit from adapted approaches to sharing personal experiences and views, for example, using Talking Mats™ (Stans et al., 2019).

Communication in context (low to high structure)

Social communication is most effectively assessed within everyday contexts and activities. Assessments can vary in structure: unstructured, such as observing a young person naturally interacting in their classroom environment; semi-structured, such as engaging a young child in a carefully selected play activity in a clinical setting where the SLT incorporates specific prompts; or highly structured, such as conversing with a young person providing targeted presses designed to elicit an expressive narrative or conversational turn-taking. Understanding a child or young person's preferences and motivations can facilitate the design of these informal assessment approaches. Profiling tools such as the SCERTS observation form

(Prizant et al., 2006) provide a structured, formal tool for gathering observations of social communication skills in the child's everyday contexts. Using a formal tool can reduce subjectivity and the lack of replication inherent in a more informal approach.

Due to the importance of the environment on communication outcomes for children and young people, evaluation of the environment is essential. This can be carried out informally or formally. The formal tools available for this purpose include the SCERTS observation form (Prizant et al., 2006) which evaluates how communication partners interact with and respond to a child or young person and the strategies, tools and environmental adaptations used, and the CIRCLE Inclusive Classroom Scale (Maciver et al., 2021), designed to assess and rate the classroom environment's inclusivity across factors such as the physical and social environment, structures and routines, motivation, and skills.

Formal assessment of communication-related skills in a clinical setting

There are many formal assessment tools for assessing specific speech and language skills/functions, both expressively and receptively. They often focus on specific aspects of speech and language, such as expressive syntax or understanding of grammatical constructs. Examples of standardised formal assessments include the Clinical Evaluation of Language Fundamentals-Fifth Edition (CELF-5) (Wiig et al., 2013) and the Diagnostic Evaluation of Articulation and Phonology (DEAP) (Dodd et al., 2002). These measures can be valuable when the initial evaluation indicates significant difficulties with speech and language as some skills can be difficult to evaluate through observation alone, such as gathering a full phonetic inventory or assessing a child's comprehension. Standardised tools can provide an objective measure of skills, this can be helpful, however, SLTs should be aware of their benefits and limitations.

It is important to consider how much these measures tell us about how the person can use the skill to communicate in everyday settings. Performance on standardised tests can be impacted by a range of factors, including the child's or young person's emotional regulation and familiarity with the tester. Few tools are neuro-affirming, with deficit-based language prevalent. It is therefore essential to use these tools thoughtfully and interpret the results in a neuro-affirming way.

By collecting and analysing data from multiple sources, using diverse methods described above, an SLT can gain a comprehensive and accurate understanding of the child's profile and communication environment.

Table 13.3 provides an overview of typical domains for assessment of the child's stage of language development based on SCERTS communication stages (Prizant et al., 2006).

A neuro-affirming approach to communication support and interventions

SLTs are working with a legacy of assessment tools, outcome measures and interventions which come from a 'neuro-normative' perspective, with comparison to typical development or compliance being the focus. The evidence we can draw on is limited and, even where there is evidence that something has worked, SLTs need to critically appraise whether the methods and outcomes are neuro-affirming and acceptable to neurodivergent people.

Focus of individual assessment based on stage of communication development

Social partner (Pre-verbal)	Language partner (Words and simple phrases)	Conversation partner (Complex language)
Motivation and preferences for communication Communication environment Skills and developmental stage		
Vocalisations Attention Sensory skills Cognitive skills, including symbol understanding Control of voluntary movements/imitation Reciprocity	Appropriate items from the previous column plus Phonology Articulation Semantics (vocabulary) Fluency and rhythm of speech Utterance length	Appropriate items from the previous column plus Syntax Morphology
Using non-verbal means to communicate Quality of communication attempts Communicative intent Understanding others' communication Interpersonal interactions and relationships Engaging in play alone or with others Attention (sharing/joint) Self-regulation within interactions	Communication in context Appropriate items from the previous column, plus Using spoken or sign language, non-verbal means or devices to communicate Using conversation and discussion skills	Appropriate items from the previous column, plus Understanding and use of higher-level conversation and discussion skills (language pragmatics) Conversational turns Topic management Non-literal language Language flexibility Narrative skills Interpersonal interactions and relationships Picking up on social cues Understanding and use of social norms and conventions

Table 13.3 Focus of individual assessment based on stage of communication development

In order to be neuro-affirming, we will need tools and outcomes designed with and by neurodivergent people, which take account of environment and context and consider the double empathy problem (Milton et al., 2022). This theory highlights that people of similar neurotypes experience more successful interactions together and with mixed neurotype pairs or groups, there is a greater chance of miscommunication. Milton clarifies that this is not because neurodivergent people are impaired but that they can have particular styles and preferences, which can be different to neurotypical people. This and other theories take a 'difference not deficit approach', while still recognising difficulties experienced.

Neuro-affirming communication support and intervention mean taking an individualised approach and using the assessment information gathered to identify developmentally relevant targets or plans based on what is important to the child or young person or their family. The focus is on helping individuals to participate in meaningful communication, with access to a means of expression relevant to them, support to understand others and to be their authentic self, without the need to mask (Sedgewick, Hull and Ellis, 2021). Therapists might support people with decision-making about the focus of intervention or support by highlighting choices and revisiting decisions over time.

Planning to support needs within an ICF Framework

The framework above can be applied when using assessment information to develop plans, interventions, supports and outcome measures.

There is no single intervention or set of interventions universally recommended or evidence-based for all neurodivergent children (Hume et al., 2021; RCSLT, 2023). The examples below highlight approaches commonly used but are not exhaustive. SLTs are encouraged to be reflective practitioners, guided by neuro-affirming principles and the framework in Figure 13.1. This ensures that interventions consider the child within their physical and social environment, emphasising predictability and desirability. Effective support focuses on changing the actions, understanding, and mindsets of those closest to the child, such as the family and educational staff.

The four framework elements are interconnected. For example, when teaching signing, it is essential to establish the individual has the necessary motor skills, consider meaningful and motivating vocabulary (e.g., names and actions), plan opportunities for practice, and address personal or environmental factors that may affect participation, such as attitudes towards signing in those proximal to the child.

Environment-focused interventions

SLTs use environment-focused and person-centred interventions to support meaningful communication. The goal is to enhance access to responsive communication partners, create opportunities for interaction in natural settings, and tailor expectations to each individual's developmental stage and preferences. Neuro-affirming SLTs emphasise changes to the physical and social environments rather than teaching children to mask anxiety or use too much energy to regulate emotions in unadapted or unpredictable situations (Johnston et al., 2024). They work collaboratively in multidisciplinary teams to address anxiety, distress, or dysregulation by modifying the environment instead of focusing solely on the individual's 'behaviour'. There is a range of available options:

- *Collaboration with educators* to implement universal and targeted adjustments and environmental modifications in the school setting, like those outlined in the CIRCLE framework (MacIver et al., 2021).
- *Parent programmes*, such as the updated Hanen More Than Words programme (Weitzman, 2024).
- *Daily and social routines* can be designed using play, mealtimes or other routines to promote predictability and encourage participation.
- *Visual support strategies* for home or school settings (Rutherford et al., 2020).
- *Alternative and Augmentative Communication (AAC)* tools, both low-tech and high-tech, with a focus on fostering autonomy and authentic communication (Gibson et al., 2021).

- *Social stories* (McCadden, 2024) can prepare communication partners for specific scenarios. SLTs can ensure these are written in accessible language and are not used to enforce compliance or behaviour change. Furthermore, they help facilitate conversations to define clear goals and assess whether these or alternative strategies are most effective.

Personal factors interventions

These focus on helping individuals, or those supporting them, to understand what motivates, engages, and enables successful communication or learning. This understanding is then used to guide adjustments that support effective communication. Again, various options exist:

- *Psychoeducation*: SLTs can provide education to help individuals understand their own communication and sensory preferences, needs, and thinking styles (Black et al., 2024). Available published materials may be based on deficit frameworks – so local adaptation may be required to ensure the experience is neuro-affirming.
- *Building neurodivergent identity*: Supporting individuals in developing a positive sense of their neurodivergent identity and foster connections with others in the neurodivergent community (Fotheringham et al., 2023).
- *Communication tools*: SLT-led tools like Talking Mats (Stans et al., 2019) can facilitate effective communication about their preferences and motivations.
- *Personal profiles*: Individuals with metacognitive skills can be guided to create and use personal profiles or communication passports to enhance communication.

These approaches empower individuals to better understand and advocate for their needs while fostering meaningful connections and autonomy.

Activity and participation-focused interventions

Neurodivergent individuals often face barriers to participation, and while SLTs play a role in addressing these challenges, for example, in cases of situational mutism (Hipolito et al., 2023), participation is limited by an inability to speak in specific contexts. Much of the existing evidence has not been shaped by the neurodiversity paradigm. Participation can be supported through a range of adjustments and a neurodevelopmental lens on the experience.

The neurodiversity paradigm complements the ICF model by highlighting how SLTs can foster meaningful participation in interactions and relationships. Rather than relying on traditional 'social skills' groups or interventions aimed at teaching neurodivergent individuals to mask or adopt neurotypical communication styles, a neuro-affirming approach recognises difficulties some individuals experience with social participation. Priorities of this approach are listed below:

- *Peer relationships-focused interventions*: Bringing together individuals with shared communication styles or interests to engage in enjoyable activities (Lofthouse, 2024).

- *Forming connections*: Support in 'finding their people' and 'allies' – communities where individuals can express themselves authentically and feel a sense of belonging.

The focus is changing from the individual, to creating environments and opportunities that celebrate diversity and promote genuine connection.

Supporting communication through mutual and self-regulation

For social and language partners (Prizant et al., 2006), regulation often depends on mutual adjustments rather than deliberate self-regulation or monitoring strategies. For conversation partners, a metacognitive approach can be helpful. Support might involve:

- *Self-advocacy*: Helping the individual understand and advocate for their own communication needs and preferences.
- *Understanding social expectations*: Providing insight into rules commonly applied in neurotypical communication, without expecting neurodivergent individuals to conform to these rules.

This approach prioritises empowerment and understanding over conformity, promoting communication that respects individual needs and authenticity.

Body functions and structure or skills-focused interventions

These can be relevant if aligned with an individual's developmental stage, trajectory, environment, motivation and routines:

- *Speech, language and communication skills*: It is important that needs in this area are not overlooked because the individual is neurodivergent. For example, targeted learning opportunities to develop skills in speech, language, communication may be highly relevant.
- *Vocabulary of body functions*: This might be to support individuals to communicate body states, such as hunger, tiredness, pain.

To ensure these interventions are neuro-affirming, they should be engaging, meaningful, and free from compliance-based or ableist approaches (Sutton, 2024).

Teaching approaches and affirming practices

The effectiveness of teaching is often determined not just by *what* skill is taught, but *how* it is taught. For instance, introducing picture exchange as a communication system for children who lack a way to request or initiate interactions is a valid goal. However, the method of implementation could lead to non-affirming practices.

For example:

- Using picture exchange with children who have not yet reached a symbolic stage of development may lead to prompt dependency.

- Certain teaching methods may invade a child's body autonomy or cause distress, such as withholding preferred items. For instance, giving only one crisp at a time to a child accustomed to having a full bag, or withholding a requested item until the child uses picture exchange, can make the child feel dysregulated.

Alternatively, adults who have a trusting relationship with the child can foster communication in affirming ways by:

- creating engaging and motivating situations where the child wants to request actions or objects
- providing a symbol-rich and accessible environment
- being responsive to the child's natural communication signals and gently pairing these signals with symbols when developmentally appropriate.

With consistent repetition and positive experiences, children can gradually learn the value of picture exchange and integrate it as one of their meaningful communication methods, without stress or coercion. More published evidence of effective neuro-affirming speech and language therapy intervention is needed.

Key principles

A neuro-affirming SLT intervention holds to 10 key principles:

1. Use neuro-affirming language and mindsets.
2. Listen to and learn from neurodivergent people.
3. Recognise different developmental trajectories instead of seeing only deficits.
4. Value all forms of communication and preferences for communication, without preferencing more neurotypical communication.
5. Recognise that just because there is evidence that an approach worked, does not mean that the outcomes from this approach are desirable or that we should do it.
6. It's not what you do but how you do it that determines whether it is neuro-affirming.
7. Taking a developmentally relevant approach.
8. Provide access to relevant communication support across the lifespan.
9. Make assessment meaningful.
10. Prioritise autonomy and independence.

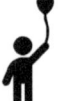

Mattie's story

Mattie is a 4-year-old boy waiting for a neurodevelopmental assessment. Plans are underway for transition to school. Concerns were raised by his parents and nursery about his language understanding and difficulty following directions outside familiar routines. He uses delayed and immediate echolalia for communication with some spontaneous language. Mattie enjoys solitary play, particularly sensory activities, and has met developmental milestones except for communication.

Initial SLT contact

A phone consultation with Mattie's parents revealed the following:

- Mattie uses around 30 spontaneous words and echolalia, such as 'Mummy outside' and 'Where's Olaf?'
- He recognises letters and numbers, reading bus numbers aloud.
- He does not use spontaneous gestures or maintain eye contact when speaking.

Parents are uncertain about his level of understanding.

Assessments

- SLT observed Mattie in nursery, focusing on language and social communication.
- SLT met with the nursery team to discuss their observations and support strategies.
- SLT conducted a formal comprehension assessment in the clinic.
- Further information gathering with parents at clinic appointment.

Outcome of assessment

- *Person and environment factors*: Mattie loves Disney's *Frozen*, active play, and climbing. He is the eldest of three children. His parents would like to attend the Hanen More Than Words programme, though shift work poses challenges. His nursery environment suits him, offering visual supports, clear routines and staff with skills to adapt and use clear language. However, his parents are unsure how to support his communication at home and currently do not use visual supports.
- *Speech and language skills*: Mattie can follow single-word instructions consistently and occasionally two-keyword instructions. He uses approximately 30 spontaneous words.
- *Activity and participation*: Mattie uses language to greet people, accept and refuse and to respond in social routines. He rarely initiates to make requests for objects or actions.
- *Intervention plan*: Offer appointments to support parents in applying strategies at home to enhance Mattie's comprehension and communication skills.
- *Collaborate* with nursery about communication support and needs for transition to school.

Summary

Supporting neurodivergent children and young people requires a holistic, individualised approach that prioritises their strengths, preferences, and developmental trajectories. The role of SLTs and other professionals is to carry out meaningful, holistic assessment and create environments and interventions that foster authentic communication, meaningful participation, and positive identity development.

There are several key strategies:

- *Person-focused interventions*, which emphasise understanding and accommodating individual preferences and needs.

- *Environment-focused adjustments*, such as fostering supportive relationships, modifying physical and social contexts, and introducing tools like AAC to enhance communication.
- *Skill-building interventions*, designed in affirming ways that respect developmental readiness and avoid coercion or compliance-based practices.
- *Participation-focused approaches*, which prioritise connection and authenticity over enforcing neurotypical norms, creating spaces where individuals feel seen, valued, and included.

By embracing the neurodiversity paradigm, and applying knowledge and skills about neurodevelopment, SLTs can lead the move beyond deficit-based models to adopt practices that affirm the unique communication experiences and contributions of neurodivergent individuals. This requires working at a universal, targeted and specialist level, with ongoing collaboration with neurodivergent people, families, educators, and multidisciplinary teams to ensure interventions are both effective and respectful.

Ultimately, the goal is to empower neurodivergent children and young people to thrive in environments that celebrate their individuality and provide the support they need to participate meaningfully in the ways they would like to do.

References

American Psychiatric Association (2013) *Diagnostic and Statistical Manual Of Mental Disorders: DSM-5*. 5th edn. Washington, DC: American Psychiatric Publishing.

Astle, D.E., Holmes, J., Kievit, R. and Gathercole, S.E. (2022) 'Annual Research Review: The transdiagnostic revolution in neurodevelopmental disorders', *Journal of Child Psychology and Psychiatry*, 63(4), 397–417.

Beardon, L. (2020) *Avoiding Anxiety in Autistic Children: A Guide for Autistic Wellbeing*. London: Hachette UK.

Bishop, D. V. M. (2003) *The Children's Communication Checklist, Version 2*. London: Pearson.

Black, M.H., Helander, J., Segers, J., Ingard, C., Bervoets, J., de Puget, V.G. and Bölte, S. (2024) 'Resilience in the face of neurodivergence: A systematic scoping review of resilience and factors promoting positive outcomes', *Clinical Psychology Review*, August 15, 102487. https://doi.org/10.1016/j.cpr.2024.102487

Blank, R., Barnett, A.L., Cairney, J., Green, D., Kirby, A., Polatajko, H., Rosenblum, S., Smits-Engelsman, B., Sugden, D., Wilson, P. and Vinçon, S. (2019) 'International clinical practice recommendations on the definition, diagnosis, assessment, intervention, and psychosocial aspects of developmental coordination disorder', *Developmental Medicine & Child Neurology*, 61(3), 242–285. https://doi.org/10.1111/dmcn.14132

Bölte, S., Alehagen, L., Black, M.H., Hasslinger, J., Wessman, E., Lundin Remnélius, K., Marschik, P.B., D'Arcy, E., Crowson, S., Freeth, M. and Seidel, A. (2024) 'The Gestalt of functioning in autism revisited: First revision of the International Classification of Functioning, Disability and Health Core Sets', *Autism*, 13623613241228896.

Bölte, S., Lawson, W.B., Marschik, P.B. and Girdler, S. (2021) 'Reconciling the seemingly irreconcilable: The WHO's ICF system integrates biological and psychosocial environmental determinants of autism and ADHD: The International Classification of Functioning (ICF) allows to model opposed biomedical and neurodiverse views of autism and ADHD within one framework', *BioEssays*, 43(9). https://doi.org/10.1002/bies.202000254

Botha, M., Chapman, R., Giwa Onaiwu, M., Kapp, S. K., Stannard Ashley, A. and Walker, N. (2024) 'The neurodiversity concept was developed collectively: An overdue correction on the origins of neurodiversity theory', *Autism*, 28(6), 1591–1594. https://doi.org/10.1177/13623613241237871

Bougeard, C., Picarel-Blanchot, F., Schmid, R., Campbell, R. and Buitelaar, J. (2021) 'Prevalence of autism spectrum disorder and co-morbidities in children and adolescents: A systematic literature review', *Frontiers in Psychiatry*, 12. https://doi.org/10.3389/fpsyt.2021.744709

Briley, P.M. and Ellis Jr, C. (2018) 'The coexistence of disabling conditions in children who stutter: Evidence from the National Health Interview Survey', *Journal of Speech, Language, and Hearing Research*, 61(12), 2895-2905. https://doi.org/10.1044/2018_JSLHR-S-17-0378

Brown, C.M., Newell, V., Sahin, E. and Hedley, D. (2024) 'Updated systematic review of suicide in autism: 2018-2024', *Current Developmental Disorders Reports*, 11, 225-256. https://doi.org/10.1007/s40474-024-00308-9

Brown, T.R., Jansen, M.O., Zhou, A.N., Moog, D., Xie, H., Liebesny, K.V., Xu, K.Y., Lin, B.Y. and Deng, W.Y. (2024) 'Co-occurring autism, ADHD, and gender dysphoria in children, adolescents, and young adults with eating disorders: An examination of pre- vs. post-COVID pandemic outbreak trends with real-time electronic health record data', *Frontiers in Psychiatry*, 15, 1402312. https://doi.org/10.3389/fpsyt.2024.1402312

Centers for Disease Control and Prevention (2023) 'Prevalence and characteristics of autism spectrum disorder among children aged 8 years–Autism and Developmental Disabilities' Monitoring Network, 11 sites, United States, 2020'. Available at: https://www.cdc.gov (accessed 29 November 2024).

Charlton, J., Gréaux, M., Kulkarni, A., Dornstauder, M. and Law, J. (2024) 'UK paediatric speech and language therapists' perceptions on the use of telehealth in current and future clinical practice: An application of the APEASE criteria', *International Journal of Language & Communication Disorders*, 59(3), 1163-1179. https://doi.org/10.1111/1460-6984.12988

Christiansen, G.B., Petersen, L.V., Chatwin, H., Yilmaz, Z., Schendel, D., Bulik, C.M., Grove, J., Brikell, I., Semark, B.D., Holde, K. and Abdulkadir, M. (2024) 'The role of co-occurring conditions and genetics in the associations of eating disorders with attention-deficit/hyperactivity disorder and autism spectrum disorder', *Molecular Psychiatry*, 1-10. https://doi.org/10.1038/s41380-024-02825-w

Crump, C., Sundquist, J. and Sundquist, K. (2023) 'Preterm or early term birth and risk of attention-deficit. hyperactivity disorder: A national cohort and co-sibling study', *Annals of Epidemiology*, 86, 119-125. https://doi.org/10.1016/j.annepidem.2023.08.007

Danielson, M.L., Claussen, A.H., Bitsko, R.H., Katz, S.M., Newsome, K., Blumberg, S.J. and Ghandour, R. (2024) 'ADHD prevalence among U.S. children and adolescents in 2022: Diagnosis, severity, co-occurring disorders, and treatment', *Journal of Clinical Child & Adolescent Psychology*, 53(3), 343-360. https://doi.org/10.1080/15374416.2024.2335625

Day A-M., Allely C., Robinson L., Turner K., Gerry, F., and Forrester A. (2024) 'The over-representation of neurodivergent children in Youth Justice Systems and The Youth Court', *Medicine, Science and the Law*, 64(4), 255-258. doi:10.1177/00258024241274073

de Broize, M., Evans, K., Whitehouse, A.J., Wray, J., Eapen, V. and Urbanowicz, A. (2022) 'Exploring the experience of seeking an autism diagnosis as an adult', *Autism in Adulthood*, 4(2), 130-140. https://doi.org/10.1089/aut.2021.0028

Department for Education and Department of Health (2015) *Special Educational Needs and Disability Code of Practice: 0 to 25 Years*. Available at: https://www.gov.uk/government/publications/send-code-of-practice-0-to-25 (accessed 19 November 2024).

Department of Education Northern Ireland (2020) *SEN Framework Review*. Available at: https://www.education-ni.gov.uk/articles/sen-review (accessed 19 November 2024).

DeThorne, L.S. and Searsmith, K. (2021) 'Autism and neurodiversity: Addressing concerns and offering implications for the school-based speech-language pathologist', *Perspectives of the ASHA Special Interest Groups*, 6(1), 184-190.

Dodd, B., Hua, Z., Crosbie, S., Holm, A. and Ozanne, A. (2002) *Diagnostic Evaluation of Articulation and Phonology (DEAP)*. London: Pearson Assessment.

Doherty, M., McCowan, S. and Shaw, S. C. (2023) 'Autistic SPACE: A novel framework for meeting the needs of autistic people in healthcare settings', *British Journal of Hospital Medicine*, 84(4), 1-9. https://doi.org/10.12968/hmed.2023.0006

Dunn, K., Rydzewska, E., Fleming, M. and Cooper, S.A. (2020) 'Prevalence of mental health conditions, sensory impairments and physical disability in people with co-occurring intellectual disabilities and autism compared with other people: A cross-sectional total population study in Scotland', *BMJ Open*, 1i0. https://doi.org/10.1136/bmjopen-2019-035280

Etyemez, S., Esler, A., Kini, A., Tsai, P. C., Dirienzo, M., Maenner, M. and Lee, L.C. (2022) 'The role of intellectual disability with autism spectrum disorder and the documented cooccurring conditions: A population-based study', *Autism Research*, 15(12), 2399-2408. https://doi.org/10.1002/aur.2831

Fotheringham, F., Cebula, K., Fletcher-Watson, S., Foley, S. and Crompton, C.J. (2023) 'Co-designing a neurodivergent student-led peer support programme for neurodivergent young people in mainstream high schools', *Neurodiversity*, 1. https://doi.org/10.1177/27546330231205770

Francés, L., Quintero, J., Fernández, A., Ruiz, A., Caules, J., Fillon, G., Hervás, A. and Soler, C.V. (2022) 'Current state of knowledge on the prevalence of neurodevelopmental disorders in childhood according to the DSM-5: A systematic review in accordance with the PRISMA criteria', *Child and Adolescent Psychiatry and Mental Health*, 16(1), 27. https://doi.org/10.1186/s13034-022-00462-1

Gaddy, C. and Crow, H. (2023) 'A primer on neurodiversity-affirming speech and language services for autistic individuals', *Perspectives of the ASHA Special Interest Groups*, 8(6), 1220–1237. https://doi.org/10.1044/2023_PERSP-23-00106

Gibson, R.C., Bouamrane, M.M. and Dunlop, M.D. (2021) 'Alternative and augmentative communication technologies for supporting adults with mild intellectual disabilities during clinical consultations: Scoping review', *JMIR Rehabilitation and Assistive Technologies*, 8(2), 19925. https://doi.org/10.2196/19925

Gillberg, C. (2010) 'The ESSENCE in child psychiatry: Early symptomatic syndromes eliciting neurodevelopmental clinical examinations', *Research in Developmental Disabilities*, 31(6), 1543–1551. https://doi.org/10.1016/j.ridd.2010.06.002

Gillberg, C. (2021) *The Essence of Autism and Other Neurodevelopmental Conditions: Rethinking Co-Morbidities, Assessment, and Intervention*. London: Jessica Kingsley Publishers.

Guilbaud, J., Vuattoux, D., Bezzan, G. and Malchair, A. (2021) 'Autism Spectrum disorder: Ethiopathogenesis and benefits of early diagnosis', *Revue Médicale de Liège*, 76(9), 672–676.

Hipolito, G., Pagnamenta, E., Stacey, H., Wright, E., Joffe, V., Murayama, K. and Creswell, C. (2023) 'A systematic review and meta-analysis of nonpharmacological interventions for children and adolescents with selective mutism', *JCPP Advances*, 3(3), 12166. https://doi.org/10.1002/jcv2.12166

Hume, K., Steinbrenner, J.R., Odom, S.L., Morin, K.L., Nowell, S.W., Tomaszewski, B., Szendrey, S., McIntyre, N.S., Yücesoy-Özkan, S. and Savage, M.N. (2021) 'Evidence-based practices for children, youth, and young adults with autism: Third generation review', *Journal of Autism and Developmental Disorders*, 1–20. https://doi.org/10.1007/s10803-020-04844-2

Johnston, L., Maciver, D., Rutherford, M., Gray, A., Curnow, E. and Utley, I. (2024) 'A brief neuro-affirming resource to support school absences for autistic learners: Development and program description', *Frontiers in Education*, 9, 1358354. https://doi.org/10.3389/feduc.2024.1358354

Kapp, S.K. (2020) *Autistic Community and the Neurodiversity Movement: Stories from the Frontline*. Cham: Springer Nature.

Keating, C.T., Hickman, L., Leung, J., Monk, R., Montgomery, A., Heath, H. and Sowden, S. (2023). 'Autism-related language preferences of English-speaking individuals across the globe: A mixed methods investigation', *Autism Research*, 16(2), 406–428. https://doi.org/10.1002/aur.2864

Keville, S., Zormati, P., Shahid, A., Osborne, C. and Ludlow, A.K. (2023) 'Parent perspectives of children with selective mutism and co-occurring autism', *International Journal of Developmental Disabilities*, 1–11. https://doi.org/10.1080/20473869.2023.2173835

Khachadourian, V., Mahjani, B., Sandin, S., Kolevzon, A., Buxbaum, J. D., Reichenberg, A., and Janecka, M. (2023) 'Comorbidities in autism spectrum disorder and their etiologies', *Translational Psychiatry*, 13(1). https://doi.org/10.1038/s41398-023-02374-w

Lang, J., Wylie, G., Haig, C., Gillberg, C. and Minnis, H. (2024) 'Towards system redesign: An exploratory analysis of neurodivergent traits in a childhood population referred for autism assessment', *PLoS One*, 19(1), e0296077. https://doi.org/10.1371/journal.pone.0296077

Lofthouse, J. (2024) 'What can we learn from autistic speech and language therapists about neuro-affirming practice?' Available at: https://www.researchgate.net/profile/Jessica-Lofthouse/publication/385746578_What_can_we_learn_from_autistic_speech_and_language_therapists_about_neuro-affirming_practice/links/6733b79269c07a4114458d69/What-can-we-learn-from-autistic-speech-and-language-therapists-about-neuro-affirming-practice.pdf (Accessed: 18 November, 2024)

Maenner, M.J., Warren, Z., Williams, A.R., Amoakohene, E., Bakian, A.V., Bilder, D.A. and Shaw, K.A. (2023) 'Prevalence and characteristics of autism spectrum disorder among children aged 8 years – Autism and Developmental Disabilities Monitoring Network, 11 Sites, United States, 2020', *MMWR: Surveillance Summaries*, 72(2), 1–14. https://doi.org/10.15585/mmwr.ss7202a1

Maciver, D., Hunter, C., Johnston, L. and Forsyth, K. (2021) 'Using stakeholder involvement, expert knowledge and naturalistic implementation to co-design a complex intervention to support children's inclusion and participation in schools: The CIRCLE framework', *Children*, 8(3). https://doi.org/10.3390/children8030217

Maciver, D., Rutherford, M., Johnston, L., Curnow, E., Boilson, M. and Murray, M. (2023) 'An interdisciplinary nationwide complex intervention for lifespan neurodevelopmental service development: Underpinning principles and realist programme theory', *Frontiers in Rehabilitation Sciences*, 3, 1060596. https://doi.org/10.3389/fresc.2022.1060596

Maciver, D., Rutherford, M., Johnston, L. and Roy, A.S. (2023) 'Prevalence of neurodevelopmental differences and autism in Scottish primary schools 2018-2022', *Autism Research*, 16(12), 2403-2414. https://doi.org/10.1002/aur.3063

Male, I., Farr, W. and Reddy, V. (2020) 'Should clinical services for children with possible ADHD, autism or related conditions be delivered in an integrated neurodevelopmental pathway?', *Integrated Healthcare Journal*, 2(1). https://doi.org/10.1136/ihj-2019-000037

McCadden, E.R. (2024) 'Social story intervention through the neurodiversity lens', *Topics in Language Disorders*, 44(4), 321-330. https://doi.org/10.1097/TLD.0000000000000355

Mencap. (2020) How common is learning disability? Available at: https://www.mencap.org.uk/learning-disability-explained/research-and-statistics/how-common-learning-disability (accessed 30 October 2024).

Miller, T.M. and Kagan, D.R. (2019) 'Moving from categorical to dimensional approaches in the assessment of neurodevelopmental disorders', *Clinical Psychology: Science and Practice*, 26(4), e12309. https://doi.org/10.1111/cpsp.12309

Milton, D., Gurbuz, E., and López, B. (2022) 'The "double empathy problem": Ten years on', *Autism*, 26(8), 1901-1903. https://doi.org/10.1177/13623613221129123

Morgan, A. (2020) Support for learning: All our children and all their potential. Scottish Government. Available at: https://www.gov.scot/publications/review-additional-support-learning-implementation/ (accessed 19 November 2024).

Norbury, C.F., Gooch, D., Wray, C., Baird, G., Charman, T., Simonoff, E., Vamvakas, G. and Pickles, A. (2016) 'The impact of nonverbal ability on prevalence and clinical presentation of language disorder: Evidence from a population study', *Journal of Child Psychology and Psychiatry*, 57(11), 1247-1257. https://doi.org/10.1111/jcpp.12573

Nyholmer, M., Wronski, M.L., Hog, L., Kuja-Halkola, R., Lichtenstein, P., Lundstrom, S., Larsson, H., Taylor, M.J., Bulik, C.M. and Dinkler, L. (2024) 'Neurodevelopmental and psychiatric conditions in 600 Swedish children with the ARFID phenotype', *medRxiv*, 2024-05. https://doi.org/10.1101/2024.05.16.24307471

Panceri, C., Sbruzzi, G., Zanella, L. W., Wiltgen, A., Procianoy, R.S., Silveira, R.C. and Valentini, N.C. (2024) 'Developmental coordination disorder in preterm children: A systematic review and meta-analysis', *European Journal of Neuroscience*, 60(3), 4128-4147. https://doi.org/10.1111/ejn.16320

Patrick, M.E., Shaw, K.A., Dietz, P.M., Baio, J., Yeargin-Allsopp, M., Bilder, D.A. and Maenner, M.J. (2021) 'Prevalence of intellectual disability among eight-year-old children from selected communities in the United States, 2014', *Disability and Health Journal*, 14(2), 101023. https://doi.org/10.1016/j.dhjo.2020.101023

Pehlivanidis, A., Papanikolaou, K., Mantas, V., Kalantzi, E., Korobili, K., Xenaki, L.A., Vassiliou, G. and Papageorgiou, C. (2020) 'Lifetime co-occurring psychiatric disorders in newly diagnosed adults with attention deficit hyperactivity disorder (ADHD) or/and autism spectrum disorder (ASD)', *BMC Psychiatry*, 20, 1-12. https://doi.org/10.1186/s12888-020-02828-1

Pellicano, E. and den Houting, J. (2022) 'Annual research review: Shifting from "normal science" to neurodiversity in autism science', *Journal of Child Psychology and Psychiatry*, 63(4), 381-396. https://doi.org/10.1111/jcpp.13534

Prizant, B.M., Wetherby, A.M., Rubin, E., Laurent, A.C. and Rydell, P.J. (2006) *The SCERTS Model: A Comprehensive Educational Approach for Children with Autism Spectrum disorders*, vol. 1. Baltimore, MD: Paul H. Brookes Publishing.

Raymaker, D.M. (2020) 'Shifting the system: AASPIRE and the loom of science and activism'. In S.K. Kapp (ed.) *Autistic Community and the Neurodiversity Movement: Stories from the Frontline*. Cham: Springer Nature, pp. 133-145.

RCSLT (Royal College of Speech and Language Therapists) (2023) 'Autism guidance: supporting children and young people with autism', 2nd edn. RCSLT. Available at: https://www.rcslt.org/members/clinical-guidance/autism/autism-guidance/ (accessed 22 November 2024).

Rong, Y., Yang, C.-J., Jin, Y., and Wang, Y. (2021) 'Prevalence of attention-deficit/hyperactivity disorder in individuals with autism spectrum disorder: A meta-analysis', *Research in Autism Spectrum Disorders*, 83. https://doi.org/10.1016/j.rasd.2021.101759

Rutherford, M., Baxter, J., Grayson, Z., Johnston, L. and O'Hare, A. (2020) 'Visual supports at home and in the community for individuals with autism spectrum disorders: A scoping review', *Autism*, 24(2), 447–469. https://doi.org/10.1177/1362361319871756

Rutherford, M. and Johnston, L. (2022) 'Rethinking autism assessment, diagnosis, and intervention within a neurodevelopmental pathway framework'. In M. Carotenuto (ed.), *Autism Spectrum Disorders: Recent Advances and New Perspectives*. IntechOpen.

Rutherford, M., Maciver, D., Johnston, L., Prior, S. and Forsyth, K. (2021) 'Development of a pathway for multidisciplinary neurodevelopmental assessment and diagnosis in children and young people', *Children*, 8(11), 1033. https://doi.org/10.3390/children8111033

Sayal, K., Prasad, V., Daley, D., Ford, T. and Coghill, D. (2018) 'ADHD in children and young people: Prevalence, care pathways, and service provision', *The Lancet Psychiatry*, 5(2), 175–186. https://doi.org/10.1016/s2215-0366(17)30167-0

Scottish Government (2004) The Education (Additional Support for Learning) (Scotland) Act 2004 (Amended 2009). Available at: https://www.legislation.gov.uk/asp/2004/4/contents (accessed 19 November 2024).

Scottish Government (2017) 'Getting it right for every child (GIRFEC)'. Available at: https://www.gov.scot/policies/girfec/(accessed 19 November 2024).

Scottish Intercollegiate Guidelines Network (2019) 'Children and young people exposed prenatally to alcohol A national clinical guideline SIGN156'. Available at: https://www.sign.ac.uk/media/1092/sign156.pdf. (accessed 19 November 2024).

Sedgewick, F., Hull, L. and Ellis, H. (2021) *Autism and Masking: How and Why People Do It, and the Impact It Can Have*. London: Jessica Kingsley Publishers.

Sonuga-Barke, E.J. (2020) ' "People get ready": Are mental disorder diagnostics ripe for a Kuhnian revolution?', *Journal of Child Psychology and Psychiatry*, 61(1), 1–3. https://doi.org/10.1111/jcpp.13181

Stans, S.E.A., Dalemans, R.J.P., De Witte, L.P. and Beurskens, A.J.H.M. (2019) 'Using Talking Mats to support conversations with communication vulnerable people: A scoping review', *Technology and Disability*, 30(4), 153–176. https://doi.org/10.3233/tad-180219

Stroupková, L., Vyhnalová, M., Kolář, S., Knedlíková, L., Packanová, I., Bittnerová, A.M., Nováková, N., Kučerová, H.P., Horák, O., Ošlejšková, H. and Theiner, P. (2024) 'Use of telehealth in autism spectrum disorder assessment in children: Evaluation of an online diagnostic protocol including the brief observation of symptoms of autism', *Journal of Autism and Developmental Disorders*. https://doi.org/10.1007/s10803-024-06524-x

Sutton, K. (2024) 'The myth of brokenness: ableism and anti-ableism in the field of speech-language pathology'. Western Washington University. Available at: https://cedar.wwu.edu/cgi/viewcontent.cgi?article=1810&context=wwu_honors (accessed 26 November 2024).

Van Bael, K., Scarfo, J., Suleyman, E., Katherveloo, J., Grimble, N. and Ball, M. (2024) 'A systematic review and meta-analysis of the relationship between subjective interoception and alexithymia: Implications for construct definitions and measurement', *PloS One*, 19(11), e0310411. https://doi.org/10.1371/journal.pone.0310411

Weitzman, E. (2024) 'Neurodiversity-affirming practice'. Available at: https://www.hanen.org/information-tips/neurodiversity-affirming-practice (accessed 25 November 2024).

Welsh Government (2021). 'Additional Learning Needs (ALN) Code for Wales 2021'. Available at: https://gov.wales/additional-learning-needs-code (accessed 19 November 2024).

Wiig, E. H., Semel, E. and Secord, W. A. (2013) *Clinical Evaluation of Language Fundamentals–Fifth Edition (CELF-5)*. Bloomington, IN: Pearson.

WHO (World Health Organization) (2007). *International Classification of Functioning, Disability and Health: Children and Youth Version: ICF-CY*. Geneva: World Health Organization.

WHO (World Health Organization) (2019). *International Classification of Diseases for Mortality and Morbidity Statistics*, 11th edn. Available at: https://icd.who.int/ (accessed 25 November 2024).

Wu, S., Zhao, J., De Villiers, J., Liu, X. L., Rolfhus, E., Sun, X., Jiang, F. (2023) 'Prevalence, co-occurring difficulties, and risk factors of developmental language disorder: First evidence for Mandarin-speaking children in a population-based study', *The Lancet Regional Health - Western Pacific*, 34, 100713. https://doi.org/10.1016/j.lanwpc.2023.100713

Xie, S., Heuvelman, H., Magnusson, C., Rai, D., Lyall, K., Newschaffer, C. J. and Abel, K. (2017) 'Prevalence of autism spectrum disorders with and without intellectual disability by gestational age at birth in the Stockholm youth cohort: A register linkage study', *Paediatric and Perinatal Epidemiology*, 31(6), 586–594. https://doi.org/10.1111/ppe.12413

Yan, X., Li, Y., Li, Q., Li, Q., Xu, G., Lu, J. and Yang, W. (2024) 'Prevalence of autism spectrum disorder among children and adolescents in the United States from 2021 to 2022', *Journal of Autism and Developmental Disorders*, 1–7. https://doi.org/10.1007/s10803-024-06390-7

14 Social, emotional and mental health needs
Trauma-informed and anxiety-aware care

Susan McCool

What you'll learn in this chapter

- Communication support needs and social, emotional and mental health (SEMH) needs often co-occur, yet the combined complexity is frequently overlooked
- Effective practice in this area means embracing complexity and nurturing relationships, in flexible and positive approaches that are trauma-informed, and which promote self-regulation. Skilled supervision is important
- A rounded understanding of a child's communication support needs requires a biopsychosocial approach, using multiple means to understand variance across contexts. The child's own views are crucial. Dynamic assessment is valuable
- Effective intervention in SEMH contexts should promote meaningful outcomes, by removing barriers to communication participation and/or promoting functional communication goals
- While there is a place for developing an individual's communication capacities, more widespread and lasting change can come from enhancing communication accessibility. This means enabling change in the people and places around children.

Key information about SEMH

Social, emotional and mental health needs

Social, emotional and mental health (SEMH) is a collective term that points to critical dimensions of child development. Neaum (2022, p. 76) usefully defines social development as 'the growth of a child's ability to relate to others appropriately, within the social context of their life'. Emotional development, meanwhile, involves 'the progression towards the capability to feel and express emotions in ways that contribute to our own and others' wellbeing'. Mental health, meanwhile, is conceived of as being at the intersection of two continua: one representing the experience of mental disorder or psychological distress, while the other encapsulates wellbeing, including aspects such as the individual's sense of meaning, self-worth and quality of life (McCool, 2024). Diagnoses include anxiety, depression, attachment disorder, psychosis and eating disorders – among others. Traditionally, distinctions were drawn between internalising disorders such as anxiety and externalising conditions such as conduct disorders or hyperactivity. Now, a more nuanced view acknowledges that distress typically underlies and/or accompanies overt behaviours. Notions of equilibrium and growth permeate most contemporary accounts of mental health. It is a dynamic concept, reflecting continual interactions between multiple factors within and beyond the individual.

Note the crucial role of relational and contextual elements in the above definitions. Children are most shaped by their relationships in everyday contexts. To flourish, every child needs crucial things from the people and places around them. And what does every child need? Safety, consistency, and a sense that they have an unconditionally valued place in their world, now and in their future. Autonomy. Responsiveness. Love. Things that are easy to say and hard for many parents and practitioners to provide.

Many children need additional support to bolster their social and emotional development and to promote mental health. SEMH needs arise from a complex mix of interacting factors. That is why a biopsychosocial approach is recommended (see Chapter 1). Children may be biologically primed to need additional support: through genetic predisposition; through exposure to neurotoxins such as alcohol at the foetal stage of development; or through the impact of early life adversity on the developing brain and nervous system. Psychological aspects such as temperament have an influence. Social challenges arising within the context around the child, too, are often significant, leading to experiences such as displacement, discrimination, poverty, trauma, and maltreatment. Children facing these additional challenges require more careful consideration, and often they need greater intensity and coordination of effort and resource. Mainstone-Cotton (2021) suggests that SEMH needs span three key everyday areas of functioning: relationships, participation, and change.

Children are dependent on adults, so their likelihood of getting what they need depends on the capacity of close contacts to provide it. In turn, this is influenced by how well resourced those key adults are, materially and emotionally. Where key adults are not adequately equipped, the chances are greatly reduced that children in their care (personally *or* professionally) will get what they need. As a result, there is escalation in urgency and scale of children's SEMH need. And so, the cycle continues, with a close inter-relationship between children's escalating needs and others' increasingly stretched capacities to recognise or meet those needs.

The landscape of specialist services for children with SEMH needs is diverse and reflects multiple different orientations. The network includes various forms of educational provision, psychological services, the care system, youth justice services and Child and Adolescent Mental Health Services (CAMHS). Despite distinct pathways and often siloed working, it should be noted that there is substantial overlap in the populations served across this varied landscape. Greater service integration would be transformative.

SEMH and speech and language therapy (SLT)

It is misguided to assume that SEMH needs arise *exclusively* within specialist services or systems. Many – perhaps most – children's needs are not formally identified, which is why it is impossible to accurately determine prevalence. Since SEMH is a core strand of child development, all practitioners should be mindful that wherever there are many children, there are many children with additional SEMH needs.

Moreover, while it sometimes suits us to focus on developmental dimensions as if they are distinct, it is important to remember that in practice, all areas of development are 'interrelated, inseparable and interdependent' (Neaum, 2022). Changes in any area will affect the others in reciprocal developmental cascades. Importantly, both language and cognition are closely intertwined with social and emotional aspects of development.

All practitioners must be alert to elevated levels of SEMH needs among children with speech, language and communication needs (SLCN). Accumulated research highlights, for instance, that around half of children with Developmental Language Disorder (DLD) have significant SEMH needs (Conti-Ramsden et al., 2019; Hentges et al., 2021; Donolato et al., 2022). Elevated levels of SEMH needs have been identified across many traditional SLT client groups, including Deaf children, those with cleft conditions, and children with developmental (non-progressive) motor disorder (McCool, 2024).

Conversely, there is a high prevalence of SLCN in populations with identified SEMH needs. Social communication differences are closely linked with vulnerability in mental health (Dall, Fellinger and Holzinger, 2022), including eating disorders (Solmi et al., 2020). Many children with anxiety diagnoses have been shown to experience challenges in oral and written language (Sbicigo et al., 2020). Situational/Selective mutism, currently categorised as an anxiety disorder, often co-occurs with wider SLCN (Hipolito and Johnson, 2021). High levels of SLCN have been identified in children who were prenatally exposed to alcohol (Kippin et al., 2021), those who have experienced maltreatment (Hyter, 2021; Palazon-Carrion and Sala-Roca, 2020) and those who are care-experienced (Maguire et al., 2021). Likewise, accumulated research underscores rates of SLCN at up to 60% among children and young people in conflict with the law (Chow et al., 2022).

Although neurodevelopmental conditions such as autism, ADHD and intellectual disability are conceptually distinct from SEMH, research confirms significantly overlapping populations. Complex communication needs pervade this landscape (McCool, 2024). Importantly, communication support needs often remain overlooked and unmet in children with SEMH - and vice versa (McCool, 2024). Services are siloed, and professionals aren't primed to identify associated needs (Hancock et al., 2023). The consequences of unmet needs are far-reaching:

- an incomplete or inaccurate understanding emerges
- intervention is insufficient, inappropriate or inaccessible
- impact of support is diminished
- disillusionment and disengagement ensue.

It is important, then, that practitioners with a focus on either SLCN or SEMH are equipped to identify and respond to interrelated needs in these key developmental domains.

Important points about SLT practice in SEMH

Embrace complexity

The developmental domains covered by SLCN and SEMH carry elements of ambiguity. There is often debate about the meaning, scope of and relationship between different components (McCool, 2024).

Changes in diagnostic classification systems mean that boundaries between different conditions are re-drawn periodically, often introducing new ways of thinking about challenges children encounter in their development (Foulkes, 2022). In part, confusion arises because of the close interrelatedness between SLCN and SEMH.

Putting children's needs first requires a pragmatic approach that embraces developmental complexity. Effective practitioners in this area are open to the prospect of working across traditional role boundaries. As ever, collaboration and transparency are key, as are training, and support to ensure that practitioners operate within their scope of competence.

Nurture relationships

Relationships are tricky, especially in the face of historic mistrust, communication challenges, insecurities, adversities and scarce resources. This applies to relationships between professionals and children, families and communities. It also applies to relationships between historically separate professional groups. Effective practice involves negotiating sometimes difficult terrain with warmth, compassion, flexibility, positivity, determination and good humour (Ungar, 2021). It means investing effort to develop and maintain positive and reciprocal relationships.

Positive framing

Unfortunately, stigma often accompanies the term SEMH, explicitly or implicitly. Negative framing abounds, in a focus on surface *behaviour* rather than underlying *distress*; and in the emphasis on *difficulties or deficits* assumed to reside within a child, rather than *needs* arising from complex origins. Effective practitioners in this area will adopt anti-discriminatory language and approaches, focused on children's needs and rights.

Trauma-informed and anxiety-aware care

Although often overlooked, past or present trauma is pervasive among people with SEMH needs. A priority of trauma-informed care is nurturing trusting relationships (O'Leary, Rupert and Lotty, 2023). Effective practitioners will employ grounding techniques, and act to minimise trauma reminders. They will understand the value of clear boundaries, while anticipating, accepting and compassionately responding to confusion or challenges around boundaries (Yehuda, 2016).

Likewise, anxiety frequently occurs in this population, as a primary or secondary characteristic. Flexibility is the watchword for effective practitioners, with an emphasis on co-creating opportunities, rather than making demands. At the same time, they will work in partnership to dismantle patterns that may unhelpfully reinforce avoidance. Truly child-centred and family-centred care is the aim, with the intention of supporting the child's enhanced participation.

Routine situational demands can trigger extreme distress or fear in some children, resulting in variable responses, including fight, flight, freeze, fawn and flop reactions. Where appropriate, practitioners will employ 'low-demand, low-arousal', defocused and de-escalatory approaches (Table 14.1).

- Sit beside rather than opposite the child
- Focus on a joint activity, not on the child
- Avoid direct questions. Instead, wonder aloud, offering tentative possibilities
- Be comfortable with silence
- Value non-spoken contributions, and show that they have been understood and accepted
- Be careful about expressions of praise – some might overwhelm specific children
- Exercise caution with traditional reward systems: these can reinforce a sense of power of authority figures and feel confrontational. Instead, jointly agree aims and responses.
- Beyond a few non-negotiable boundaries, compromise and negotiate
- Keep focused on what really matters
- Small steps . . .
- Circle back as required

Table 14.1 Low-demand, low-arousal strategies

Promote self-regulation

Supporting the growth of self-regulation is within the scope of SLT practice (Binns, Hutchinson and Cardy, 2019). Enhanced self-regulation allows the child to plan, focus, and stay engaged in the face of distraction or challenge. Many children require support, via dynamic co-regulatory interactions, to form stronger foundations in self-regulation. Binns, Hutchinson and Cardy (2019) provide a framework of useful strategies which SLTs can integrate in their work, including environmental modifications, modelling, co-construction and strategic questioning. The aim is to mitigate stressors and scaffold children towards increasingly autonomous use of relevant skills.

Supported professional development

Practitioners engaged in the realities of supporting children's combined communication and SEMH needs must be adequately equipped for the job. This means ensuring that they develop – and maintain – the required knowledge, skills and attitudes to practice effectively. It also involves reflecting deeply on one's practice.

Skilled supervision provides essential support for reflection and development in SEMH practice (Cross, 2025). Supervision enhances practice, mitigates the risk of indirect trauma, and sustains personal and professional vitality.

Understanding children's SLCN in the SEMH context

What are we trying to achieve?

The attempt to understand children's communication needs in the SEMH context may focus on populations or individuals. For example, it can be worthwhile for services to reflect on common needs among their service users, with the intention of changing routine practice to benefit all.

Equally, there are occasions that merit detailed consideration of individual functioning, and this section focuses on that. As ever, the primary purpose of assessment activity is to understand how best to support a child. In this context, several intentions may drive this process. It may be relevant to establish if diagnosable conditions play a part. Additionally, it is valuable to explore all aspects contributing to a child's situation, to make sense of the child's unique experience, and to provide them with a sense of being understood. Moreover, it provides a solid baseline against which to measure the benefits brought about by the support offered.

The relationship between SLCN and SEMH is complex, variable and multifactorial. While communication needs may be primary in some children, the reverse may be true in others. Needs in both areas simultaneously may arise from shared underlying factors or may be influenced by a range of moderating and mediating variables. Cognition, executive functioning and emotional regulation also play important roles. To fully account for this complexity, a biopsychosocial approach (see Chapter 1) is recommended for a rounded appreciation of all elements (Clegg, 2020; McCool, 2024).

A wide-ranging understanding of the full multiplicity of factors is called a formulation. It takes account of factors both past and present, including those within and beyond the child. It encapsulates not only perceived challenges, but also strengths and potential solutions. Importantly, it also considers variation across contexts, times, communication partners, situational demands and medication status, for example.

Above all, the understanding gained should be functional: it should establish the 'goodness of fit' between what the child needs for optimal function in both SLCN and SEMH and what is typically available to them in their everyday contexts. It will ascertain the causes and consequences of any mismatch between the child's needs and the support available. It will ascertain, in a dynamic way, the capacity for change in both the child and their environment. As an outcome, this process will establish the nature of support needed to bring change about in the optimum way.

A full appreciation will consider all aspects of speech, language and communication. Certain aspects, though, are likely to merit special consideration in the SEMH context:

- social communication/ pragmatics, including all aspects of narrative
- comprehension of language, including questions, abstract and non-literal language
- the child's self-monitoring and signalling of comprehension breakdown
- expressive language, including semantics (especially emotions vocabulary) and syntax (especially as used in sequencing, cause and effect and formulating questions)
- conversational participation, balance and repair.

How do we do it?

A comprehensive outlook should draw on multiple methods of gathering information, to give insights from varied perspectives. Complexities and sensitivities in the SEMH context highlight limitations in some methods and benefits of others. Structured observation, for example, has its limitations. Being observed tends to change the way people behave. Extra sensitivity is also warranted in the SEMH context, especially in circumstances where people have experienced trauma or have heightened anxiety. In any case, it would be impractical to observe across all relevant contexts. Nonetheless, watchful and reflective practitioners can often glean valuable understanding from informally observed glimpses of interaction between the child and key others.

Standardised assessments also have drawbacks in the SEMH context. The standardisation sample may not sufficiently reflect the child's background. Children who are highly sensitive to perceived judgement can find testing intolerable. Unreliable results can emerge in children with uneven profiles, or who find it difficult to engage with the formal structure. Where test administration is deemed necessary, assessors often employ allowable adjustments such as movement breaks and tangible rewards. Sometimes, in the interests of probing children's capacities, adjustments go beyond those permissible: thus, if testing beyond the ceiling item or providing extra prompts, reporting should highlight that numerical results are invalid.

Various assessments attempt to gauge social communication and pragmatic language in a 'semi-structured' way, typically by setting up 'role-playing' style scenarios between the child and clinician. Caution is advised, for not only do these poorly emulate any 'real-life' situation but also, for some children, encountering trusted adults behaving in unusual and unpredictable ways can be anxiety-inducing or even a trauma reminder (Yehuda, 2016). Alternative methods, therefore, often become the basis of a sound appreciation of a child's SLCN in the SEMH context. These include checklists/conversations, discourse analysis and dynamic assessment.

It is crucial to tap into the child's own perspectives of their SLCN and their priorities for change. First, it is important to establish trust, as the child may have built up various means of concealing communication challenges from themselves and others, as a protective mechanism in response to repeated distressing encounters. Rating scales and checklists can be very useful, especially if they can be adapted to overcome potential communication barriers. Examples can be found in McCool (2024) and Branagan et al. (2020). The child's comprehension should be supported throughout, via the reduction and simplification of language, and selective use of visual supports (see Table 14.2). The same strategies should be used to reduce the reliance on verbal responses from the child. Talking Mats deserves mention as a valuable approach to increase accessibility of all manner of discussion topics.

---

1. Ask what would make your communication better . . .
2. And do it!
3. Be alert that the person may not signal a lack of understanding
4. Use the person's name frequently, especially at the start of utterances
5. Say your message in the simplest way
6. Split it into small chunks
7. Pause between chunks
8. Use clear, everyday words
9. Stress key words
10. Flag up the important bits
11. Flag up order: first . . . then . . .
12. Use communication supports (see Table 14.3)
13. Offer clear explanation and justification for using communication support tools
14. Co-create the design, use and evaluation of communication support tools
15. Be straightforward – avoid ambiguous language, such as inference and irony
16. Be direct – avoid euphemisms and acronyms
17. Be concrete – avoid hypotheticals and conditionals
18. Use active language, for example, 'Mia ate the apple', not 'the apple was eaten by Mia'
19. Repeat key points in different ways
20. Check understanding by asking the person to repeat in their own way (words or pictures)

Table 14.2 20 adjustments to support communication

A multi-dimensional understanding of SLCN also relies on the valuable perspectives of parents/ caregivers, teachers and relevant others. Checklists can be useful if interpreted with caution, for example, the standardised Children's Communication Checklist 2 (Bishop, 2003). Informal checklists and rating scales are more adaptable and can be used flexibly to support meaningful conversations, see McCool (2024) and Branagan et al. (2020) for examples.

Discourse analysis involves sampling the child's conversations, narratives and explanatory language and analysing grammar and/ or pragmatics (Kellaghan, 2020). Dynamic assessment provides real-world information about how the child responds to variations in the kind of support offered and its intensity (Hasson and Joffe, 2007).

Overall, a rounded understanding of SLCN, gained through dynamic engagement, can usefully guide decision-making. It helps identify the real priorities of all the relevant parties. It helps select effective approaches (and avoid those that are not). Further, it signals how to adapt the communication accessibility of any SEMH support offered, optimising its potential benefits.

Supporting children's needs in SEMH

This section outlines the main SLT roles for supporting children's communication in the SEHM context. A comprehensive strategy often simultaneously targets more than one of the following inter-related aspects: the communication environment, communication partners, and/or an individual's communication capabilities (see the EPIC model, Chapter 1).

Key principles inform this work. Goals should arise from, and therefore be meaningful to, the people who are intended to benefit. As such, objectives can include mitigating challenges as well as promoting positive outcomes. Aims include promoting functional communication for developing and sustaining real-world relationships, and removing or reducing communication barriers (Hobson et al., 2022).

Optimum impact can come from working with a child's contacts and contexts to boost communication accessibility. Far-reaching value comes from helping children to understand and be understood – both in their everyday lives, and when receiving support for SEMH needs.

Roles in enhancing the communication environment

SLTs have a role in promoting inclusive communication within universal settings such as mainstream schools. Lots of children who have SEMH needs are never identified as such and many others are supported within non-specialist settings. Strategies range from raising awareness through social media campaigns to the introduction of accreditation schemes whereby schools and other settings can attain and maintain 'communication-friendly' status.

SLTs also have a pivotal role in promoting accessible communication in services tailored specifically to children's SEMH needs. The Royal College of Speech and Language Therapists in the UK (RCSLT, 2022) has created a resource to inform SLTs' work in this area, highlighting 'Five Good Communication Standards' which SEMH services can use to evaluate and enhance their approach:

1. There is a detailed and easily accessible record of how best to communicate with each child.
2. Practitioners value and competently implement those recommendations.
3. The service fosters relationships and opportunities that allow communication to flourish.
4. Each child is supported to understand and express their wellbeing needs.
5. Each child is meaningfully involved in decision-making about all aspects of their care, including indicating how well significant people communicate with them.

Helping services meet and uphold these Standards requires SLTs to focus on the communication approach of key people. We turn next to that aspect of practice.

Roles in supporting and advising communication partners

SLTs have a role in advocating for the importance of SLCN in SEMH contexts. SLTs doing this advocacy work are agents of change. People find change uncomfortable. Clearly, then, to be effective, SLTs need to be skilled in persuasion, negotiation and collaboration. Raising awareness is often a valuable first step. Colleagues' engagement may be gained through the prospect of achieving a more rounded understanding of children and how to help them, prompting more effective intervention and leading to enhanced satisfaction all round. Parents and other informal communication partners may be drawn by the hope of greater connection with the child, and in helping their situation.

A crucial role for SLTs is to enable colleagues to apply appropriate judgements, skills and strategies to support children's communication. SEMH assessment processes and therapeutic work are often talk-based and conducted in a relational context that relies on assumed communication adeptness. SEMH interventions are often delivered in socially demanding group settings or following manualised approaches that assume foundational communication competencies. Adaptation is often required to make intervention optimally accessible for children with SLCN (see Tables 14.2 and 14.3). Staff can be equipped with the required communication-support competencies via coaching and mentoring, bespoke training, or being signposted to open online training and resources (see Recommended resources).

Scales, diagrams and charts
- Likert scales and rating scales
- Emotion thermometers/ traffic lights/ ladders
- Pyramids/ icebergs
- Timelines
- Flowcharts

Table 14.3 Examples of communication support tools (can be combined)

(Continued)

Symbols (and examples of their use)
- Talking Mats supported conversations
- Choice boards
- Visual timetable
- Now & Next cards
- Emoticons
- Written words (colour-coded)
- Social Stories™

Drawings, doodles and cartoons
- Visually Supported Conversations/ Comic Strip Conversations (speech bubbles/ thought bubbles, colours denote emotions)

Pictures, photographs and videos
- Blob resources
- Emotions cards
- Sequences
- Cause and effect

Prompts cards
- e.g. Could you break that down into chunks, please?
- e.g. I need some time out, please.

Table 14.3 (Continued)

A key SLT role is to promote more effective communication between a child and their close contacts, so that they may sustain positive relationships. Regular communication partners can be helped to understand any less conventional ways in which a specific child communicates (such as behavioural indications of underlying distress or confusion). Communication partners, including parents, professionals and peers, can be supported in learning how to adapt their own approach to ensure easier and more effective communication.

Roles in supporting individual children's communication capacities

Identifying children who may have specific communication support needs is often a central role for SLTs, who can contribute valuable SLCN perspectives to SEMH team discussions of the likely needs of newly referred children, or to reviews of existing cases. Alternatively (or additionally) screening processes may be set up.

Through in-depth exploratory activity, SLTs can support a rounded understanding of individual children's SLCN needs. As an outcome, there will be a clear account of the adjustments, tools and techniques that best support each child's communication participation.

SLTs enable the child's 'voice' to be heard, gaining valuable insights into a child's perspectives and aspirations, and guiding everyone around the child to integrate the child's own views about their strengths and priorities for change. Importantly, amplifying the child's experience also serves an important safeguarding function in this uniquely vulnerable population.

There may also be varied roles in supporting and developing individual children's capacities. This may involve empowering the child to use their existing capacities more effectively, such as having the confidence to ask for the support they need. Or it could be equipping the child with useful strategies if they run into communication challenges, such as flagging up a lack of understanding, or finding ways to repair a breakdown in conversation. Where speaking situations provoke intense fears in children, sensitive application of behavioural techniques such as hierarchical exposure, stimulus fading and cognitive restructuring (among others) complements work to modify the approach of those around the child (Hipolito and Johnson, 2021). Working as part of a team, SLTs also play pivotal roles in assessing and managing eating, drinking and swallowing disorders in the SEMH population (Irish Association of Speech and Language Therapists, 2022), including Avoidant Restrictive Food Intake Disorder (ARFID).

Equally, there can be a place for equipping a child with enhanced language and communication skills. While goals can be established covering any relevant aspect of speech, language or communication, some targets frequently occur because they have an immediate functional impact:

- Vocabulary targets covering language related to emotions, bodily states, relationships, behaviours, thinking and 'the language of intervention' can enhance accessibility of SEMH processes and supports (Branagan et al., 2020)
- Enhancing language skills in narrative coherence, and for handling cause & effect and sequencing can address challenges common among trauma-experienced children (Yehuda, 2016) and those with other SEMH needs
- Support for social communication skills can assist in developing and maintaining peer and other relationships (McCool, 2024).

A flexible resource which offers comprehensive guidance for assessment and intervention in all these aspects is Language for Behaviour and Emotions (Branagan et al., 2020).

The evidence base

Intervention research is lacking (Hancock et al., 2023). Since traditional controlled studies are less applicable in this varied and vulnerable population, there is scope for more descriptive case series and cohort studies. As a starting point, McCool (2024) provides ten illustrative case examples based on the work of several specialist SLTs. Future research could usefully investigate the effectiveness of communication modifications in enhancing the accessibility of talk-based interventions in this population (Hancock et al., 2023).

Expert opinion is another important dimension of evidence-based practice. The intervention approach outlined in this chapter is supported by qualitative research incorporating the views of SLTs and mental health professionals (Hancock et al., 2023).

Equally, the views of service users and carers are pivotal elements of evidence-based practice. This chapter's functional and relational emphasis is fully supported by qualitative research with parents of children with combined SLCN and SEMH (Hobson et al., 2022). While more research seeking the views of this specific population of children would be welcome, indirect evidence supports this chapter's focus on peer relationships (Janik Blaskova and Gibson, 2021) and wellbeing (Lyons and Roulstone, 2018).

Leon's story*

Leon, 15 years old, had experienced substantial developmental trauma including neglect and abuse. Now in secure care, Leon's extreme anxiety was evident in his refusal to leave his room and as a trigger for destructive behaviour. Leon's siblings had tampered with his food in his younger years – and now he was reluctant to take prescribed medication. The SLT became involved to address the team's concerns about Leon's capacity to make informed decisions about his care. Informal observation and skilled use of Talking Mats highlighted Leon's significant difficulty in understanding what had been said. For example, he didn't understand what 'anxiety' meant. He also struggled to find the words to describe his thoughts and feelings coherently. Visual support tools were developed to facilitate discussion of key concepts, and the SLT suggested simplified language to talk, for example, about what happens in our head and body when we're anxious. Clinical colleagues described these adaptations as transformational. When initially presented with visuals to support his understanding of anxiety Leon simply said, 'How did you know? This is me.' He asked if he could keep the visuals and referred to them frequently during intervention sessions. Crucially, he consented to take key prescribed medication, which marked a turning point in his treatment and care.

Note: *Brid Corrigan, Principal SLT (CAMHS), is thanked and credited as the source of this case example.

 Summary

This chapter has described SEMH as a developmental strand closely tied to cognition, self-regulation – and communication. All children rely on adults for optimum SEMH development, but many need additional support. To engage with and benefit from SEMH help, a substantial proportion of children need communication support. Unfortunately, this need is often missed. SLTs have important roles in identifying where communication support would be valuable and in working with others to plan and implement integrated support. Currently, communication needs in the SEMH population are often undetected, reducing the impact of SEMH interventions. Evidence from professionals, parents and children shows that greater communication support would be valued. There is therefore much scope to increase recognition of the SLT's essential contribution, and to enhance service integration and collaboration.

 Recommended Resources

Clinical resource and reference guide about SLCN and mental health, produced by Orygen and Speech Pathology Australia. Available at: https://www.orygen.org.au/Training/Resources/Neurodevelopmental-disorders/Clinical-practice-points/Speech,-language-and-communication-needs-in-youth

Factsheets on SEMH produced by the Royal College of Speech and Language Therapists. Available at: https://www.rcslt.org/speech-and-language-therapy/clinical-information/social-emotional-and-mental-health/#section-2

Mind Your Words (free, open-access e-learning from the Royal College of Speech and Language Therapists). Available at: https://www.rcslt.org/learning/mind-your-words/

References

Binns, A.V., Hutchinson, L.R. and Cardy, J.O. (2019) 'The speech-language pathologist's role in supporting the development of self-regulation: a review and tutorial', *Journal of Communication Disorders*, 78, 1-17. https://doi.org/10.1016/j.jcomdis.2018.12.005

Bishop, D.V.M. (2003) *The Children's Communication Checklist-2*. London: Pearson.

Branagan, A., Cross, M. and Parsons, S. (2020) *Language for Behaviour and Emotions: A Practical Guide to Working with Children and Young People*. Abingdon: Routledge.

Chow, J.C., Wallace, E.S., Senter, R., Kumm, S. and Mason, C.Q. (2022) 'A systematic review and meta-analysis of the language skills of young offenders', *Journal of Speech, Language and Hearing Research*, 65(3), 1166-1182. https://doi.org/10.1017/S0954579421000328

Clegg, J. (2020) 'Children's communication and their mental health', in C. Jagoe and I.P. Walsh (eds), *Communication and Mental Health Disorders*. Havant: J & R Press, pp. 27-51.

Conti-Ramsden, G., Mok, P., Durkin, K., Pickles, A., Toseeb, U. and Botting, N. (2019) 'Do emotional difficulties and peer problems occur together from childhood to adolescence? The case of children with a history of developmental language disorder (DLD)', *European Child and Adolescent Psychiatry*, 28(7), 993-1004. https://doi.org.10.1007/s00787-018-1261-6

Cross, M. (2025) 'A life jacket in stormy seas: Supervision for speech and language therapists working with young people who have mental health challenges', in S. Sparkes, S. Simpson and D. Harding (eds), *Supervision in Speech and Language Therapy: Personal Stories and Professional Wisdom*. Abingdon: Routledge, pp. 80-93.

Dall, M., Fellinger, J. and Holzinger, D. (2022) 'The link between social communication and mental health from childhood to young adulthood: a systematic review', *Frontiers in Psychiatry*, 13. https://doi.org/10.3389/fpsyt.2022.944815

Donolato, E., Cardillo, R., Mammarella, I.C. and Melby-Lervag, M. (2022) 'Research review: language and specific learning disorders in children and their co-occurrence with internalizing and externalizing problems: A systematic review and meta-analysis', *The Journal of Child Psychology and Psychiatry*, 63(5), 507-518. https://doi.org/10.1111/jcpp13536

Foulkes, L. (2022) *What Mental Illness Really Is (and What It Isn't)*. London: Penguin Random House

Hancock, A., Northcott, S., Hobson, H. and Clarke, M. (2023) 'Speech, language and communication needs and mental health: the experiences of speech and language therapists and mental health professionals', *International Journal of Language and Communication Disorders*, 58(1), 52-66. https://doi.org/10.1111/1460-6984.12767

Hasson, N. and Joffe, V. (2007) 'The case for dynamic assessment in speech and language therapy', *Child Language Teaching and Therapy*, 23(1), 9-25. https://doi.org/10.1177/02565659007072142

Hentges, R.F., Devereux, C., Graham, S.A. and Madigan, S. (2021) 'Child language difficulties and internalizing and externalizing symptoms: A meta-analysis', *Child Development*, 92(4), e691-e715. https://doi.org/10.1111/cdev.13540

Hipolito, G. and Johnson, M. (2021) 'Selective mutism'. In L. Cummings (ed.), *Handbook of Pragmatic Language Disorders: Complex and Underserved Populations*. Cham: Springer Nature, pp. 247-281. https://doi.org/10.1007?978-3-030-74985-9

Hobson, H., Kalsi, M., Cotton, L., Forster, M. and Toseeb, U. (2022) 'Supporting the mental health of children with speech, language and communication needs: The views and experiences of parents', *Autism & Developmental Language Impairments*, 7. https://doi.org/10.1177/23969415211011137

Howes, R. (2023) *Reflective Clinical Supervision in Speech and Language Therapy: Strengthening Supervision Skills*. London: Routledge.

Hyter, Y. (2021) 'Childhood maltreatment consequences on social pragmatic communication: A systematic review of the literature', *Perspectives of the ASHA Special Interest Groups*, 6(2), 262-287. https://doi.org/10.1044/2021_PERSP-20-00222

Irish Association of Speech and Language Therapists (2022) 'Role of Speech and Language Therapy in Eating Disorders'. Available at: https://www.iaslt.ie/media/y31lz3o2/role-of-slt-in-eating-disorders-5th-sept-2022.pdf (accessed 16 October 2024).

Janik Blaskova, L. and Gibson, J.L. (2021) 'Reviewing the link between language abilities and peer relations in children with developmental language disorder: The importance of children's own perspectives', *Autism & Developmental Language Impairments*, 6. https://doi.org/10.1177/23969415211021515

Kellaghan, S. (2020) 'Pragmatic language and social conversational skills intervention for children with mental health disorders', in C. Jagoe and I.P. Walsh (eds), *Communication and Mental Health Disorders*. Havant: J & R Press, pp. 91–127.

Kippin, N.R., Leitao, S., Watkins, R., and Finlay-Jones, A. (2021)'Oral and written communication skills of adolescents with prenatal alcohol exposure (PAE) compared with those with no/ low PAE: A systematic review', *International Journal of Language and Communication Disorders*, 56(4), 694–718. https://doi.org/10.1111/1460-6984.12644

Lyons, R. and Roulstone, S. (2018) 'Well-being and resilience in children with speech and language disorders', *Journal of Speech, Language and Hearing Research*, 61(2), 324–344. https://doi.org.10.1044/2017_JSLHR-L-16-0391

Maguire, D., McCormack, D., Downes, C., Teggart, T., and Fosker, T. (2021) 'The impact of care-related factors on the language and communication needs of looked after and adopted children/young people', *Developmental Child Welfare*, 3(3), 235–255. https://doi.org/10.1177/25161032211021436

Mainstone-Cotton, S. (2021) *Supporting Children with Social, Emotional and Mental Health Needs in the Early Years: Practical Solutions and Strategies for Every Setting*. Abingdon: Routledge.

McCool, S. (2024) *Working with Child and Adolescent Mental Health: The Central Role of Language and Communication*. London: Routledge.

Neaum, S. (2022) *Child Development for Early Years Students and Practitioners*. 5th edn. Exeter: Learning Matters.

O'Leary, N., Rupert, A.C., and Lotty, M. (2023) 'Understanding the why: The integration of trauma-informed care into speech and language therapy practice', *Advances in Communication and Swallowing*, 26(2), 81–87. https://doi.org/10.3233/ACS-220017

Palazon-Carrion, E. and Sala-Roca, J. (2020) 'Communication and language in abused and institutionalized children: A scoping review', *Children and Youth Services Review*, 112. https://doi.org/10.1016//j.childyouth.2020104904

Royal College of Speech and Language Therapists (2022) 'Supporting children and young people with SEMH: the five good communication standards'. Available at: https://www.rcslt.org/wp-content/uploads/2022/04/RCSLT-supporting-SEMH-5-good-communication-standards.pdf (accessed 10 October 2024).

Sbicigo, J.B., Toazza, R., Becker, N., Ecker, K., Manfro, G.G. and Salles, J.F.D. (2020) 'Memory and language impairments are associated with anxiety disorder severity in childhood', *Trends in Psychiatry and Psychotherapy*, 42(2), 161–170. https://doi.org/10.1590/2237-6089-0051

Solmi, F., Bentivegna, F., Bould, H., Mandy, W., Kothari, R. and Rai, D. et al. (2020) 'Trajectories of autistic social traits in childhood and adolescence and disordered eating behaviours at 14 years: A UK general population cohort study', *Journal of Child Psychology and Psychiatry*, 62(1), 75–85. https://doi.org/10.1111/jcpp.13255

Ungar, M. (2021) *Working with Children and Youth with Complex Needs: 20 Skills to Build Resilience*. 2nd edn. London: Routledge.

Yehuda, N. (2016) *Communicating Trauma: Clinical Presentations and Interventions with Traumatized Children*. New York: Routledge.

PART V

Selected populations with specialist needs

15 Deaf children

Sarah Beazley and Judy Halden

What you'll learn in this chapter

- How commonly deafness occurs in children
- The nature of deafness (types, onset, causes and levels) and amplification devices
- Ways to check hearing levels and amplification devices
- The key role of linguistic and auditory input, and of early communication support
- A way to look at communication used with, and by, a deaf child, which considers context, conversation, language, agency and multisensory signals
- Some support approaches for environmental adaptations and conversation skill development
- Therapy ideas around meaning, grammar and speech that target challenges faced by deaf children
- A short case example to highlight ways you might work with a deaf child.

Key information about deafness

The term 'deaf' is used to describe children with all types of reduced hearing levels and in order to avoid the term 'loss', as this is not how it is always experienced. You may find the term 'Deaf' too, as an indicator of cultural and/or linguistic belonging (Friedner and Kusters, 2020). Sensitivity to changing terms around hearing levels of differing types, degrees and onset is important, but the choice of which term is used needs to remain with the individual and, for younger children, with their families.

Here the frequency of deafness in children is described, and the types, onset, causes and levels of hearing. A brief description of the technological aids that might support deaf children is also provided.

Frequency of deafness in children

There are more than 34 million deaf children in the world, the majority of whom live in low-income countries (WHO, 2024). In the UK, there are 50,000 deaf children and young people (NDCS, 2021) with around 90% born to hearing parents (Mitchell and Karchmer, 2004; Greenhalgh et al., 2023).

DOI: 10.4324/9781003671626-21

Types of deafness

- *Conductive*: affecting the outer ear through to the middle ear.
- *Sensori-neural*: affecting the inner ear and beyond (retro-cochlear). The inner part of the ear contains tiny hair cells that change sounds into electric signals. These may not develop fully or become damaged. Retro cochlear deafness affects the auditory nerve or central auditory system and leads to auditory neuropathy spectrum disorders (ANSD). This can affect 1–10% of deaf people and it presents in very variable ways from mild to severe reductions in hearing level and with differing responses to amplification devices (De Siati et al., 2020). Atypical language development out of proportion with sound detection abilities may result. Multidisciplinary teamwork is needed to confirm the diagnosis and look at options. If you notice a child's speech perception is poorer than expected from an audiogram, share that information with the audiologist. Therapy support may need to draw on approaches for children with reduced hearing and those used with developmental language disorders.
- *Mixed*: affecting either the outer and/or middle ear, as well as some part of the inner ear or beyond.

Onset

The incidence of children born deaf is 4/1000 live births and rises to approximately 20% from 12 years old (Kenna, 2015). The onset time of deafness will have a bearing on outcomes for the development of language and is described as follows:

- *congenital*: developed in utero, leading to deafness at birth;
- *acquired*: developed postnatally. This may be pre-lingual, i.e. before the acquisition of speech and language; or post-lingual, i.e. after the acquisition of speech and language.

The earlier that hearing levels are reduced, the greater the impact on language as a child will have less exposure to the home language. This highlights the importance of early diagnosis.

Aetiology

Deafness may be caused through:

- complications during pregnancy, including maternal infections, such as cytomegalovirus (CMV), rubella, herpes;
- prematurity, which increases the likelihood of infections;
- genetic disorders, such as Pendred syndrome (PDS), which is the most common syndromic form of deafness (Tesolin et al., 2021) and involves inner ear malformations. Other syndromes that cause deafness include Down Syndrome, CHARGE, Ushers, Treacher Collins, Waardenburg and Goldenhaar Syndromes. Around 50% of childhood deafness in the UK is caused by genetic changes (NDCS, n.d.).
- toxins from oto-toxic drugs used to treat meningitis and some cancers;
- unknown causes.

Levels of deafness

Levels of deafness are measured in decibels (dB) and are described as follows in the UK (BATOD, 2023):

- mild: 20-40 dB;
- moderate: 41-70 dB;
- severe: 71-95 dB;
- profound: more than 95 dB.

Averages are taken, using responses to pure tone audiometry in the better ear and can provide us with information about the distribution of different types of hearing levels in children. For example, in the UK, children with reduced hearing in only one ear make up 21%; those with mild reductions, 26%; those with moderate reductions, 31%; those with severe reductions (9%) and those with profound hearing level reductions, 12% (NDCS, 2021).

Personal amplification devices

Hearing aids (HAs), cochlear implants (CIs) and auditory brainstem implants (ABI)

Although no device can restore hearing to typical levels, these can support deaf children in making the most of their hearing potential. Digital signal processing has improved HAs significantly in recent years. Both analogue and digital HAs work by amplifying sound waves which are then transmitted from the outer ear through the middle ear to the inner ear. There they are converted into signals that the brain can process, passed up to the auditory cortex via the auditory nerve through both electrical and neurological transduction.

CIs work by conducting an electrical signal directly to the brain via the auditory nerve, bypassing the outer and middle ear altogether. The receiver is implanted surgically into the cochlea. The speech processor, worn behind the ear, transmits and converts sound waves into an electrical signal which is then passed to the receiver.

ABIs use technology similar to that of a CI but instead of electrical stimulation within the cochlea, it stimulates the cochlear nucleus in the brainstem. It thus bypasses the auditory nerve in cases where the nerves are extensively damaged, narrow or absent.

The decision to provide an implant or HA will depend on local guidelines. For example, in the UK, the National Institute for Health and Care (NICE) recommends simultaneous bilateral CIs for children with severe to profound deafness who do not receive adequate benefit from HAs (NICE, 2019).

Advantages are:

- they provide children with access to a wider range of environmental and speech sounds;
- they enable children to hear warnings, e.g. traffic noise, sirens;
- they provide better access to spoken language.

Disadvantages are:
- they have an optimum listening range of between 1-2 metres;
- they may not provide clear signals in background noise;
- they do not provide full hearing, and outcomes vary;
- equipment maintenance is required;
- implant surgery carries risks, as does any surgery.

Bone conduction listening devices

These are amplification devices that transmit sound through the skull to the inner ear and can be suitable for children with conditions that prevent the use of conventional HAs, particularly for blockages or structural anomalies of the middle ear. These can be bone-anchored HAs (BAHAs) or middle ear implants (MEIs).

Remote listening devices

Remote listening devices allow personal aids to connect to other equipment such as microphones, smartphones, tablets, and computers. These help to reduce the difficulties encountered when listening over distance.

The multidisciplinary team (MDT)

Families with deaf children can be overwhelmed with advice from a range of different professionals in health and education, such as audiologists, ENT (ear/nose/throat) consultants, speech and language therapists (SLTs), teachers of deaf children (ToDCs) and sign language support workers. Wherever possible, practices that transcend discipline-specific approaches and take account of different circumstances will enable more positive support for families (O'Neill et al., 2019; Hughes, 2022; NDCS, 2024a).

Important points about SLT practice with deaf children

As an SLT, you may meet children identified as deaf in pre-school settings, in mainstream schools and colleges, or within specialist provisions. You may also meet children who are not yet diagnosed, and you have an important role in checking this potentially unrecognized need.

In addition to good practice around collaborative working with a child and family, and the MDT to support independence in communication, some important points around SLT practice with deaf children include hearing level checks, amplification device checks, linguistic and auditory input, and early communication development.

Hearing level checks

You need to keep hearing levels in mind when you are working with any child, whether identified as deaf or not. Fluctuating or acquired changes in hearing levels may not be picked up through routine audiological assessment.

Around a third of the world's countries have universal newborn hearing screening (UNHS) in place (Neumann et al., 2020) which has enabled early introduction of aids and intervention to support deaf children in their early years. However, children may pass UNHS with mild reductions in hearing level or may pass but have changes in hearing postnatally. Families and professionals need to keep alert to potential reductions in hearing level, and delayed speech and language is seen as a significant possible indicator (Duan et al., 2022).

The points below provide some observations you can make of a child's hearing levels. You can note responses to:

- environmental sounds:
  o How do they react to sounds that are loud/quiet?
  o How do they react to sounds that are near/far?
  o How do they react to sounds that are from different directions?
- visual and tactile stimuli:
  o Do they watch faces/lips intently?
  o Do they startle when people come into line of vision?
  o Do they need touch to gain their attention?
- spoken communication input:
  o Do they respond to different voices or tones (warnings, calming)?
  o Do they respond to their name?
  o Are they alert to speech at a distance?
  o Do they show awareness of talking behind them?

In addition to initial observations, you need to check regularly that a child's hearing is functioning at a baseline you have established with them. This might be, for example, picking out names from a closed set such as of friends' names, or using the Ling Sound Test (Ling, 2012), which uses a small range of English vowels and consonants, to check perception across the speech spectrum. The approach has been developed for other languages, considering the specific frequency ranges required (Sun et al., 2018; Ondáš et al., 2022; Onen et al., 2022). Such regular checks allow you to pick up changes or problems with an amplification device.

Check amplification devices

There are some simple checks you can do to ensure a child is gaining appropriately from their amplification device. You can find helpful guides on manufacturers' websites or national support organizations (NDCS, 2024b). The child and/or family may have a good working knowledge of the device, and others in the MDT such as ToDCs or audiologists can also support you. It is important that a device is functioning fully, and it is more fruitful to spend time getting it right than continuing a session with amplification that is not working correctly.

You can check that the device is:

- available and on the child's ear;
- in the correct ear (marked with a red dot for right, outside or in the battery drawer);
- properly inserted (ask the child or others to show you if needed);
- switched on, with the battery working;
- not whistling (whistling indicates feedback caused by sound leaking out, usually due to poor mould fitting).

You can look to see if:

- the ear mould is blocked, protruding, not fitting well;
- the tubing is kinked, hard, cracked or showing condensation;
- the link between the aid and the tubing is insecurely connected.

You can check how a device is working through comments from a child; and observing consistent responses to sounds.

It is important to determine a child's understanding of their own hearing and knowledge of strategies to manage amplification devices and listening situations. For example:

- in which contexts do they hear best/worst?
- can they manage any amplification device(s) independently>
- can they seek support?

Input of language and environmental context

Language deprivation is identified as the biggest risk for deaf children (Howerton-Fox and Falk, 2019). This arises through limited access either to spoken language (due to reduced hearing levels) or to signed language (due to hearing parents' lack of familiarity).

Approaches to supporting communication often prioritize either signed or spoken language but there is no evidence yet for a definitive way to support social and educational outcomes. Communication opportunities happen in context and depend on conversational partners, who will vary in their confidence and competence in talking/signing with a deaf child. Deaf children often access a complex blend of multisensory linguistic and communicative information (Hall and Dills, 2020).

As an SLT you need to know the local resources available for deaf children and their families, such as sign language support, implant teams, visiting ToDCs. You should also consider the multisensory input that might be available to the child and the family.

This includes thinking about the communication environment and about yourself as a communicator. For example, it may help to reflect on how you move and how lip-readable you are, as well as your spoken/signed language presentation. Work with a child/family to determine the best lighting for them in different rooms, to notice background noise, to consider the impact of the number of people, and share ideas about what can or cannot be changed.

Early communication development

You may be asked to see families with deaf babies under 12 months old, especially if you work in a region of the world where UNHS is established. This will require you to use your knowledge of early communication between babies and caregivers (Beazley and Halden, 2025). There is a risk that the process of parent-infant interaction might stall due to a deaf child not hearing a caregiver's input at the same time as attending to an object or event and/or to the caregiver talking as if they can be fully heard or limiting talk, assuming the child cannot understand.

Visual-tactile strategies for this early stage have emerged from research looking at how deaf parents establish communication with their deaf babies, and this may help you in supporting maintenance of the infant's natural attention to multisensory signals (Roos et al., 2016).

Understanding deaf children's needs

Some 40% of deaf children are identified with additional difficulties (Inscoe and Bones, 2016). Given this high percentage, it is important for a SLT to check whether all skills, such as those of motor, play and cognitive development are emerging evenly and as expected. In this section we focus on support relating specifically to reduced hearing levels.

Communication and language needs

As language deprivation remains the greatest risk for deaf children, their most important need is that of maximized input. While technology continues to improve access to audition, access to language and communication is still limited by the range of hearing, and the quality and quantity of input from conversational partners. Input is a key feature across the framework in Figure 15.1 that we use as a guide to the areas of communication we can monitor with deaf children and their families.

Context

The physical and linguistic environment will significantly influence the input to which a deaf child is exposed. Lighting, background noise, distance from speakers, reverberation, number

```
C        Conversational skills (discourse and pragmatics)              O
                ▸ the purpose of a conversation          I
O               ▸ the rules of conversation                             U
                ▸ awareness of the listeners             N
N               ▸ non-verbal signals                                    T
                                                         P
T                                                                       P
         Language skills (language/modality)             U
E                                                                       U
                ▸ semantics/meaning                      T
X               ▸ grammar                                               T
                ▸ intelligibility spoken/signed
T
```

⟵——————— deaf individual's agency ———————⟶

⟵——————— access to multi-sensory communication ———————⟶

Figure 15.1 A framework for looking at communication

of people, topic clarity and factors such as the familiarity of conversational partners with a child or with deafness in general, all create different contexts which influence access to auditory and visual information. It is important you note such factors to determine their impact on a deaf child's opportunities to develop communication across various settings.

Conversation

Despite good speech and language outcomes in test situations, deaf children struggle to function in areas that are important to them, such as accessing information and participating socially (Rijke et al., 2021). They have fewer opportunities to learn why people communicate, and how conversations start, are maintained, repaired, and finished. The parallel skills of interpreting non-verbal signals of communication and becoming aware of listeners' needs may also be less developed because of language deprivation stemming from reduced hearing levels.

We naturally put in strategies to avoid conversational breakdown and such tactics have been observed when adults talk to young deaf children, using more directives, less high-level language, fewer mental states references, shorter utterances and persisting features of infant-directed speech than with hearing children of the same age (Dirks et al., 2020; Lovcevic et al., 2022; Brock and Hampton, 2023). This unbalanced sharing of conversational responsibility reduces deaf children's chances to be active communicators.

Observing the dynamic input of caregivers, siblings, peers and extended family as they converse with deaf children will help you to support development of discourse and pragmatic skills which have been described as 'the missing piece' in maximizing their potential and wellbeing (Szarkowski et al., 2020).

Language

Deaf children often present with delays and gaps in vocabulary, grammar and speech due to incomplete auditory access restricting overhearing opportunities and limiting the saliency of grammatical and acoustic phonetic features (Golestani, Jalilevand and Kamali, 2018; Carrigan and Coppola 2020; Holt, Bruggeman and Demuth, 2023). You will also need to consider the cumulative effect of limited language access and carefully discriminate disorder from delay or difference (Hall, 2020).

Delayed spoken grammar and vocabulary can be perceived by peers as immature, which may impact on social inclusion of deaf children (Batten, Oakes and Alexander, 2014). Small differences in intelligibility are quickly judged and can leave deaf people embarrassed, vulnerable and distressed (Kyle, 1993; Freeman et al., 2017).

Word endings can be difficult for deaf children to perceive, especially those using high frequency sounds such as /s/ for English plurals or possessives. These outward signs of language skill must build on foundations of input, and you need to monitor all linguistic aspects surrounding a deaf child. For example, caregiver use of sensory/cognitive/affective verbs that support the development of theory of mind, or peer repair strategies with a deaf child in school.

Agency

Deaf children can be active participants in learning about language and communication. However, through a combination of restricted access to language and changes in the quantity and quality of others' input, they may have limited awareness of communication unless directed to them (Cole and Flexer, 2019). You can support their learning about the value of understanding others and being understood, and of observing communication between others as they develop skills in becoming an independent communicator.

Multisensory communication

Deaf children can have very differing experiences of language; some with access to spoken language(s) through early audiological input and interventions; others with access to a national sign language; and still others with very limited or no language exposure until they reach school (Howerton-Fox and Falk, 2019). They often access a complex blend of multisensory information that varies across conversational partners (Hall and Dills, 2020).

As deaf children do not get full access to spoken language in the way that hearing people do, account should be taken of multisensory learning needs. Where children are using mixed modalities to communicate, you will need to learn about bimodal transcription (Parker, 1999; Pichler et al., 2010; Beazley and Halden, 2025).

Assessments

Using the framework in Figure 15.1, you can build up a picture of the support you can offer a deaf child and those around them. Various approaches can help you, including the use of published assessments, questionnaires and checklists.

Published assessments

There is a wide range of published assessments available, including useful resources from the CI and HA companies, and from charities focusing on deafness. Examples include Personal Understanding of Deafness (PUD) (BATOD, n.d.) and Success from the Start (NDCS, 2020).

You may want to use formal assessments that look in detail at aspects of language, but many are not standardized with deaf children, and results and scores must be used with caution. Some tests have been designed for deaf children who sign and require testers competent in the language.

Questionnaires

Seeking the views of deaf children and their conversation partners is an important part of working in partnership to identify approaches and strategies for expanding communication skills. For example, you could develop questions for a teacher about a deaf child's functional understanding in school, for a parent about the use of amplification devices, or for a deaf teenager about their listening experiences in school.

Purpose		Deaf child	Conversation partner
Conversation	looking after own needs		
	sharing topics		
	directing		
Narrative	reporting and commenting on experiences, events		
	recounting		
	imagining		
Expository	explaining and reflecting on a process		
	predicting		
Other	projecting into feelings of others		

Table 15.1 Purpose of communication checklist

Checklists

We have developed a range of checklists (Beazley and Halden, 2025) to support our observations in the areas shown in Figure 15.1, one of which, looking at reasons for communication, is shown in Table 15.1.

Supporting deaf children's needs

Overview of approaches to management/intervention

Many management approaches that are used widely in SLT can be included in your support, but we highlight here some additional or specific ideas for working with deaf children.

Targeting the child's environment

Given that language deprivation is the greatest risk for deaf children (Howerton-Fox and Falk, 2019), you need to support the input of conversation and language. This can start with you, a family and, over time, the child, assessing the context and making adjustments to improve opportunities to access auditory and visual information and to avoid listening fatigue (Davis and Hornsby, 2023). For example, a remote listening device such as a radio aid might help a small child to be more aware of the interactive chat in the family car; an educational sign language interpreter could enable access to the curriculum for a deaf student; and holding a baby close and facing the speaker would provide greater opportunity for perception of multisensory communication.

Supporting conversation

Information and strategies are needed for both a deaf child and those around them.

Conversational control

Conversations where others choose the topics, and ask frequent questions to avoid conversational breakdown, can feel quite stilted and often indicate that a child has had limited opportunity to notice and experience conversational breakdown or to learn how to avoid or repair such instances. To counter natural adaptations that others make in response to a deaf child's perceived capacities, and to meet the goal of mutual understanding, some coaching of conversational partners can provide experience for a deaf child in conversation management skills (Wood et al., 1986; Ambrose et al., 2015). For example, guided barrier games with opportunities for an adult to explain when they have not understood can inform a child about a potential breakdown.

Reasons for communication

Reduced auditory access can diminish chances to determine why people talk, whether this is for consolidating friendships or describing events. Deaf children may need support in understanding how to shape language for different purposes or to adapt communication for different listeners and settings.

Conversation structure

Opportunities to observe and learn about how conversations work between hearing people can provide valuable information for deaf children. For example, the starts and ends of conversations often occur beyond the range of their hearing with or without amplification and, especially at home, greetings and farewells can happen out of sight as someone leaves the house or returns. Learning about greetings and knowing who is at home in a family can develop social communication and support inference, for example, seeing someone is wet and linking it to a rain shower when they were out.

Non-verbal signals that orchestrate conversations differ in groups of hearing or deaf people. Learning to watch for back-channel signals of understanding as a speaker will help expand repair strategies. Awareness that speech reading is being misinterpreted as staring might give a deaf child a chance to explain they are a lipreader.

Meaning

You can support a deaf child in becoming an active listener even when conversation is not directed at them by building opportunities for observing others talking. Games such as 'I went to the shop' are ideal, or activities where a child checks that instructions given by a speaker have been followed correctly by a listener in a drawing or building task.

The ability to overhear is key in acquiring new vocabulary within social settings. Many semantics programmes will be helpful in filling vocabulary gaps that deaf children often experience.

When you are working with children using both signed and spoken language, semantic structure might help to support communication development. For example, indication of the place, time or manner relating to an action or experience can be shown by a child with sign or speech and the combination might allow you to determine holistic communication development.

Grammar

Grammar support needs to be language-specific, with communicative impact of spoken forms separated from written grammar activities. Linking grammar to pragmatics work can help a deaf child recognize that spoken clauses are often elided, unfinished or finished by someone else within the collaborative context of conversations. Elision can link to learning about listener perspective, which is useful for some deaf children who have had reduced opportunities in using spoken language.

Narrative is driven by verbs, both active ones and those relating to internal experiences, and you can provide support in learning how to structure these for listeners and use them in multiclause sequences. For example, learning how to combine clauses such as 'I like apples. Apples are crunchy' could illustrate varied meanings across clauses using different connectors such as of cause, time, contrast. 'I like apples *because* they are crunchy, *if* they are crunchy, *when* they are crunchy'.

Grammar can also be linked to speech work, for example, using auditory training (Beazley and Halden, 2025) to provide opportunities to observe word endings and learn their function. High frequency speech sounds such as /s/ might only be heard in ideal conditions, but therapy can build awareness of their function in spoken language.

In small groups, you can use the topic/situation/functions approach, which allows you to break down clauses into component parts and build them up again into a communicative context, with lots of chances for repetition. For example:

Topic = travel
Situation = getting to school
Functions = time present, 3rd person singular and reporting information: *Sam cycles, Bobby walks, Nilam gets a lift.*

Speech

Any support of speech must be based on appropriate levels of transcription which may need to include vowels and non-segmental features (e.g. breath patterns, rhythm, resonance and pitch), and on good understanding of a deaf child's access to speech sounds. Input needs to take account of the acoustic phonetics and lip-patterns of the language in which you are working, to plan opportunities for listening through well prepared auditory training with inclusion/reduction of visual prompts (Beazley and Halden, 2025). You may need to seek support from specialist SLTs with experience of working with deaf children.

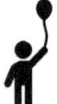

Amari's story

Amari was diagnosed with moderate reduction in hearing levels in both ears at 2 years old. 'Speech' development was described as slow and by 6 years, Amari did not appear to understand others fully, despite appropriate aiding and the use of a remote listening device.

Assessment

Comments from others: Family and teachers commented that Amari did not know how to pay attention, make friends or share conversations.

Therapist's observations: Others sometimes spoke to Amari from a distance or facing away. Amari's hearing aids were not always in or on. Others sometimes simplified grammar and vocabulary when talking to Amari, or over-mouthed words. Noise levels could be high in some parts of school and home. Despite vocabulary, grammar and phonology assessment indicating only mild delays, Amari found conversation difficult, sometimes holding onto topics, struggling to sequence narratives and being unaware of communication breakdowns. Amari was not always aware of who was talking.

Comments from Amari: 'I like talking to mum' and 'my hearing aids don't always work'.

What should we do in practice?

The SLT needs to work within the MDT to support Amari, the family, school staff and peers as follows.

Hearing levels

- Check if an audiology review is due.
- Check listening devices work consistently across the day.
- Check hearing has not deteriorated, e.g., through colds/ear infections.

The environment

- Check noise levels across settings and any adaptations needed.
- Check attention-gaining strategies being used, adding in visual alerts as needed, e.g. lights on/off before speaking.
- Check positioning for maximum access, e.g., nearer speakers, good lighting on faces.
- Check and develop Amari's skills in managing the listening environment.
- Conduct amplification device checks and see if Amari knows what to do/who to ask for help.
- Check best positions for communicating with people individually/in groups/in larger noisy environments.
- Check the value of tuning in to everyday conversations.
- Check the signals that indicate others want to speak (McTear, 1985).

The SLT can use professional knowledge to monitor and develop communication with and by Amari which could involve:

- communication awareness training for those around Amari, including input from Amari;
- support for pragmatic skills:
  - opportunities to observe how conversations start, topics are shared, and repairs are achieved within mutually negotiated interactions. A range of speaker and listener subskills would need to be built up and expanded (Beazley and Halden, 2025);

- o parallel learning about non-verbal features that support spoken communication, such as eye contact, facial expression;
- support for discourse skills:
  - o learning how information can be sequenced to support listeners, initially using story boards/grids/maps or retelling familiar stories;
  - o practising giving instructions, e.g. explaining recipes, describing experiments.

Summary

This chapter has introduced the main principles you need to know when working with deaf children, particularly on the technology you may have to manage and the significance of focusing on input in your support. You can widen your understanding and practical knowledge through more experienced colleagues but also by working in close partnership with deaf children and their families.

References

Ambrose, S.E., Walker, E.A., Unflat-Berry, L.M., Oleson, J.J. and Moeller, M.P. (2015) 'Quantity and quality of caregivers' linguistic input to 18-month and 3-year-old children who are hard of hearing', *Ear and Hearing*, 36, 48S-59S. doi: 10.1097/AUD.0000000000000209

BATOD (British Association of Teachers of Deaf Children) (2023) 'Describing deafness'. Available at: https://www.batod.org.uk/resource/2-1-describing-deafness/ (accessed 8 December 2024).

BATOD (British Association of Teachers of Deaf Children and Young People) (n.d.) 'P.U.D. (Personal Understanding of Deafness)'. Available at: https://www.batod.org.uk/wp-content/uploads/2024/02/PUD-Final.pdf (accessed 13 November 2024).

Batten, G., Oakes, P.M. and Alexander, T. (2014) 'Factors associated with social interactions between deaf children and their hearing peers: A systematic literature review', *Journal of Deaf Studies and Deaf Education*, 19(3), 285-302. https://doi.org/10.1093/deafed/ent052

Beazley, S. and Halden, J. (2025). *Working with Deaf Children and Young People: A Guide for Practitioners*. Abingdon: Routledge.

Brock, A.S. and Hampton, C.E. (2023) 'The linguistic input of fathers of children who are deaf or hard of hearing', *Perspectives of the ASHA Special Interest Groups*, 8(4), 683-692.

Carrigan, E. and Coppola, M. (2020) 'Delayed language exposure has a negative impact on receptive vocabulary skills in deaf and hard of hearing children despite early use of hearing technology'. In *Proceedings of the 44th Boston University conference on language development*. Boston: Cascadilla Press, pp. 63-76.

Cole, E.B. and Flexer, C. (2019) *Children with Hearing Loss: Developing Listening and Talking, Birth to Six*. 4th edn. San Diego, CA: Plural Publishing.

Davis, H. and Hornsby, B. (2023) 'Listening-related fatigue in deaf and hard of hearing students: understanding and managing the "fatigue factor"'. *Research Proceedings of the 2023 Global Listening and Spoken Language Virtual Symposium, Volta Review*, 23(1), 21-34.

De Siati, R.D., Rosenzweig, F., Gersdorff, G., Gregoire, A., Rombaux, P. and Deggouj, N. (2020) 'Auditory neuropathy spectrum disorders: From diagnosis to treatment: literature review and case reports', *Journal of Clinical Medicine*, 9(4), 1074.

Dirks, E., Stevens, A., Sigrid, K.O.K., Frijns, J. and Rieffe, C. (2020) 'Talk with me! Parental linguistic input to toddlers with moderate hearing loss', *Journal of Child Language*, 47(1), 186-204.

Duan, M., Xie, W., Persson, L., Hellstrom, S. and Uhlén, I. (2022) 'Postnatal hearing loss: A study of children who passed neonatal TEOAE hearing screening bilaterally', *Acta oto-laryngologica*, 142(1), 61-66.

Freeman, V., Pisoni, D.B., Kronenberger, W.G. and Castellanos, I. (2017) 'Speech intelligibility and psychosocial functioning in deaf children and teens with cochlear implants', *Journal of Deaf Studies and Deaf Education*, 22(3), 278-289.

Friedner, M. and Kusters, A. (2020) 'Deaf anthropology', *Annual Review of Anthropology*, 49(1), 31-47.

Golestani, S.D., Jalilevand, N. and Kamali, M. (2018) 'A comparison of morpho-syntactic abilities in deaf children with cochlear implant and 5-year-old normal-hearing children', *International Journal of Pediatric Otorhinolaryngology*, 110, 27–30.

Greenhalgh, K., Mahler, N., Zimmer-Gembeck, M.J. and Shanley, D.C. (2023) 'Childhood hearing loss: An uncertain context for parenting', *Deafness and Education International*, 25(2), 121–139.

Hall M.L. (2020) 'The input matters: Assessing cumulative language access in deaf and hard of hearing individuals and populations', *Frontiers in Psychology*, 11, 1407. doi: 10.3389/fpsyg.2020.01407.

Hall, M.L. and Dills, S. (2020) 'The limits of "communication mode" as a construct', *Journal of Deaf Studies and Deaf Education*, 25(4), 383–397.

Holt, R., Bruggeman, L. and Demuth, K. (2023) 'Effects of hearing loss and audio-visual cues on children's speech processing speed', *Speech Communication*, 146, 11–21.

Howerton-Fox, A. and Falk, J.L. (2019) 'Deaf children as "English learners": The psycholinguistic turn in deaf education', *Education Sciences*, 9(2), 133.

Hughes, J. (2022) 'Getting it right from the start . . .: What makes good support for families of deaf children?' *International Journal of Birth and Parent Education*, 9(3), 14.

Inscoe, J.R. and Bones, C. (2016) 'Additional difficulties associated with aetiologies of deafness: Outcomes from a parent questionnaire of 540 children using cochlear implants', *Cochlear Implants International*, 17(1), 21–30.

Kenna, M.A. (2015) 'Acquired hearing loss in children', *Otolaryngologic Clinics of North America*, 48(6), 933–953.

Kyle, J.G. (1993) 'Integration of deaf children', *European Journal of Special Needs Education*, 8(3), 201–220.

Ling. D. (2012) 'What is the Six Sound Test and why is it so important in auditory verbal therapy and education?' In W. Estabrooks (ed.), *101 Frequently Asked Questions about Auditory-Verbal Practice*. Washington, DC: Alexander Graham Bell Association for the Deaf and Hard of Hearing, pp. 58–62.

Lovcevic, I., Burnham, D. and Kalashnikova, M. (2022) 'Language development in infants with hearing loss: Benefits of infant-directed speech', *Infant Behavior and Development*, 67, 101699.

McTear, M. (1985) *Children's Conversation*. Oxford: Blackwell.

Mitchell, R.E. and Karchmer, M.A. (2004) 'Chasing the mythical ten percent: Parental hearing status of deaf and hard of hearing students in the United States', *Sign Language Studies*, 4(2), 138–163.

NDCS (National Deaf Children's Society) (2020) 'Success from the start: A developmental resource for families of deaf children aged 0 to 3'. Available at: https://www.ndcs.org.uk/successfromthestart (accessed 13 November 2024).

NDCS (National Deaf Children's Society) (2021) 'Information about deaf children and young people in the UK'. Available at: https://www.ndcs.org.uk/media/6809/dcyp-in-the-uk-info-sheet.pdf (accessed 9 December 2024).

NDCS (National Deaf Children's Society) (2024a) 'Charity highlights support for parents of deaf children'. Available at: https://www.ndcs.org.uk/about-us/news-and-media/latest-news/charity-highlights-support-for-parents-of-deaf-children/ (accessed 5 November 2024).

NDCS (National Deaf Children's Society) (2024b) 'Taking care of hearing aids'. Available at: https://www.ndcs.org.uk/information-and-support/childhood-deafness/hearing-aids-and-implants/hearing-aids/care/ (accessed 1 November 2024).

NDCS (National Deaf Children's Society) (n.d.) 'How genes can cause deafness.' Available at: https://www.ndcs.org.uk/information-and-support/childhood-deafness/causes-of-deafness/genetics/genes/ (accessed 5 November 2024).

Neumann, K., Euler, H.A., Chadha, S. and White, K.R. (2020) 'A survey on the global status of newborn and infant hearing screening', *Journal of Early Hearing Detection and Intervention*, 5(2), 63–84.

NICE (National Institute for Health and Care) (2019) 'Cochlear implants for children and adults with severe to profound deafness: Technology appraisal guidance'. Available at: https://www.nice.org.uk/guidance/ta566/chapter/1-Recommendations (accessed 9 December 2024).

O'Neill, R., Bowie, J., Foulkes, H., Cameron, A., Meara, R. and Camedda, D. (2019) 'Families living on a low income bringing up deaf children'. Edinburgh: Scottish Sensory Centre. Available at: http://www.ssc.education.ed.ac.uk/research/tellingit/tellingit_final.pdf

Ondáš, S., Pleva, M., Juhár, J., Kiktová, E., Zimmermann, J. and Šoltésová, V. (2022) 'Modified Ling Six Sound Test Audiometry Application'. In *12th International Conference on Advanced Computer Information Technologies (ACIT)*, pp. 549–553.

Onen, Ç., Mengu, G., Altinyay, S. and Kemaloglu, Y.K. (2022) 'Determination of the acoustic properties of Turkish Ling Six Sounds used in speech tests', *Speech, Language and Hearing*, 25(3), 377–387.

Parker, A. (1999) *PETAL: Phonological Evaluation and Transcription of Audio-Visual Language*. Bicester: Winslow.

Pichler, D.C., Hochgesang, J.A., Lillo-Martin, D. and de Quadros, R.M. (2010) 'Conventions for sign and speech transcription of child bimodal bilingual corpora in ELAN', *Language, Interaction and Acquisition*, 1(1), 11–40.

Rijke, W.J., Vermeulen, A.M., Wendrich, K., Mylanus, E., Langereis, M.C. and van der Wilt, G.J. (2021) 'Capability of deaf children with a cochlear implant', *Disability and Rehabilitation*, 43(14), 1989–1994.

Roos, C., Cramér-Wolrath, E. and Falkman, K.W. (2016) 'Intersubjective interaction between deaf parents/deaf infants during the infant's first 18 months', *Journal of Deaf studies and Deaf education*, 21(1), 11–22.

Sun, W., Zhang, H., Li, A. and Liu, S. (2018) 'The establishment of frequency range of the "Ling Six Sounds" test in standard Chinese', *Journal of Audiology and Speech Pathology*, pp. 120–125.

Szarkowski, A., Young, A., Matthews, D. and Meinzen-Derr, J. (2020) 'Pragmatics development in deaf and hard of hearing children: A call to action', *Pediatrics*, 146(Supplement_3), S310–S315.

Tesolin, P., Fiorino, S., Lenarduzzi, S., Rubinato, E., Cattaruzzi, E., Ammar, L., Castro, V., Orzan, E., Granata, C., Dell'Orco, D. and Morgan, A. (2021) 'Pendred syndrome, or not Pendred syndrome? That is the question', *Genes*, 12(10), 1569.

WHO (World Health Organization) (2024) 'Deafness and hearing loss'. Available at: https://www.who.int/news-room/fact-sheets/detail/deafness-and-hearing-loss (accessed 8 December 2024).

Wood, D., Wood, H., Griffiths, A. and Howarth, S. (1986) *Teaching and Talking with Deaf Children*. Chichester: John Wiley.

16 Cleft lip and palate

Stephanie van Eeden and Julie Davies

What you'll learn in this chapter

- What is cleft lip and palate?
- How it affects speech, language, and communication development
- Impact on life outcomes
- Current care pathways
- Current research and considerations for treatment.

Key information about cleft lip and palate

Cleft lip and palate is the most common congenital orofacial anomaly, with an estimated prevalence of 10 per 10,000 live births worldwide (IPDTOC, 2011). This equates to approximately 1000 babies born with a cleft in the United Kingdom every year (Royal College of Surgeons, 2024). There are different phenotypes of cleft (see Figure 16.1). These include a cleft of the lip only, a cleft of the lip and palate (which can be on one side (unilateral) or both sides (bilateral)), and a cleft of the palate only (which can affect both the hard and soft palate or the soft palate only). Babies born with a cleft involving the palate are at risk of speech and language difficulties and in the UK will be seen by a specialist speech and language therapist (SLT) linked to a regional cleft centre throughout their childhood. In this chapter we will therefore refer to cleft palate +/- lip (CP±L). Around 30% of cleft diagnoses involve an additional diagnosis (Stanier and Moore, 2004). CP±L can therefore be part of a syndrome such as 22q11 deletion syndrome or van de Woude syndrome. Discussion of syndromic clefting is beyond the scope of this chapter and readers should consult Shprintzen (2001) for further information.

Clefting of the lip and the palate occurs in utero at different embryonic stages. Clefting of the upper lip occurs between the fourth and seventh week in utero. This may impact the fusion of the anterior palate, leading to the combined diagnosis of cleft lip and palate. Clefting of the posterior palate in isolation occurs later in gestation, between the sixth and ninth week. In addition to diagnoses of overt cleft lip or palate, it is possible to have a submucous cleft palate where there is a cleft of the palate but with intact mucosa covering it. Diagnosis of a cleft involving the lip is typically made antenatally; diagnosis of a cleft involving

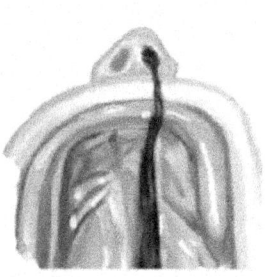
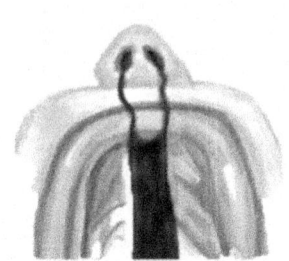
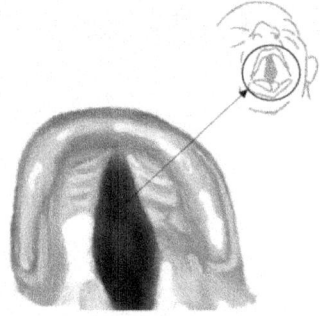

UNILATERAL CLEFT LIP AND PALATE   BILATERAL CLEFT LIP AND PALATE   ISOLATED CLEFT OF HARD AND SOFT PALATE

Figure 16.1 Diagrams of different cleft diagnoses
Source: © 2024 by Francesca Delvin is licensed under CC BY-NC-SA 4.0C.

the palate only is usually made shortly after birth. Some children may be referred in early childhood with an intact palate but with speech that sounds nasal and may subsequently be diagnosed with non-cleft velopharyngeal incompetence (VPI) (Kummer, Marshall and Wilson, 2015). The assessment and management of speech and language difficulties discussed in this chapter are relevant to all those diagnosed with either CP±L or non-cleft VPI.

 Important points about SLT practice in cleft lip and palate

Why is the palate important for speech?

To create the amount of pressure within the oral cavity that is needed to produce clear oral speech sounds, the soft palate must lift and close off against the pharyngeal wall, ensuring no unnecessary nasal escape of air when talking (see Figure 16.2). This is necessary for all sounds in the English language apart from /m, n, ŋ/. The inability to seal off the nasal cavity from the oral cavity means that the intraoral pressure needed to create oral speech sounds is compromised until the soft palate is repaired surgically. This usually occurs before the age of 12 months. In some children this first surgery is not successful, and this can lead to VPI and compensatory articulation errors. Feeding is also affected by a cleft of the palate as the infant is unable to seal off the nasal from the oral cavity. Cleft nurse specialists will help parents, providing specialist bottles and advice regarding assistive feeding.

SLT practice in CP±L therefore traditionally focuses on resonance problems and speech sound disorder (SSD) characterised by articulatory difficulties. These will be discussed below. However, recent research has highlighted wider consequences of being born with CP±L. Many of these require the knowledge and help of a SLT.

It's not just about speech

Children with CP±L are at greater risk of language difficulties. This has often been linked to early hearing loss, or delayed babble development due to the structural anomaly (Chapman et al., 2001; Baylis et al., 2020). However, recent studies have shown that there may

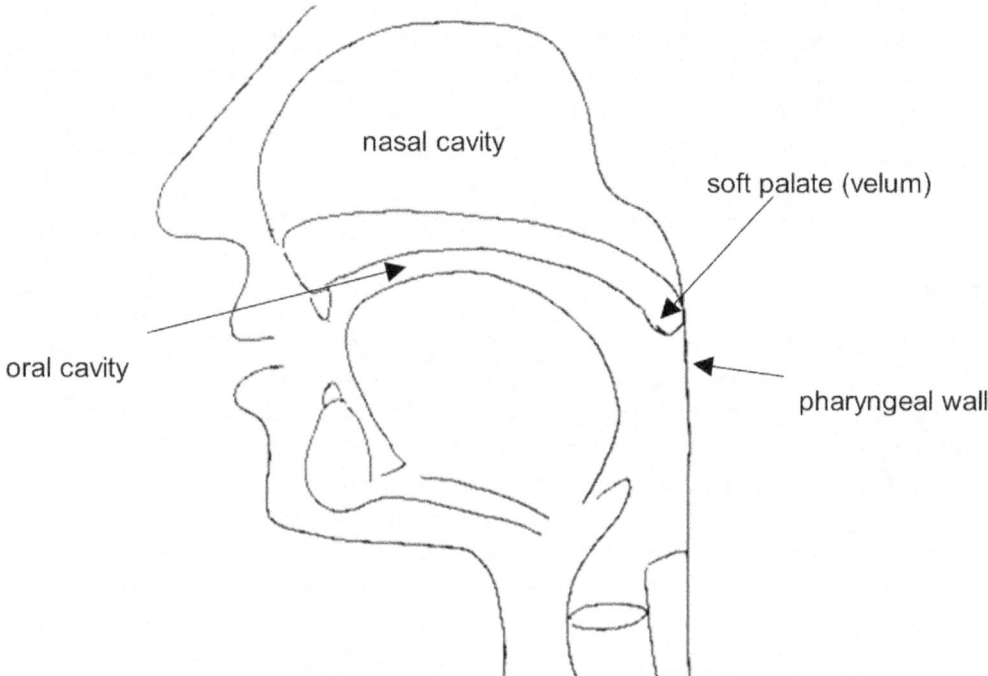

Figure 16.2 Lateral view of the head showing key structures for velopharyngeal function

be continued difficulties with oral and written language in middle childhood (Lancaster et al., 2020; 2022) and into adulthood (Conrad et al., 2014; Ardouin, Davis and Stock, 2021). In addition, attention difficulties are prevalent (Lemos and Feniman, 2010; Huang et al., 2024), along with difficulties processing sounds, especially in noisy environments (Banumathi and Jain, 2023). These skills have a complex relationship with speech and language development (van Eeden, 2023), which may in turn play a part in the reported lower educational outcomes compared to peers for children with CP+/-L (Fitzsimons et al., 2018; Grewal et al., 2021).

The multidisciplinary team

CP±L is a condition which can have lifelong consequences. In childhood and early adulthood multiple hospital appointments are required. During this period priorities can change for patients and families. Therefore, treatment and service delivery plans need to be flexible. All children born with CP±L will be treated by a multidisciplinary team (MDT). Across the UK and Ireland there are 17 regional teams. The cleft specialist SLT is a core member of this team, which includes surgeons, specialist nurses, paediatric dentists, orthodontists, audiologists, and clinical psychologists. The complex development of speech and language in children with CP±L means that SLTs must work closely with colleagues to achieve optimum outcomes. Routine reviews with the specialist SLT are typically held post primary palate repair, at 18-24 months, 3 years, 5 years, 10 years and 15 years. In the early years, the SLT may work alongside the cleft nurse specialist to meet the needs of families. If there are ongoing issues with VPI, the SLT will work closely with the cleft surgeon to investigate the causes and plan treatment options. In later years, the SLT may work alongside clinical psychologists working on issues around the impact of having speech and language difficulties. At all times, if difficulties with speech sounds or language are detected, the cleft specialist SLT will liaise with colleagues in community SLT teams to provide optimum care as close to home as possible.

Understanding children's needs in cleft lip and palate

Speech

Speech difficulties in CP±L can be twofold. The SLT working with children with CP±L will need to assess both velopharyngeal function and speech sound development.

For good velopharyngeal function, the soft palate must lift against the pharyngeal wall which moves in a sphincteric manner to create a tight seal (see Figure 16.2). VPI can occur if the muscles in the soft palate (velum) are anterior to where they need to be and so do not reach the pharyngeal wall or if there is a large velopharyngeal space behind the palate. Further surgery is indicated in either case. The role of the specialist SLT here is to assess speech for features of VPI. This assessment is both perceptual and instrumental. An oral examination will also be performed to observe any obvious structural anomalies (NB: this is particularly pertinent when assessing speech in suspected non-cleft VPI as the SLT may observe signs of a submucous cleft palate or other structural anomalies such as a bifid uvula - see Figure 16.3).

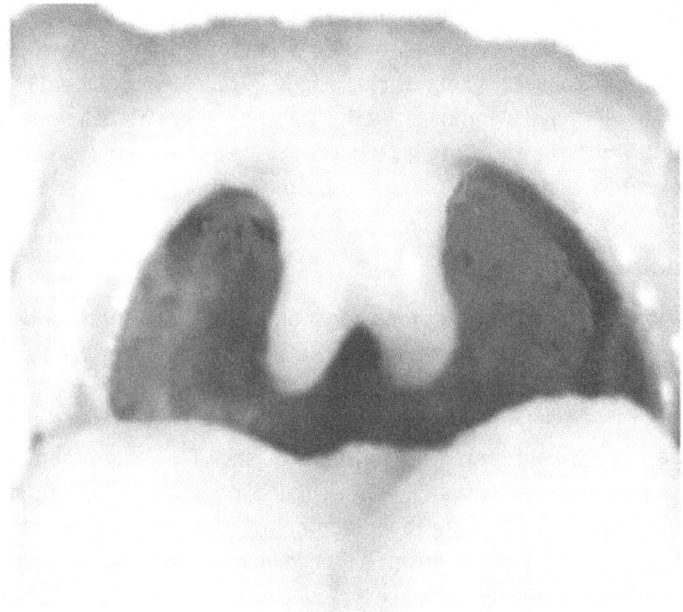

Figure 16.3 Bifid uvula

Perceptual assessments, like the Great Ormond Street Speech Assessment (GOS.SP.ASS) (Sell, Harding and Grunwell, 1999), involve listening to rote speech and repetition of sentences. Cleft specialist SLTs will listen for the following:

- *Resonance*: the balance of resonance in English should be oral. Specialist SLTs listen for nasal-sounding speech on vowels and voiced consonants. This is recorded on a scale reflecting mild, moderate or severe hypernasality. For example, hypernasality detected on close, high vowels such as /i/ and /u/ would be classed as mild; if hypernasality is also noted on open vowels such as /ɑ/ and voiced consonants are nasalised, this would be classed as moderate; severe hypernasality is recorded when all vowels are hypernasal and high pressure consonants are produced as nasals (e.g., /d/→[n]; /b/→[m]).
- *Nasal airflow*: a functioning velopharyngeal mechanism should prevent air from escaping on consonant production. Specialist SLTs listen for nasal escape on voiceless consonants, which may be quiet (nasal emission) or noisy (nasal turbulence).
- *High pressure consonants*: if VPI is present, plosive and fricative consonants may be affected, resulting in weak or nasalised production.

The specialist SLT will also note any changes to voice quality (which may also be an indication of VPI) and observe signs of nasal or facial grimace which can often accompany nasal airflow difficulties.

If a perceptual assessment indicates features of VPI, instrumental assessment will be conducted. Palatal function investigations can either be done through a videofluoroscopy or a nasendoscopy (Golding-Kushner et al., 1990). A lateral videofluoroscopy provides an x-ray image of the moving palate, allowing the SLT and surgeon to view the extent and cause of any gap between the palate and the pharyngeal wall. Nasendoscopy involves a small camera being passed through one nostril into the nasal cavity and down to view the velopharyngeal port. This allows the SLT and surgeon to observe different patterns of movement to achieve closure. If there is a gap between the palate and the pharyngeal wall causing VPI, bubbles of air will be observed. The need for further surgery to correct speech in children with CP±L varies, but latest estimates in the UK are that 27% have either had or need further surgery by the age of 5 years (Royal College of Surgeons, 2024).

Perceptual assessment is also used to assess speech sound development. Speech sound disorder (SSD) in CP±L is commonly considered an articulation disorder related to a structural anomaly. Articulation errors typically observed in children with CP±L are called active cleft speech characteristics (CSCs) and are categorised according to articulatory placement. For example, anterior CSCs include dental, lateral, or palatal placement of consonants; posterior CSCs include backing to velar or uvular placement; and non-oral CSCs include any articulation which bypasses the oral cavity, e.g. pharyngeal or glottal placement, or active nasal fricatives where air is redirected into the nasal cavity despite no structural abnormality leading to this. About 35% of children with CP±L aged 5 years have ongoing difficulties with speech sound production (Royal College of Surgeons, 2024). SSD in children with CP±L can be severe and require frequent and consistent therapy to achieve intelligible speech. In addition to CSCs, studies have highlighted an increase in prevalence of developmental errors in children with CP±L, suggesting a more linguistic basis to some SSD in this population (Willadsen et al., 2019; Nachmani et al., 2022). SLTs need to consider this both in assessment and treatment (van Eeden, McKean and Stringer, 2025).

Language

It is common to observe language delay in young children with CP±L. Studies using parental report of vocabulary development have reported 100-200 fewer words in the expressive vocabularies of children aged 2 to 3 years with CP±L compared to non-cleft peers (Scherer and D'Antonio, 1995; Scherer et al., 2008; Hardin-Jones and Chapman, 2014). Mean length of utterance in children aged 2 to 3 years is also reported to be reduced by between 0.5 and 1.0 compared to non-cleft peers (Scherer and D'Antonio, 1995; Morris and Ozanne, 2003; Eshghi et al., 2022). There is further evidence of persistent language difficulties in a proportion of children with CP±L. Lancaster et al. (2020) reported average scores 0.57 standard deviations lower compared to non-cleft peers in standardised assessments of expressive language and 0.59 lower in receptive language.

In regional cleft lip and palate centres, language assessment is typically only carried out as a screen in the preschool years by specialist SLTs. If language development is a concern, a referral to community SLT teams is made. Despite a call for greater understanding of language development in this population a quarter of a century ago (Kuehn and Moller, 2000), there is still no consensus on which assessments to use, with informal assessment most frequently reported (van Eeden, Pearce and Stringer, 2021). We know that language development and speech development are linked (Bishop and Adams, 1990), so even with speech as the focus of outcome in CP±L, SLTs should not ignore the role language plays in helping to develop age-appropriate speech. Furthermore, we should not ignore the risk of low language levels for poor achievement at school (Adlof and Hogan, 2019).

Supporting children's needs in cleft lip and palate

Research shows that over 50% of children born with CP±L require intervention from a SLT during their childhood (Hardin-Jones and Jones, 2005; Peterson-Falzone et al., 2009). Therapy for children born with CP±L can begin in infancy and continue throughout their childhood. Effective therapy often requires intensive intervention (Alighieri et al., 2021) and liaison and collaboration with many professionals both within and outside of the MDT, including community SLTs, parents, teachers, and assistants. The following section will provide an overview of common management and interventions.

Babble intervention

Early intervention for children with CP±L aged 6-18 months is often recommended by cleft teams. There are links to some video resources used by UK teams in the Recommended resources section at the end of the chapter. Further research into the effectiveness of early intervention is needed, however (Lane, Harding and Wren, 2022).

Early communication interventions

Naturalistic, holistic approaches that focus on vocabulary rather than speech sounds have been found to promote speech and language in the cleft and non-cleft population (Kaiser, Yoder and Keetz, 1992; Scherer, 1999; Kaiser and Roberts, 2013). Examples of this type of intervention are focused stimulation (Ellis Weismer and Robertson, 2006) and milieu teaching (Kaiser, Yoder and Keetz, 1992). Although similar, they differ slightly. Focused stimulation involves modelling language while highlighting a particular sound. There is no pressure on the child to copy but they are given opportunities to use and hear the sound during a natural conversation. In contrast, milieu teaching involves prompting the child to copy the sound as well as listening to repeated models of the sound. Enhanced Milieu Teaching (EMT) is a modification of milieu teaching where the focus is on also increasing utterance length.

Research studies investigating naturalistic approaches with children under 3 years with CP±L have found positive outcomes. Enhanced milieu teaching and focused stimulation have both been found to increase phonetic inventories and increase percentage consonants correct (PCC) in children born with cleft with reduced utterances (Scherer, 1999; Scherer, Williams and Proctor-Williams, 2008; Ha, 2015; Kaiser et al., 2017). For children who already have at least 20 words and speak 7-10 words per minute, Enhanced Milieu teaching plus phonological emphasis (EMT+PE) has been found to increase consonant inventories and speech accuracy as well as remediate CSCs (Scherer et al., 2020). The phonological emphasis involves using speech recasting strategies when prompting the child, for example:

Child: Kak.
Adult: Yes, ca**t**.

Non-direct speech intervention

One common indirect therapy approach used with children with CP±L is Multisensory Input Modelling (MSIM) (Addenbrookes Hospital, 2000). It is designed for children around the age of 18-24 months. Based on the Stackhouse and Wells (1997) psycholinguistic framework, MSIM is an approach where the SLT produces a high number of models of the target sound, with the aim of creating new speech motor programmes (Calladine and Vance, 2019). The theory is that the child will respond positively when they are not required to produce a sound as there is no risk of failure. Output tasks can be added to the input model, which is useful for children who have a breakdown around the motor programming level. The SLT in this case models and provides the child with specific verbal feedback when they spontaneously attempt the word. When the child produces it incorrectly the SLT highlights the difference 'I do it with my lips', and provides frequent positive praise and encouragement throughout the session.

Direct speech intervention

There are many direct articulation and phonological therapy interventions, which work on speech errors in older children with CP±L. This section discusses approaches widely used within speech sound disorder (SSD) which work well with children presenting with CSCs (Kummer, 2011).

Traditional articulation therapy is commonly used (Van Riper and Emerick, 1990; Alighieri et al., 2020). In this approach, the SLT helps the child elicit the target sound first in isolation, then nonsense syllables, then words and then sentences. A common misarticulation for children with CP±L is the active nasal fricative for /s/. Using articulation therapy the SLT may achieve an oral /s/ production in isolation from an alveolar plosive, asking the child to make a 'train slowing down' sound from the /t/ (i.e. [tsss]), creating a 'new' sound. Once the oral /s/ is isolated from the introductory /t/, proficiency in an /s/ in isolation can be built on before moving to the nonsense syllable level and so forth.

Phonological therapy approaches used with children with CP±L include minimal pair therapy (Barlow and Gierut, 2002), Metaphon (Howell and Dean, 1994), maximal oppositions (Gierut, 1989) and multiple oppositions (Williams, 2000). Full discussion of each of these approaches is beyond the scope of this chapter (see Chapter 7), but maximal and multiple opposition work well for SSD where consonant inventories are severely collapsed to one or two phonemes as is often observed in children with CP±L.

Telemedicine

Telemedicine can use the above approaches with older children while providing therapy remotely, online. For SLTs working with children with CP±L there has been a mixed response to telemedicine. Sweeney et al. (2020) compared parent-led online intervention with SLT-led face-to-face intervention and found no difference in the effectiveness of either approach. Similarly, Pamplona and Ysunza (2020) looked at group therapy using telemedicine during COVID-19 and found that all made progress with their speech sound production. Whitehead et al. (2012), however, cautioned against using telemedicine as a reliable method for assessing cleft-type features of speech and, although it may be a useful additional tool for some, its effectiveness is determined by the parent's confidence in using technology, their internet access, and their acceptance that therapy delivered this way is effective (Southby et al., 2022).

Biofeedback intervention

There are two main approaches to biofeedback commonly used with children with CP±L: electropalatography (EPG) and ultrasound biofeedback (U-VBF).

EPG works by detecting tongue-to-palate contact during speech through a custom-made plate fitted with sensors, placed on the roof of the speaker's mouth. The resulting patterns of tongue contact are displayed in real time on a computer or tablet screen (Gibbon et al., 2001). It is often used by SLTs to treat entrenched lingual speech errors, for example, /t/ produced as [k], that are resistant to traditional therapy techniques. It is typically used with school-aged children and adults. Its benefit is that it provides the speaker with real-time information as to where their tongue is making contact with their palate. Therapy is clinician-led, and typically follows the traditional articulation therapy approach. Generalisation using EPG therapy has been reported as problematic (Gibbon and Paterson, 2006), but encouraging findings in this regard have been reported when using EPG following usage-based phonological theory, in particular, when using a gradient approach to achieve accurate consonant production and incorporate an average of 250 tokens of the target sound in one therapy session (Patrick et al., 2024).

Ultrasound biofeedback (U-VBF) is a relatively new technique for treating children with speech disorders (Sugden et al., 2019). With U-VBF the child sees a real-time image of their tongue moving, and through guidance from their SLT, the speaker learns a new articulatory placement. There is currently a pilot study running that will compare U-VBF with traditional articulation therapy in children with CP±L. The results from this study will inform the design of a full randomised control trial of U-VBF with children with CSCs (Cleland et al., 2022).

Working through others

Working with other professionals

Working with children with CP±L is complex and often requires collaboration and liaison with many professionals, for example, community SLTs, SLT assistants, teachers, and teaching assistants. Community SLTs working in schools have highlighted the need for continuing professional development in cleft, therefore it is highly likely that teachers and assistants will also feel ill-equipped to work on speech with children with CP±L (Kotlarek and Krueger, 2023). Kotlarek and Krueger provide a comprehensive tutorial on the general principles of speech intervention for children with cleft, strategies to elicit correct placement, evidence-based therapy approaches, and the red flags indicating that discussion needs to take place with the supervising SLT.

Working through parents

Many therapy approaches such as focused stimulation and milieu teaching do not need to be conducted by a SLT. Previous research has shown that having a parent involved in their child's therapy can result in improved therapy outcomes compared to clinician-led only interventions (Pamplona and Ysunza, 2000; Kaiser and Hancock, 2003). Parent-led focused stimulation particularly has been reported in the literature to result in significant speech gains with children with cleft (Scherer, Williams and Proctor-Williams, 2008; Ha, 2015). Parents being trained in direct therapy intervention for speech sound disorders by the SLT is also successful. Sweeney et al. (2020) compared traditional therapy with parent-led therapy supervised by a SLT and showed both groups made significant improvements in speech.

However, parents may face challenges when working with SLTs. These include lack of time to implement therapy at home, finding activities difficult and therefore feeling uncomfortable leading the therapy at home, or not understanding the benefits of therapy (Pappas and McLeod, 2008). In a collaborative practice model outlined by Klatte et al. (2020), they suggest that when the SLT takes the time to engage in conversations which explore parental reasoning, it fosters a shared understanding of each party's preferences, expectations, roles, and responsibilities. This mutual understanding can enhance parents' motivation to engage with their child. They discuss how resources such as information, time, support, and skills may need to be aligned, potentially through the SLT co-designing activities with the parent that are specifically tailored to their child. This co-design would then lead to an agreement on how the intervention will be delivered to meet the unique needs and preferences of each family.

COM-B: a behaviour change model

Successful therapy is all about behaviour change. Behaviour change can be targeted towards the clinician's behaviour, the child, the intervention itself, or the parent (or other agent of therapy as discussed above) (Roberts and Kaiser, 2012; Alias and Ramly, 2021; Shrubsole et al., 2021; Bootsma et al., 2022). COM-B is a promising behaviour change tool/framework which can identify the key parts of an intervention, the reason why therapy is not being successful, or a way of collaborating with parents to tailor therapy specifically to their child.

COM-B stands for Capability, Opportunity, and Motivation – Behaviour (Michie, Van Stralen and West, 2011). Capability is further divided into physical capability and psychological capability (e.g., do they have the knowledge?). Opportunity is divided into physical opportunity (e.g., do they have the time and resources?) and social opportunity (e.g., do they have the shared beliefs or values?). Motivation is divided into reflective motivation (e.g., the ability to plan) and automatic motivation (e.g., the desire, emotion, and impulse). COM-B is increasingly being used in a range of SLT disorders (Toft and Stringer, 2017; Law et al., 2021) and provides tools which could identify reasons for non-attendance which often affect therapy outcomes (Keyworth et al., 2020). This model may prove particularly useful when working with children with CP±L. This is because treatment for SSD in this population can be long-term and so difficult to maintain motivation; it may involve different professionals along the care pathway and therefore be disrupted by other priorities; these issues can often lead to non-attendance. An example of working with a parent of a child with CP±L using the COM-B model is outlined in the case study of Kieran.

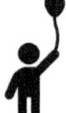

Kieran's story

This case study combines behaviour change theory with traditional SLT using the COM-B framework. Kieran was a 3-year-old boy born with an isolated cleft palate. On assessment Kieran was noted to back his anterior oral pressure consonants /t/ and /d/ to [k] and [g] respectively. The aim of therapy was therefore to target and remediate his backing pattern.

A personalised COM-B questionnaire (Keyworth et al., 2020) revealed that Kieran's mother lacked psychological capability, automatic motivation, and physical/environmental opportunity to effectively support her child's therapy (Figure 16.4). Traditional speech and language therapy was combined with the COM-B behaviour change model to identify ways that Kieran's mother could support her son with therapy practice at home. The intervention took place over eight sessions.

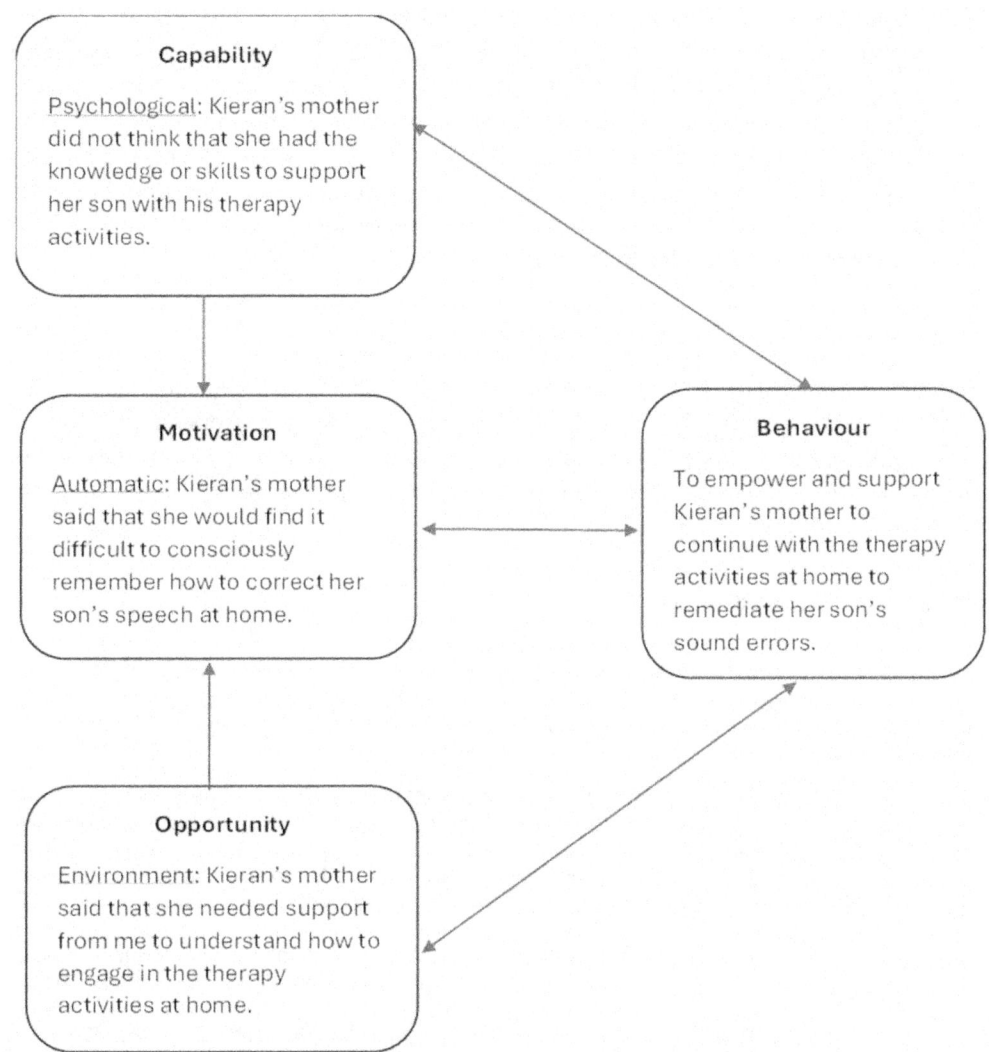

Figure 16.4 Formulation of therapy plan using the COM-B model

Intervention sessions focused on:

- *Capability* by educating Kieran's mother about the therapy's rationale (e.g. explaining the difference between front and back sounds and why children with cleft often favour sounds at the back of their mouths).
- *Opportunity* by building confidence through involvement with the therapy activities, setting weekly goals collaboratively and ensuring they were realistic and aligned with her lifestyle.
- *Motivation* by devising therapy materials tailored to Kieran's interests and reviewing progress each week, addressing challenges and successes together.

SLT intervention led to *behaviour* change reflected in these outcomes: Kieran's mother reported increased confidence in managing therapy activities and her son's behaviour by week four; she could identify speech errors and effectively support her son, leading to noticeable improvements in his speech; Kieran's backing pattern was fully remediated after 8 weeks.

The COM-B framework, integrated with traditional SLT, proved effective in enhancing parental confidence and engagement, leading to successful speech development in Kieran. This approach highlights the importance of combining behavioural change strategies with therapy to improve outcomes for children and their families.

Summary

Children born with CP±L are at risk of speech and language difficulties. Speech sound disorder (SSD) is most prevalent. Children will be treated by specialist SLTs working within a MDT at a regional cleft centre as well as by community SLTs closer to home. SLTs use a variety of treatment approaches across childhood with this population and research into the effectiveness of treatment is ongoing.

Recommended resources

The South West Cleft Service: https://youtu.be/ExoABfaUMzU
The Welsh Centre for Cleft Lip and Palate: https://www.youtube.com/watch?v=CSXAV47sMtc

References

Addenbrookes Hospital (2000). 'The use of multi-sensory input modelling to stimulate speech output processing. A teaching and demonstration video'. Available at, Cleft.NET.East Box 46, Cambridge University Hospitals Foundation Trust, Cambridge.

Adlof, S.M. and Hogan, T.P. (2019) 'If we don't look, we won't see: Measuring language development to inform literacy instruction', *Policy Insights from the Behavioral and Brain Sciences*, 6(2), 210-217. https://doi.org/10.1177/2372732219839075.

Alias, A. and Ramly, U. (2021) 'Parental involvement in speech activities of speech delayed child at home', in *2nd International Conference on Technology and Educational Science (ICTES 2020)*. Paris: Atlantis Press, pp. 217-222.

Alighieri, C., Bettens, K., Bruneel, L., D'haeseleer, E., Van Gaever, E., and Van Lierde, K. (2020) 'Effectiveness of speech intervention in patients with a cleft palate: comparison of motor-phonetic versus linguistic-phonological speech approaches', *Journal of Speech, Language, and Hearing Research*, 63(12), 3909-3933. https://doi.org/10.1044/2020_JSLHR-20-00129.

Alighieri, C., Van Lierde, K., De Caesemaeker, A.-S., Demuynck, K., Bruneel, L., D'haeseleer, E., and Bettens, K. (2021) 'Is high-intensity speech intervention better? A comparison of high-intensity intervention versus low-intensity intervention in children with a cleft palate', *Journal of Speech, Language, and Hearing Research*, 64(9), 3398-3415.

Ardouin, K., Davis, S. and Stock, N.M. (2021) 'Physical health in adults born with cleft lip and/or palate: A whole of life survey in the United Kingdom', *The Cleft Palate-Craniofacial Journal*, 58(2), 153-162.

Banumathi, C. and Jain, C. (2023) 'A systematic review of auditory processing abilities in children with non-syndromic cleft lip and/or palate', *Journal of All India Institute of Speech and Hearing*, 42(1). https://journals.lww.com/josh/fulltext/2023/42010/a_systematic_review_of_auditory_processing.2.aspx.

Barlow, J.A. and Gierut, J.A. (2002) 'Minimal pair approaches to phonological remediation.', *Seminars in Speech and Language*, 23(1), 57-68. https://doi.org/10.1055/s-2002-24969.

Baylis, A., Vallino, L.D., Powell, J. and Zajac, D.J. (2020) 'Lexical selectivity of 2-year-old children with and without repaired cleft palate based on parent report', *Cleft Palate-Craniofacial Journal*, 57(9), 1117-1124. https://doi.org/10.1177/1055665620915060.

Bishop, D.V.M. and Adams, C. (1990) 'A prospective study of the relationship between specific language impairment, phonological disorders and reading retardation', *Journal of Child Psychology and Psychiatry and Allied Disciplines*, 31(7), 1027-1050. https://doi.org/10.1111/j.1469-7610.1990.tb00844.x.

Bootsma, J.N., Phoenix, M., Geytenbeek, J.J.M., Stadskleiv, K., Gorter, J.W., Fiske, S., and Cunningham, B.J. (2022) 'Implementing the language comprehension test C-BiLLT: a qualitative description study using the COM-B model of behaviour change', *BMC Health Services Research*, 22(1), 1421.

Calladine, S. and Vance, M. (2019) 'A psycholinguistic approach to therapy with very young children born with cleft palate'. In A. Harding-Bell (ed.), *Case Studies in Cleft Palate Speech: Data Analysis and Principled Intervention*. Havant: J&R Press Ltd, pp. 330-360.

Chapman, K.L., Hardin-Jones, M., Schulte, J. and Halter, K.A. (2001) 'Vocal development of 9-month-old babies with cleft palate', *Journal of Speech, Language, and Hearing Research*, 44(6), 1268-1283. https://doi.org/10.1044/1092-4388(2001/099).

Cleland, J., Crampin, L., Campbell, L. and Dokovova, M. (2022) 'Protocol for SonoSpeech Cleft Pilot: a mixed-methods pilot randomized control trial of ultrasound visual biofeedback versus standard intervention for children with cleft lip and palate', *Pilot and Feasibility Studies*, 8(1), 93.

Conrad, A.L., McCoy, T., DeVolder, I., Richman, L.C. and Nopoulos, P. . (2014) 'Reading in subjects with an oral cleft: Speech, hearing and neuropsychological skills.', *Neuropsychology*, 28(3), 415-22. https://doi.org/10.1037/neu0000024.

Ellis Weismer, S. and Robertson, S. (2006) 'Focused stimulation approach to language intervention'. In R.J. McCauley, M. G. Fey and R. B. Gillam (eds), *Treatment of Language Disorders in Children*, Baltimore, MD: Paul Brookes Publishing, pp. 175-202.

Eshghi, M., Adatorwovor, R., Preisser, J.S., Crais, E.R. and Zajac, D.J. (2022).'Lexicogrammatical skills in 2-year-old children with and without repaired cleft palate', *Clinical Linguistics and Phonetics*, 36(6): 528-546 https://doi.org/10.1080/02699206.2021.1941263.

Fitzsimons, K.J., Copley, L.P., Setakis, E., Charman, S.C., Deacon, S.A., Dearden, L., and van der Meulen, J.H. (2018) 'Early academic achievement in children with isolated clefts: a population-based study in England', *Archives of Disease in Childhood*, 103, 356-362. https://doi.org/10.1136/archdischild-2017-313777.

Gibbon, F., Hardcastle, W. J., Crampin, L., Reynolds, B., Razzell, R. and Wilson, J. (2001) 'Visual feedback therapy using electropalatography (EPG) for articulation disorders associated with cleft palate', *Asia Pacific Journal of Speech, Language and Hearing*, 6(1), 53-58.

Gibbon, F. and Paterson, L. (2006) 'A survey of speech and language therapists' views on electropalatography therapy outcomes in Scotland', *Child Language Teaching and Therapy*, 22(3), 275-292.

Gierut, J.A. (1989) 'Maximal opposition approach to phonological treatment', *Journal of Speech and Hearing Disorders*, 54(1), 9-19.

Golding-Kushner, K.J., Ravelo, V., Argamaso, M.D., Cotton, R.T., Grames, L.M., Henningsson, G., Jones, D.L., Karnell, M.P., Klaiman, P.G. . . ., and Skolnick, L. (1990) 'Standardization for the reporting of nasopharyngoscopy and multiview videofluoroscopy: A report from an International Working Group', *Cleft Palate Journal*, 27(4), 337-348. https://doi.org/10.1597/1545-1569_1990_027_0337_sftron_2.3.co_2.

Grewal, S.S., Ponduri, S., Leary, S.D., Wren, Y., Thompson, J.M.D., Ireland, A.J., Ness, A.R. and Sandy, J.R. (2021) 'Educational attainment of children born with unilateral cleft lip and palate in the United Kingdom', *Cleft Palate-Craniofacial Journal*, 58(5), 587-596. https://doi.org/10.1177/1055665620959989.

Ha, S. (2015) 'Effectiveness of a parent-implemented intervention program for young children with cleft palate', *International Journal of Pediatric Otorhinolaryngology*, 79(5), 707-715.

Hardin-Jones, M.A. and Chapman, K.L. (2014) 'Early lexical characteristics of toddlers with cleft lip and palate', *The Cleft Palate-Craniofacial Journal*. American Cleft Palate Craniofacial Association, 51(6), 622-631. https://doi.org/10.1597/13-076.

Hardin-Jones, M.A. and Jones, D.L. (2005) 'Speech production of preschoolers with cleft palate', *Cleft Palate-Craniofacial Journal*, 42(1), 7-13.

Howell, J. and Dean, E. (1994) *Treating Phonological Disorders in Children : Metaphon-Theory to Practice*. 2nd edn. London: Whurr Publishsers.

Huang, H-H., Hsu, J-W., Huang, K-L., Su T-P., Chen, T-J., Tsai, S-J. and Chen, M-H. (2024) 'Congenital cleft lip and palate and elevated risks of major psychiatric disorders: A nationwide longitudinal study', *Clinical Child Psychology and Psychiatry*, 29(2), 637-647.

IPDTOC (International Perinatal Database of Typical Orofacial Clefts) (2011) 'Prevalence at birth of cleft lip with or without cleft palate: data from the International Perinatal Database of Typical Oral Clefts). *The Cleft Palate-Craniofacial Journal*, 48(1), 66-81. https://doi.org/10.1597/09-217.

Kaiser, A.P. and Hancock, T.B. (2003) 'Teaching parents new skills to support their young children's development', *Infants and Young Children*, 16(1), 9-21.

Kaiser, A.P. and Roberts, M.Y. (2013) 'Parent-implemented enhanced milieu teaching with preschool children who have intellectual disabilities', *Journal of Speech, Language, and Hearing Research*, 56(1), 295-309. https://doi.org/10.1044/1092-4388(2012/11-0231).

Kaiser, A.P., Scherer, N.J., Frey, J.R. and Roberts, M.Y. (2017) 'The effects of enhanced milieu teaching with phonological emphasis on the speech and language skills of young children with cleft palate: a pilot study', *American Journal of Speech-Language pathology*, 26(3), 806-818.

Kaiser, A.P., Yoder, P.J. and Keetz, A. (1992) 'Evaluating milieu teaching', in S.F. Warren and J. Reichle (eds) *Cause and Effects in Communication And Language Intervention*. Baltimore, MD: Paul H. Brookes Publishing Co., pp. 9-47.

Keyworth, C., Epton, T., Goldthorpe, J., Calam, R. and Armitage, C.J. (2020) 'Acceptability, reliability, and validity of a brief measure of capabilities, opportunities, and motivations ("COM-B")', *British Journal of Health Psychology*, 25(3), 474-501.

Klatte, I.S., Lyons, R., Davies, K., Harding, S., Marshall, J., McKean, C. and Roulstone, S. (2020) 'Collaboration between parents and SLTs produces optimal outcomes for children attending speech and language therapy: Gathering the evidence', *International Journal of Language and Communication Disorders*, 55(4), 618-628.

Kotlarek, K.J. and Krueger, B.I. (2023) 'Treatment of speech sound errors in cleft palate: A tutorial for speech-language pathology assistants', *Language, Speech, and Hearing Services in Schools*, 54(1), 171-188. https://doi.org/10.1044/2022_LSHSS-22-00071

Kuehn, D.P., and Moller, K.T. (2000) 'Speech and language issues in the cleft palate population: The state of the art', *The Cleft Palate Craniofacial Journal*, 37(4), 1-35. doi:10.1597/1545-1569_2000_037_0348_saliit_2.3.co_2

Kummer, A.W. (2011) 'Speech therapy for errors secondary to cleft palate and velopharyngeal dysfunction', *Seminars in Speech and Language*, 32(2), 191-198. https://doi.org/10.1055/S-0031-1277721/ID/41.

Kummer, A.W., Marshall, J.L. and Wilson, M.M. (2015) 'Non-cleft causes of velopharyngeal dysfunction: Implications for treatment', *International Journal of Pediatric Otorhinolaryngology*. https://doi.org/10.1016/j.ijporl.2014.12.036.

Lancaster, H.S., Lien, K.M., Chow, J.C., Frey, J.R., Scherer, N.J. and Kaiser, A.P. (2020) 'Early speech and language development in children with nonsyndromic cleft lip and/or palate: A meta-analysis', *Journal of Speech, Language, and Hearing Research*, 63(1), 14-31. https://doi.org/10.1044/2019_JSLHR-19-00162.

Lancaster, H.S., Lien, K., Haas, J., Ellis, P. and Scherer, N. (2022) 'Reading development in children with nonsyndromic cleft palate with or without cleft lip: meta-analysis and systematic review', *The Cleft Palate-Craniofacial Journal*, 59(9), 1155-1166. https://doi.org/10.1177/10556656211039871.

Lane, H., Harding, S. and Wren, Y. (2022) 'A systematic review of early speech interventions for children with cleft palate', *International Journal of Language and Communication Disorders*, 57(1), 226-245. https://doi.org/10.1111/1460-6984.12683.

Law, J., Dornstauder, M., Charlton, J. and Greaux, M. (2021) 'Tele-practice for children and young people with communication disabilities: Employing the COM-B model to review the intervention literature and inform guidance for practitioners', *International Journal of Language and Communication Disorders*, https://doi.org/10.1111/1460-6984.12592.

Lemos, I.C.C. and Feniman, M.R. (2010) 'Sustained Auditory Attention Ability Test (SAAAT) in seven-year-old children with cleft lip and palate', *Brazilian Journal of Otorhinolaryngology*, 76, 199-205.

Michie, S., Van Stralen, M.M. and West, R. (2011) 'The behaviour change wheel: A new method for characterising and designing behaviour change interventions', *Implementation science*, 6, 1-12.

Morris, H. and Ozanne, A. (2003) 'Phonetic, phonological, and language skills of children with a cleft palate', *The Cleft Palate-Craniofacial Journal*, 40, 460-470. https://doi.org/10.1597/1545-1569(2003)040<0460:PPALSO>2.0.CO;2.

Nachmani, A., Biadsee, A., Masalha, M. and Kassem, F. (2022) 'Compensatory articulation errors in patients with velopharyngeal dysfunction and palatal anomalies', *Journal of Speech, Language, and Hearing Research*, 65(7), 2518-2539. https://doi.org/10.1044/2022_JSLHR-21-00679.

Pamplona, A.Y. and Ysunza, P.A. (2000) 'Active participation of mothers during speech therapy improved language development of children with cleft palate', *Scandinavian Journal of Plastic and Reconstructive Surgery and Hand Surgery*, 34(3), 231-236.

Pamplona, M. and Ysunza, P.A. (2020) 'Speech pathology telepractice for children with cleft palate in the times of COVID-19 pandemic', *International Journal of Pediatric Otorhinolaryngology*, 138, 110318.

Pappas, N.W. and McLeod, S. (2008) *Working with Families in Speech-Language Pathology*. San Diego: Plural Publishing.

Patrick, K., Fricke, S., Rutter, B. and Cleland, J. (2024) 'Clinical application of usage-based phonology: Treatment of cleft palate speech using usage-based electropalotography', *International Journal of Speech-Language Pathology*, 26(4), 595–610.

Peterson-Falzone, S.J., Hardin-Jones, M.A. and Karnell, M.P. (2009) *Cleft Palate Speech*. 4th edn. St. Louis, MO: Mosby.

Roberts, M.Y. and Kaiser, A.P. (2012) 'Assessing the effects of a parent-implemented language intervention for children with language impairments using empirical benchmarks: A pilot study', *Journal of Speech Language and Hearing Research*, 55, 1655–1671.

Royal College of Surgeons (2024) 'Cleft Registry and Audit NEtwork Database 2024 Annual Report'. Available at: https://www.crane-database.org.uk/wp-content/uploads/2024/12/CRANE-2024-Annual-Report_V1_final.pdf (accessed 7 March 2025).

Scherer, N.J. (1999) 'The speech and language status of toddlers with cleft lip and/or palate following early vocabulary intervention', *American Journal of Speech-Language Pathology*, 8(1), 81–93.

Scherer, N.J. and D'Antonio, L.L. (1995) 'Parent questionnaire for screening early language development in children with cleft palate', *Cleft Palate-Craniofacial Journal*, 32(1), 7–13. https://doi.org/10.1597/1545-1569(1995)032<0007:PQFSEL>2.3.CO;2.

Scherer, N.J., Kaiser, A.P., Frey, J.R., Lancaster, H.S., Lien, K. and Roberts, M. (2020) 'Effects of a naturalistic intervention on the speech outcomes of young children with cleft palate', *International Journal of Speech-Language Pathology*, 22(5), 549–558.

Scherer, N.J., Williams, A.L. and Proctor-Williams, K. (2008) 'Early and later vocalization skills in children with and without cleft palate', *International Journal of Pediatric Otorhinolaryngology*, 72(6), 827–840. https://doi.org/10.1016/j.ijporl.2008.02.010.

Sell, D., Harding, A. and Grunwell, P. (1999) 'GOS.SP.ASS.'98: an assessment for speech disorders associated with cleft palate and/or velopharyngeal dysfunction (revised)', *International Journal of Language and Communication Disorders*, 34(1), 17–33. https://doi.org/10.1080/136828299247595.

Shprintzen, R.J. (2001) 'Genetics in craniofacial disorders and clefting: Then and now', in S.E. Gerber (ed.), *Handbook of Genetic Communicative Disorders*. San Diego: Academic Press, pp. 129–149. https://doi.org/10.1016/B978-012280605-6/50009-3.

Shrubsole, K., Pitt, R., Till, K., Finch, E. and Ryan, B. (2021) 'Speech language pathologists' practice with children of parents with an acquired communication disability: A preliminary study', *Brain Impairment*, 22(2), 135–151.

Southby, L., Harding, S., Davies, A., Lane, H., Chandler, H. and Wren, Y. (2022) 'Parent/caregiver views of the effectiveness of speech-language pathology for children born with cleft palate delivered via telemedicine during COVID-19', *Language, Speech, and Hearing Services in Schools*, 53(2), 307–316.

Stackhouse, J. and Wells, B. (1997) *Children's Speech and Literacy Difficulties: A Psycholinguistic Framework*. London: Whurr.

Stanier, P. and Moore, G.E. (2004) 'Genetics of cleft lip and palate: syndromic genes contribute to the incidence of non-syndromic clefts', *Human Molecular Genetics*, 13(90001), 73R–81. https://doi.org/10.1093/hmg/ddh052.

Sugden, E., Lloyd, S., Lam, J. and Cleland, J. (2019) 'Systematic review of ultrasound visual biofeedback in intervention for speech sound disorders', *International Journal of Language and Communication Disorders*. https://doi.org/10.1111/1460-6984.12478.

Sweeney, T., Hegarty, F., Powell, K., Deasy, L., O'Regan, M. and Sell, D. (2020) 'Randomized controlled trial comparing parent led therapist supervised articulation therapy (PLAT) with routine intervention for children with speech disorders associated with cleft palate', *International Journal of Language and Communication Disorders*, 55(5), 639–660.

Toft, K. and Stringer, H. (2017) 'Behaviour change technique taxonomy: a method of describing head and neck cancer dysphagia intervention delivery', *Current Opinion in Otolaryngology and Head and Neck Surgery*, 25(3), 182–187.

van Eeden, S. (2023) 'The relationship between auditory behaviours and speech and language development in children with cleft lip and palate', *Current Opinion in Otolaryngology and Head and Neck Surgery*, 31(3), 165–170. https://doi.org/10.1097/MOO.0000000000000883.

van Eeden, S., McKean, C. and Stringer, H. (2025) 'Rethinking speech sound disorder (SSD) in non-syndromic cleft lip and palate: The importance of recognizing phonological and language difficulties.', *International Journal of Language and Communication Disorders*, 60(1), e13151. https://doi.org/10.1111/1460-6984.13151.

van Eeden, S., Pearce, E. and Stringer, H. (2021) 'How and why are the early language skills of children with cleft palate +/- lip assessed and are these measures adequate?', in *Annual Scientific Meeting of the Craniofacial Society of Great Britain and Ireland*. Cardiff. http://dx.doi.org/10.13140/RG.2.2.32290.71363/1.

van Riper, C.G. and Emerick, L.L. (1990) *Speech Correction: An Introduction to Speech Pathology and Audiology*. 8th edn. Hoboken, NJ: Prentice-Hall Inc.

Wehby, G.L., Collett, B.R., Barron, S., Romitti, P. and Ansley, T. (2015) 'Children with oral clefts are at greater risk for persistent low achievement in school than classmates', *Archives of Disease in Childhood*, 100, 1148-1154. http://dx.doi.org/10.1136/archdischild-2015-308358.

Whitehead, E., Dorfman, V., Tremper, G., Kramer, A., Sigler, A. and Gosman, A. (2012) 'Telemedicine as a means of effective speech evaluation for patients with cleft palate', *Annals of Plastic Surgery*, 68(4), 415-417.

Willadsen, E., Lohmander, A., Persson, C., Boers, M., Kisling-Møller, M., Havstam, C., Elander, A. and Andersen, M. (2019) 'Scandcleft Project, Trial 1: Comparison of speech outcome in relation to timing of hard palate closure in 5-year-olds with UCLP', *The Cleft Palate-Craniofacial Journal*, 56(10), 1276-1286. https://doi.org/10.1177/1055665619854632.

Williams, A.L. (2000) 'Multiple oppositions: Theoretical foundations for an alternative contrastive intervention approach', *American Journal of Speech-Language Pathology*, 9(4), 282-288.

17 Acquired brain injury (ABI)

Katherine Buckeridge, Helen Cullimore, Lucy Cuthbertson and Rhiannon Halfpenny

What you'll learn in this chapter

- What a childhood acquired brain injury (ABI) is and the different types of ABI
- How childhood ABI differs from developmental disorders and adult ABI
- The role of the SLT in the rehabilitation pathway and transition from hospital to the community setting
- How acquired impairments affect a child's communication and swallowing skills
- An overview of the assessments, interventions and outcome measures relevant to children with ABI
- The short-term and longer-term needs of children with ABI.

Key information about ABI

Childhood acquired brain injury (ABI) is a term used to describe damage to the brain occurring after birth following a period of normal development. ABI is one of the main causes of childhood disability in the UK, affecting approximately 40,000 children per year (NHS England, 2013). Nowadays, more children are surviving severe ABI due to improvements in emergency and Intensive Care (Forsyth et al., 2012).

There are two types of ABI:

1. *Traumatic brain injury (TBI)* occurs when a child has sustained a sudden impact to the head from an outside force caused by a road traffic accident, fall, sport injury, object or deliberate act. The severity of TBI is usually measured by the Glasgow Coma Scale (GCS) (Teasdale and Jennett, 1974). TBI is the most common form of ABI affecting 35,000 children per year.
2. *Non-traumatic brain injury* is less common and refers to injury to the brain caused by other reasons, for example, stroke, brain haemorrhage, brain tumour, lack of oxygen (such as near drowning or choking), epilepsy, meningitis or encephalitis.

Individuals may experience changes to their physical skills, eating and drinking, cognition, executive function, speech language and communication (SLC), behaviour, attention, proprioception, hearing and vision. All these issues can impact on quality of life (QoL), school integration, peer and family relationships and social situations.

Factors affecting recovery from ABI include:

- the type of ABI and its severity and location within the brain
- the child's age at the time of the ABI
- the child's pre-existing conditions or disorders
- environmental factors such as family function, access to rehabilitation, and sociodemographic characteristics (Anderson et al., 2012).

The Kennard principle suggested that children would make a better recovery if the brain injury occurred when they were young due to greater plasticity than older children or adults (Dennis, 2010), but it is now thought they experience a 'neurocognitive stall'. This means that children who make a good initial recovery fall further behind their peers as cognitive, social and motor skill development slows down over time (Chapman, 2006). As a result, some problems may not become apparent until adolescence, when new deficits emerge with time.

When an ABI occurs during adolescence, which is a time of emotional and physical change, this can alter an individual's identity (how they define themselves) and there may be a sense of loss for the person they were previously (Kakonge et al., 2022). Some adolescents lack self-awareness of their impairments following ABI, a factor which can affect rehabilitation outcomes.

ABI is a life-long condition. Children with ABI develop into adults with ABI. Transition to adulthood exposes many barriers that become more obvious when the structure of school life falls away. The long-term consequences of an ABI can hinder social outcomes, employment prospects and QoL. Having a brain injury increases the risk of offending; there is a higher prevalence of TBI for those held in youth custody than in the general population (Linden et al., 2024).

Important points about SLT practice in ABI

SLTs need to understand why working with children with ABI differs from working with those with neurodevelopmental conditions or developmental disorders. They should consider the following points:

- Children with ABI are vulnerable to acquiring the same impairments as adults. However, unlike adults, they have experienced a disruption to the developing brain and so require a bespoke approach from specialist SLTs who are familiar with both the childhood skill trajectory and acquired disorders. The key areas of involvement for SLTs are speech, language and communication, eating and drinking, mouthcare and saliva management.
- As the specialist in dysphagia and communication, the SLT will be the main source of information regarding these areas. This role could include educating the child about what has happened to them, advising a parent about safe eating, drinking and swallowing, demonstrating evidence-based aphasia strategies or advising class teachers about how to modify the curriculum.

- ABI is complex and multi-faceted, so SLTs will tend to work particularly in the early stages of recovery as part of a multidisciplinary team (MDT) team with a wide range of medical staff, caregivers and allied health professionals (AHPs). Working within a cohesive MDT benefits SLTs in assessment and diagnosis, and offers the opportunity to share information, prioritise work streams and receive supervision.
- There are valuable opportunities for working with other AHPs, as disciplines will overlap when addressing communication, cognition, behaviour, sensory and motor skills. Close liaison will be needed with the psychology team, which usually has a significant role in supporting a child and their family, following such a sudden and life-changing event.
- The empowerment of family and caregivers has been cited as one of the most important factors in rehabilitation outcomes (Linden et al., 2024). Throughout the rehabilitation process SLTs will need to form affiliative partnerships with family members who will be experiencing different phases of grief. The timing of any information given needs to be sensitive to family needs, the recovery trajectory and prognosis.
- Childhood brain injuries can sometimes be acquired in circumstances that are found to be non-accidental, so the therapist will have a role in adhering to any safeguarding processes that have been put in place whilst delivering rehabilitation.

The role of the SLT in the rehabilitation pathway

A journal article by Keetley et al. (2021) provides an example of different patient rehabilitation pathways at a UK hospital for children diagnosed with ABI. It highlights the role of the SLT in this complex process. There are usually three main phases to a child's rehabilitation pathway: acute, post-acute and community, but not all children will access each of these. SLTs who work in neuro-oncology will also be involved in supporting end-of-life care.

Acute

The SLT has a role in the care of a child as soon as possible post injury (Royal College of Physicians and British Society of Rehabilitation Medicine, 2003). At this stage, the child may be on the Paediatric Intensive Care Unit (PICU), High Dependency Unit (HDU) or acute neurological ward. In this early stage, SLT input can guide families on what to expect and what they can and are already doing to help. The SLT can emphasise any positive signs, the expected fluctuations at this stage and the value of a day-to-day approach. The SLT can informally assess communication and swallowing via observation and reports from family and staff. This is particularly important when sedation medications are being weaned, and underlying skills start to emerge. It can also reveal impairments, such as movement disorders, weakness or lack of responsiveness which may indicate a potential state of Prolonged Disorder of Consciousness (PDOC) that is, 'any disorder of consciousness that has continued for at least four weeks following sudden onset brain injury' (Scolding, Owen and Keown, 2021, p. 1656).

Post-acute rehabilitation

This stage of rehabilitation refers to the time when a child is medically stable, but in need of intensive specialist therapies, medical and educational input to maximise recovery. The availability of inpatient rehabilitation for children following ABI varies across the regions of the UK. Flexibility in therapy is required as it may be necessary to tailor rehabilitation around medical needs, such as daily radiotherapy for a brain tumour. In this stage of rehabilitation, a child can be significantly impacted by fatigue so therapy sessions need to be scheduled to include rest periods, which may also be needed on an ad-hoc basis. Informal and formal assessment will provide diagnosis of acquired communication and swallowing impairments, in comparison with a child's baseline pre-injury.

Discharge to community services

Following brain injury, children are far more likely to be discharged to their home environment than adults but tend to have less access to specialist therapeutic services to support their rehabilitation. Discharge Planning Meetings are an essential step in the sharing of information between inpatient neurorehabilitation teams and community services. Often the burden of navigating services in the community falls to parents and caregivers in the longer term (Diener et al., 2022), so signposting support is an important part of the SLT role. A referral should be made to community services as soon as ongoing speech and language therapy is indicated. Community SLTs may lack experience of children with ABI as this population tends to be a minority within caseloads.

Return to school

Planning for a child's return to school is a team effort and this can be fraught with challenges. Some children may not be able to return to their previous setting and a placement with a Special Educational Needs (SEN) school or college may be required. SEN establishments can be valuable in their small class sizes, high staff-to-pupil ratio, staff skill set and access to therapies and facilities when a child has significant physical and learning needs. SLTs should be involved in the process of securing support for a child's needs, for example, providing evidence for an Education Health and Care Plan (EHCP) application and providing guidance to educators. It vital that children with ABI have access to SLT assessment and intervention throughout their education and during periods of transition such as changing schools or when undertaking qualifications.

Transition to adult services

When an individual is between 16 and 18 years of age, it is important to instigate a smooth transition to adult services where SLTs can support interventions that focus on life skills relevant to adulthood, such as access to higher education, independence, employment and relationships. SLTs may be consulted about whether a young person has mental capacity to make decisions about their life (Mental Capacity Act 2005).

Understanding children's needs in ABI

Communication

A small number of children will remain non-speaking following ABI, requiring augmentative and alternative communication (AAC) but most will recover the ability to speak. However, their language skills tend to be poorer than non-brain injured peers, despite a trajectory of improving skills. Children with ABI often have subtle impairments affecting everyday communication but which are not easily identifiable on standardised assessments. They may have difficulty with naming, sentence repetition, sentence construction, word knowledge, social interaction and pragmatics (Catroppa and Anderson, 2004; Nippold et al., 2007; Togher, McDonald and Code, 2014; Breau et al., 2015). Acquired language disorders in children with ABI may be referred to as dysphasia or aphasia (O'Hare, 2016). Aphasia affects both spoken and written understanding of language and expression (Blosser and DePompei, 2003). When verbal or non-verbal communication is affected by disruption of cognition, this is called cognitive-communication disorder (CCD) (American Speech-Language Association, 2005, p. 2). However, the term CCD is used inconsistently in relation to children so standardisation of terminology has been recommended (Crumlish et al., 2022).

Children with ABI may have dysarthria (a motor speech disorder), dyspraxia (motor planning problems) and difficulties with articulation, respiration and phonation. Dysarthria can persist for up to fifteen years post ABI (Morgan, 2014). Dyspraxia and dysarthria can particularly affect children with Posterior Fossa Syndrome (PFS). This is typically only seen in children following resection of a brain tumour in the posterior fossa region of the brain. It is characterised by a combination of symptoms which can include loss of speech (referred to as cerebellar mutism), irritability, low tone (hypotonia) and uncoordinated and uncontrolled movements (ataxia). Children will sometimes emerge from surgery speaking in sentences and then stop or have significantly reduced spoken language. Some progressive brain tumours, such as a diffuse midline glioma, are associated with cranial nerve involvement and deterioration of bulbar functioning, impacting on the clarity of speech.

Clinicians should consider several general principles when assessing a child's speech, language and communication following ABI.

- It is important to consider baseline communication skills from the case history and the length of time since the injury, the cause of the injury, location and severity. This allows a hypothesis to be formed about what you might expect and how to assess for it.
- Referral to an audiologist or an ophthalmologist may be needed for further investigation of hearing and vision impairments impacting on communication. With a clearer understanding of the child's communication needs, relevant referral to agencies beyond the immediate rehabilitation team can be made, for example, an AAC Service.
- Informal assessment in the early phase is essential to capture a child's responses, their reliability and repeatability. Objective measure using video analysis and observational charts can be completed by all those who interact with the child over a set period. The value of observation with no stimuli can reveal behaviours such as involuntary movements and attempts to initiate interaction. The findings from a Disorders of Consciousness (DOC) assessment can be used to advise others on the optimum environment and approach.

Area	Assessment	Description (age range stated by authors in brackets)
Disorders of consciousness	Coma Recovery Scale-Revised (CRS-R) (Giacino et al., 2020)	Assesses level of consciousness and monitors behavioural recovery. It is relatively quick to administer and can be repeated based on clinical need (children and adults)
	Coma Recovery Scale for Pediatrics (CRS-P) (Slomine et al., 2019)	This should be used when assessing children who have not yet completed language and motor development (1-5 years)
	Sensory Modality Assessment and Rehabilitation Technique (SMART) (Gill-Thwaites, et al., 2004)	Provides a detailed objective assessment for Prolonged DOC. The assessment process is therapeutic and provides objective diagnostic information. Must be used by a trained SMART assessor (adults)
	Wessex Head Injury Matrix (WHIM) (Shiel et al., 2000)	Used to assess and monitor recovery of cognitive function (16 years and older)
		These assessments are usually administered in conjunction with the MDT
Comprehension	British Picture Vocabulary Scale-3 (BPVS-III) (Dunn, 2011)	Assesses comprehension of single spoken words by picture selection (3 to 16 years)
	Test for Reception of Grammar-2 (TROG-2) (Bishop, 2003a)	The test measures understanding of English grammatical contrasts (4 years to adults)
Expression	Bus Story Test (Renfrew Language Scales) (Renfrew, 2010)	Information content, sentence length and grammatical usage assessment via retelling of a story (3 to 8 years)
	Renfrew Action Picture Test (RAPT) (Renfrew, 2019)	This screening test assesses words used to convey information i.e. nouns, verbs, prepositions (3 to 8 years 5 months)
	Renfrew Expressive Vocabulary Test (REV) (Renfrew 2023)	Used to assess naming of nouns, adjectives and verbs (3-11 years 11 months)

Table 17.1 Key assessments used by SLTs in the UK for childhood ABI

Area	Assessment	Description (age range stated by authors in brackets)
Language	Test of Adolescent/Adult Word Finding-2 (TAWF-2) (German, 2013)	A single-word expressive language test that measures word finding abilities of adolescents and adults (12–80 years)
	Test of Word Finding-3 (TWF-3) (German, 2014)	A single-word expressive language test that measures a child's word-finding ability (4 years 6 months–12 years 11 months)
	Clinical Evaluation of Language Fundamentals 5 (CELF 5) (Wiig et al., 2017)	A comprehensive measure of language performance for children and young adults. Assesses semantics, morphology, syntax, and pragmatics (5–21 years 11 months)
	CELF-5 Metalinguistics (Wiig and Secord, 2014)	Tests higher-level language skills (Inference, conversation, multiple meanings, figurative language). The assessment results can inform rehabilitation of functional communication skills (9 to 21 years)
	Clinical Evaluation of Language Fundamentals Preschool-3 (CELF Preschool-3 UK) (Wiig et al., 2024)	Assesses comprehension and production of verbal language skills, play and attention (birth to 7 years 11 months)
	Preschool Language Scales-5 UK (PLS-5) (Zimmerman et al. 2011)	Designed for pre-school children. Assesses a broad range of expressive and receptive language skills (3–6 years 11 months)
	Test of Adolescent and Adult Language-4 (TOAL 4) (Hammill et al., 2007)	Designed to measure the spoken and written language in adolescents and young adults (12–24 years 11 months)
Aphasia	Boston Naming Test (BNT) (Kaplan et al., 2004)	A naming test commonly used to diagnose and assess aphasia and explore the underlying cause of word finding difficulties i.e. language vs cognition (25–88 years)
	Comprehensive Aphasia Test (CAT) (Swinburn et al., 2023)	A test for use with people who have acquired aphasia. It provides a relatively quick assessment of key areas in aphasia (adults)
	Psycholinguistic Assessments of Language in Aphasia (PALPA) (Kay et al., 1992)	Provides a comprehensive assessment of aphasia based on a language processing model (adults)

Table 17.1 (Continued)

Area	Assessment	Description (age range stated by authors in brackets)
Communication questionnaires	Children's Communication Checklist-2 (CCC-2) (Bishop, 2003b)	A screening tool to be completed by a parent or caregiver for children who are likely to have a language or pragmatic impairment (4-16 years)
	Communication Checklist- self report (CC-SR) (Bishop et al., 2009)	A self-report instrument for older children and adults with communication impairments (10 to 80 years)
	La Trobe Communication Questionnaire (Douglas et al., 2010)	A measure of perceived communicative ability that assesses communication ability of adults and adolescents with ABI, based on information gathered from the patient and close others (13 to 64 years)
Cognitive communication	Functional Assessment of Verbal Reasoning and Executive Strategies (FAVRES) (MacDonald and Johnson, 2005)	Assesses verbal reasoning, complex comprehension, discourse, and executive functioning during performance on functional tasks (adults)
	Mount Wilga High Level Language Test (Revised) (Simpson, 2006)	A non-standardised tool used to screen higher-level language skills and other aspects of cognition in people with neurological conditions (adults)
	Pediatric Test of Brain Injury (PTBI) (Hotz et al., 2010)	Assesses neurocognitive, language and literacy skills. It is the only criterion-referenced, standardised test that assesses the skills children need to return to school and function in the general education curriculum following ABI (6-16 years)
Phonology	CLEAR Phonology Screening Assessment (Kehoe, 2001)	Tests each phoneme individually in word initial, medial and final positions (3 to 9 years)
	Diagnostic Evaluation of Articulation and Phonology (DEAP) (Dodd et al., 2006)	Detects and differentiates between articulation problems, delayed phonology and consistent versus inconsistent phonological disorder (3-6 years 11 months)
	South Tyneside Assessment of Phonology 2 (STAP 2) (Armstrong and Ainley, 2007)	Provides a profile of a child's phonological system. It assesses a children's phonological system at word level (5-12 years)

Table 17.1 (Continued)

Area	Assessment	Description (age range stated by authors in brackets)
Neurological speech impairments	Barry-Albright Dystonia Scale (BAD) (Barry et al., 1999)	A 5-point, criterion-based, ordinal scale used to assess dystonia in eyes, mouth, neck, trunk, and limbs (children and young people)
	Dyskinesia Impairment Scale (DIS-II) (Vanmechelen et al., 2023)	This was designed to measure dystonia and choreoathetosis in dyskinetic cerebral palsy. It analyses speech deficits as a component of complex movement disorder (5 years to young adults)
	Frenchay Dysarthria Assessment-2 (FDA-2) (Enderby and Palmer, 2008)	Thorough analysis of dysarthria, informs an impairment-based therapy programme and diagnosis of dysarthria type (12 years to adults)

Table 17.1 (Continued)

- Use of published assessments needs to be carefully considered and discussed within the rehabilitation team so that the timing is appropriate and justified. Any standardised assessment must occur after the child's spontaneous phase of recovery has plateaued. It is essential that the child is out of Post Traumatic Amnesia (PTA), as assessment during this fluctuating and transient phase of recovery will not provide a true picture of skills.
- It should be noted that most SLT assessments used clinically have not been criterion-referenced or standardised for the paediatric ABI population. Developmental assessments are not always sensitive to the specific profiles seen post ABI, so there is a danger of masking functional communication difficulty. A child with an ABI who scores well on standardised assessment may not be able to perform to the same level in a busy classroom, when they are already tired and overwhelmed by the journey to school.
- There are a wide range of paediatric and adult assessments to choose from when assessing a child's skills post ABI. Some of these are reviewed in papers by Gilardone et al. (2023), Crumlish et al. (2022) and McCauley et al. (2012). The assessment selected by the SLT will depend on the specific impairment, rehabilitation phase or transition planned. More experienced colleagues in childhood ABI will offer guidance regarding the best assessment to select. Table 17.1 summarises some of the assessments commonly used by SLTs in the UK, but it is not exhaustive.

Dysphagia

Dysphagia (difficulty swallowing) occurs in up to 68% of children following severe ABI (Morgan et al., 2003) and can have negative nutritional, respiratory and psychosocial consequences. Factors that may predict the presence of dysphagia include a low post injury GCS, intubation longer than 1.5 days, upper and/or lower limb motor impairments and cognitive impairments (Morgan, 2010).

Children with dysphagia are more likely to need an intensive care admission and require longer and more intensive post-injury rehabilitation compared to children without dysphagia. Based on best practice guidelines from Australia, an initial assessment of swallowing should occur within two days post-extubation and/or when the child is alert enough, stable and able to be safely positioned. If dysphagia is present, then the child should be seen at least weekly for review in the early stages post injury during their inpatient admission and when indicated post discharge (Mei et al., 2018). Silent aspiration is common and instrumental assessment of swallowing may be needed for some children, to fully understand their swallowing physiology, characterise aspiration risk and help guide therapeutic interventions.

It is important to understand the specific nature of the brain injury, including the areas of the brain affected and the extent of the damage alongside a child's pre-injury level of functioning to begin to form a hypothesis about their swallowing. A detailed case history, including pre-existing skills, site and onset of injury, as well as an oral-motor examination should form part of every swallowing assessment for a child post ABI. Clinicians should use the specialist knowledge of the team around them including the neurologists, neurosurgeons and paediatricians to aid their understanding of the child's injury.

Functional resolution of dysphagia is typically seen within the first two to three months post-injury (Mendell and Arvedson, 2016), however persistent dysphagia in young people with ABI has been documented (Cornwell et al., 2003; Morgan, Ward and Murdock, 2004) and is associated with negative quality of life consequences (Lefton-Greif et al., 2014). Most children with ABI will show improvement over time. However, children with certain types of brain tumours who need ongoing treatment in the form of radiotherapy, chemotherapy or surgery may experience further change or deterioration in swallowing. Ongoing rehabilitation or treatments are also likely to disrupt typical mealtime experiences for children and families.

Further information about the assessment and management of eating, drinking and swallowing in children can be found in Chapter 18, with some specific features related to childhood ABI outlined below.

- *Sensory changes* can occur after ABI, including a child's perception of smell and flavour, which may impact a child's desire to eat and drink, or their dietary preferences post injury.
- *Cognitive impairments* may lead to difficulties with attention, agitation, impulsivity, disinhibition or self-monitoring which can have a negative impact on a child's ability to safely eat and drink. Impairments may include overfilling the mouth with food, reduced chewing of harder textures, difficulties maintaining a stable position for eating and drinking or significant agitation which impacts a child's desire to eat and drink. Children with cognitive impairments may not recognise their difficulties which creates further challenges in relation to safe management of dysphagia via textural modification, postural or pacing strategies. Children with a mild dysphagia may present with significant nutritional and safety risks if a dysphagia co-occurs alongside cognitive impairments.
- *Fatigue* is extremely common following brain injury and can negatively impact physical and cognitive functioning. Fatigue may exacerbate dysphagia, leading to oral-motor or cognitive decline as a mealtime progresses. This can impact the safety and efficiency of swallowing over the course of a mealtime, or at different times in the day.
- *Changes to mobility, posture and independence*. Where a brain injury simultaneously impacts a child's limb functioning or postural control, they may move from being independent during mealtimes, to being reliant on others to support them to eat and drink. This can lead to feelings of frustration or loss as they come to terms with this change.
- *Nutrition* is essential to meet the often-increased metabolic demands placed on the body following ABI to reduce the risk of malnutrition related complications, such as infection and poor wound repair (Chowdhury, 2024). Children may require non-oral methods to supplement or completely replace their nutrition. If a child is likely to require a non-oral means of nutrition for a long period, then referral for a percutaneous endoscopic gastrostomy (PEG) tube should be considered. When children are having ongoing treatments such as chemotherapy, they may benefit from non-oral methods of nutrition for factors unrelated to swallowing, such as mucositis or nausea. Teamwork, including the child and their caregivers, will help support decision making regarding this.
- *Oral health* Poor oral health is common following brain injury. SLTs have a role in providing advice and education surrounding the benefits of mouthcare to improve QoL, provide comfort and reduce the risk of organism colonisation contributing to aspiration pneumonia (Gurgel-Juarez et al., 2020).

Supporting children's needs in ABI

Communication

There can be significant variation in the extent of communication impairment experienced by individuals. Some children may no longer be able to use spoken language to communicate whilst others may only have occasional word finding difficulties. Management of aphasia in a child with ABI needs to reflect the interruption to their already developing language skills and potential to learn new language functions in the future (Gilardone et al., 2023). Most research studies reflect the higher prevalence of TBI compared to children who have stroke, illness or cancer. Evaluation and comparison of studies can be difficult due to the different ways they categorise injury severity or use diagnostic labels. Furthermore, the range of variables previously described can influence the results. Studies of lived experience can provide insight into how communication is affected in everyday life for children following ABI (Buckeridge et al., 2020; Lo, Waite and Rose, 2023).

As the evidence base is limited for children with aphasia or dysarthria, SLTs select from a variety of approaches and interventions, drawn from the adult and child developmental fields. SLTs will also consult literature in the wider field of neurodisability (Beresford et al., 2018; Novak et al., 2020). Guidance is provided in other chapters of this book such as language development, speech sound disorders, stammering, voice and AAC which will be relevant to the management of children with ABI. Clinicians have reported that collaborative music therapy in rehabilitation settings has led to improvement in speech, communication and social interaction in children with ABI, but this approach may be difficult to replicate in community settings. As with most areas of childhood ABI, further research is needed (Burns and O'Connor, 2023).

While it is beyond the scope of this chapter to explore every possible intervention in depth, the following outlines some key principles when working with children with ABI.

Principles of intervention

- The main goal of therapy should be to enhance the child's ability to communicate effectively in a range of settings, with people who are important to them. This may include therapy aimed at *rehabilitating* lost skills, *habilitating* skills not yet learned, or use of strategies to *compensate* for difficulties.
- When designing therapy materials, it is important to include things that interest the young person and are appropriate to them. Teenagers may get frustrated if you are asking them to do activities that are intended for a much younger child.
- Children who are multilingual may communicate better in one language than another, or struggle to use all their languages following ABI. Interpreters should be used if the child or family does not speak the same language as the treating therapists.
- Interventions should be targeted to the child's strengths and needs. The International Classification of Functioning (ICF) and the F-words (Rosenbaum and Gorter, 2012) can help SLTs to plan meaningful interventions by focusing not only on what a child needs help with but considers the support network that is in place to help a child engage in activities they enjoy and those fostering participation.

- It is important to involve the people who care for the child in their treatment. ABI education aims to increase understanding of communication and how this can break down. Throughout the rehabilitation journey, parents and caregivers are encouraged to reflect on what they are already doing to support interaction with the child and supported with strategies to enhance communication. ABI education could include a range of people who are important to the child in the community, including friends.

Specific areas of intervention

- *Early communication*: Losing the ability to speak can often be a source of anxiety and frustration, so establishing a clear and functional means of communication should be a goal of early treatment planning. Establishing clear and consistent yes/no responses using symbols, gestures or vocalisations is often an early goal.
- *Alternative and Augmentative Communication (AAC)*: Following ABI, some children use writing, drawing, pictures, symbols, gestures and signing in place of or to augment speech when intelligibility is affected (O'Hare, 2016). For children whose speech may deteriorate (e.g. in some forms of brain tumour), AAC should be considered at the earliest opportunity. Symbols can be used to support writing.
- *Dysarthria:* Most treatment methods were developed for adults and include exercises and strategies to help improve breath support, volume, articulation and prosody when speaking. Similar approaches have been shown to be effective for children with cerebral palsy (CP) and can be considered when working with children with acquired dysarthria (Pennington et al., 2013).
- *Acquired apraxia of speech*: Treatment may include articulatory kinematic approaches to improve clarity of speech by using motor programming and planning principles. The recommended interventions for children with apraxia include Rapid Syllable Transition Treatment (ReST) which targets 'consistency and accuracy of sounds, sequencing, and prosody' (McCabe, Thomas and Murray, 2020, p. 821) and the Nuffield Centre Dyspraxia Programme (Williams and Stephens, 2004). AAC may be used by some children when speech intelligibility is poor. Non speech oro-motor exercises are not recommended (RCSLT, 2024)
- *Language*: These interventions target specific deficits in relation to receptive and expressive language including reading and writing. Techniques include labelling items (Rispoli et al., 2010), word webs (Best et al., 2018) or semantic and phonological cueing strategies. The latter are indicated as most effective (Meteyard and Bose, 2018) and may help when a child has word retrieval difficulties. Written word reading, writing and comprehension tasks target literacy difficulties. SLTs will need to target any higher-level language impairment (difficulties with making inference, prediction, etc.) by linking therapy to the curriculum.
- *Cognitive communication disorder (CCD)*: Interventions may aim to *restore* impaired cognitive functions or *compensate* for deficits to support executive functions such as planning and organisation. CCD interventions are often functional in nature and use real-world, meaningful situations, e.g. supporting a young person to plan and execute a trip to the cinema independently. Treatment effects are more successful when the intervention includes family and peers (Laane and Cook, 2020).

- *Social communication*: Intervention may target conversational turn-taking, staying on topic and curtailing verbosity (Rispoli et al. 2010), as well as supporting family and peers to understand and best respond to differences in social communication. Again, strategies are best practised with familiar communication partners initially. The Talkabout series by Alex Kelly (see Recommended resources) can provide a useful framework when working with children who have pragmatic difficulties following ABI.

Dysphagia

The aims of intervention should be to maximise safe oral intake whilst minimising associated risks such as of choking, aspiration, malnutrition or negative psychosocial and participation impacts. Eating and drinking is a social, pleasurable and cultural experience for many people and therefore supporting return to these aspects of mealtimes should be a priority in treatment planning. Specific ABI-related interventions are discussed below, but further information will be found in Chapter 18.

- *Cognition*: Education of children and caregivers should aim to improve awareness of a child's eating and drinking needs. Specific strategies can be implemented, for example, children who impulsively overfill their mouth may benefit from pacing strategies and visual reminders to take one bite of food at a time. Cognition-related impairments may be further exacerbated by noisy and distracting environments, so adjusting the location of mealtimes may be needed. Consider the possible unintended consequences of this however, such as a loss of social interaction with peers if a mealtime is moved from the dining-area into a quiet classroom.
- *Fatigue*: Frequent mealtimes may be recommended or supplementary tube feeds to allow smaller meals with a 'top-up' of nutrition.
- *Swallowing exercises*: The effortful swallow, Mendelsohn manoeuvre and super-supraglottic swallow could be considered in older children with pre-existing adult-like physiology, where cognition and language comprehension allow correct execution (Morgan, 2011). However, there is limited evidence base for their use in children.
- *Oral care*: Use of a non-foaming toothpaste or suctioning during mouthcare may be needed for children with dysphagia. Further information about mouthcare, related to specific age groups and populations, can be found on the Mouthcare Matters website (see Recommended resources).

Setting therapy goals

The role of the SLT entails discussing rehabilitation goals with the team around the child, as the child may have needs in every domain. In the early stages of rehabilitation, the child and family's wishes are often expressed more generally, such as to walk, to talk, to eat or to go back to school. The SLT will need to counsel the family sensitively about interim steps, leading to session goals, short-term goals, and long-term goals for the future. As in other fields of SLT, it is important that goals are clearly stated with a specific statement of what is to be achieved, that is measurable, observable and time limited. Goal Attainment Scaling

(Turner-Stokes et al., 2009) is a person-centred approach to setting rehabilitation goals which has been adopted for use in childhood ABI rehabilitation (Kelly et al., 2019).

A review of the literature has highlighted how participation in personally meaningful activities and creating achievable goals helps a child adjusts to their post-injury identity (Perkins et al., 2022). Examples of setting goals on this basis would be:

- A facial weakness meant that biting and chewing a chocolate bar was not possible. An interim step of melting two cubes of chocolate, to be sucked off a spoon, was a realistic and achievable compromise.
- Sending text messages to their grandmother was not possible due to aphasia but saying, 'hi' on a daily videocall was.
- Although receptive language was good, verbal communication was not possible, so a bespoke low-tech eye gaze system was established so the child could express opinions about their care.

Measuring therapy outcomes

Recording whether goals have been achieved, and reflecting on why not, is good practice. It helps the SLT to consider whether there are factors influencing goal attainment such as the child's physical or emotional state, level of motivation, resilience and social environment. As no two children with a brain injury will be the same, predicting a child's rehabilitation outcomes is notoriously difficult. Therapy outcome measures can effectively capture the complex profiles of children with ABI and measure improvements during rehabilitation (Moll et al., 2022). The SLT may also contribute to national databases such as the UK Rehabilitation Outcomes Collaborative (UK ROC) database (UK Specialist Rehabilitation Outcomes Collaborative, 2013).

Dorothy's story

Dorothy is a 4-year-old who suffered a severe traumatic brain injury after falling from a window. Dorothy was taken to the nearest Paediatric Major Trauma Centre. Scans confirmed a severe diffuse axonal injury and a left temporal skull fracture with underlying contusion.

Dorothy was managed on the Paediatric Intensive Care Unit (PICU) with neuroprotection. A nasogastric tube (NGT) was sited. Dorothy was extubated on day three and was referred to speech and language therapy for swallowing and communication assessment. There had been no birth or developmental concerns. Parents gave a detailed history of Dorothy's personality, preferences and usual routine. Dorothy had acquired right limb weakness and poor head control. Dorothy was confirmed to have no acquired hearing impairments but had some right-sided visual neglect. Dorothy had acquired a severe receptive and expressive aphasia.

Multidisciplinary work with Dorothy and her family allowed optimum positioning, medication and routine, with therapy tailored to her interests. Dorothy was provided with a sensory programme to prevent oral aversion and promote early swallowing rehabilitation. Dorothy resumed full oral intake and the NGT was removed a month post-injury. A programme emphasised the importance of reduced stimulation, protected rest times and communication strategies.

Multidisciplinary input was provided to enable Dorothy to obtain neurorehabilitation goals. Dorothy's receptive aphasia improved but was affected by auditory memory and attention. Dorothy continued to have a moderate expressive aphasia. A mild right-sided limb weakness remained. At discharge planning meetings, emphasis was placed on the unknown trajectory of change. A graded return to school was planned. Staff training and ongoing family support were arranged. An Education and Health Care Plan (EHCP) was initiated. Dorothy was discharged from hospital six months after the accident.

Summary

This chapter can only touch on the many strands involved in working with children with ABI. However, the overview shows that it is a fascinating area of SLT. Diagnosis and management are challenging due to the interplay of injury to a developing brain and the idiosyncratic and emotive nature of each case. Even the most experienced SLT will find it challenging to generate a hypothesis about the relationship between the brain injury and their observations. This is because no two children with ABI are alike; each comes into the rehabilitation setting with their unique set of circumstances and past experiences. This presents the SLT with a superb opportunity to learn something new with every child they encounter. While the child is at the centre of rehabilitation, a holistic approach involving family is vital, from the acute stage through to transition into the community and many years after. It is an important part of the SLT role to help a child and their family adapt to life following ABI and after a period of spontaneous recovery, well planned interventions often lead to improvements in QoL. Rehabilitation settings can be an intense place for the SLT to work but they are also incredibly rewarding. Not many client groups offer the prospect of working in a skilled MDT with medical professionals, AHPs and caregivers. SLTs with expertise in childhood ABI are also essential and valued in community teams so that children can be supported to continue with their long-term rehabilitation goals once they return home.

Recommended resources

British Paediatric Neurology Association (BPNA). Available at: https://bpna.org.uk/
Child Brain Injury Trust. Available at: https://childbraininjurytrust.org.uk/
Children's Trust. Available at: https://www.thechildrenstrust.org.uk/Educating Children and Young
Educating Children and Young People with Acquired Brain Injury by Sue Walker and Beth Wicks (2018): https://www.routledge.com/Educating-Children-and-Young-People-with-Acquired-Brain-Injury/Walker-Wicks/p/book/9781138211025
Encephalitis. Available at: https://www.encephalitis.info/
European Paediatric Neurology Society (EPNS). Available at: https://www.epns.info/
Head injury: assessment and early management NICE guideline [NG232]. Available at: https://www.nice.org.uk/guidance/ng232
Headway. Available at: https://www.headway.org.uk/
Hypoxic-Ischaemic Encephalopathy (H.I.E.). Available at: https://www.peeps-hie.org/
Meningitis. Available at: https://www.meningitisnow.org/
Mouth Care Matters, Available at: https://mouthcarematters.hee.nhs.uk/
RCLST Brain injury guidance. Available at: https://www.rcslt.org/members/clinical-guidance/brain-injury/brain-injury-guidance/
RCSLT Podcast Sound Waves. Available at: https://soundcloud.com/rcslt/paediatric-stroke-childhood-brain-injury-a-patient-and-therapist-perspective

Stroke Association. Available at: https://www.stroke.org.uk/
Stroke in childhood, clinical guideline for diagnosis, management and rehabilitation. Available at: https://www.rcpch.ac.uk/resources/stroke-in-childhood-clinical-guideline
Talkabout Series. Available at: http://alexkelly.biz/alexs-work-and-talkabout/

References

American Speech-Language Association (2005) 'Roles of speech-language pathologists in the identification, diagnosis, and treatment of individuals with cognitive-communication disorders: Position statement'. Available at: https://www.asha.org/policy/ (accessed 28 November 2024).
Anderson, V., Godfrey, C., Rosenfield, J.V. and Catroppa, C. (2012) '10 years outcome from childhood traumatic brain injury', *International Journal of Developmental Neuroscience*, 30(3), 217-24. DOI: 10.1016/j.ijdevneu.2011.09.008
Armstrong, S. and Ainley, M. (2007) *South Tyneside Assessment of Phonology (STAP 2)*. 2nd edn. Newcastle: Stass Publications.
Barry, M.J., VanSwearingen, J.M. and Albright, A.L. (1999) *Barry-Albright Dystonia Scale (BAD)*. Washington, DC: APA PsycTests.
Beresford, B., Clarke, S. and Maddison, J. (2018) 'Therapy interventions for children with neurodisabilities: A qualitative scoping study', *Health Technology Assessment*. 22(3). DOI: 10.3310/hta22030
Best, W., Hughes, L. M., Masterson, J., Thomas, M., Fedor, A., Roncoli, S., … Kapikian, A. . (2018) 'Intervention for children with word-finding difficulties: A parallel group randomised control trial', *International Journal of Speech-Language Pathology*, 20(7), 708-719. DOI: 10.1080/17549507.2017.1348541
Bishop, D. (2003a) *Test for Reception of Grammar (TROG-2)*. 2nd edn. Harlow: Pearson Clinical Assessments.
Bishop, D. (2003b) *The Children's Communication Checklist (CCC-2)*, version 2. Harlow: Pearson Clinical Assessments.
Bishop, D., Whitehouse, A. and Sharp M. (2009) *Communication Checklist-self report (CC-SR)*. Harlow: Pearson Clinical Assessments.
Blosser, J.L. and DePompei, R. (2003) *Pediatric Traumatic Brain Injury Proactive Intervention*. 2nd edn. Toronto: Delmar Learning.
Breau, L.M., Clark, B., Scott, O., Wilkes, C., Reynolds, S., Ricci, F., Sonnenberg, L. Zwaigenbaum, L., Rashid, M. and Goez, H.R. (2015) 'Social communication features in children following moderate to severe acquired brain injury: A cross-sectional pilot study', *Journal of Child Neurology*, 30(5), 588-594. DOI: 10.1177/0883073814528282
Buckeridge, K., Clarke, C. and Sellers, D. (2020) 'Adolescents' experiences of communication following acquired brain injury', *International Journal of Language and Communication Disorders*, 55(1), 97-109. DOI: 10.1111/1460-6984.12506
Burns, J. and O'Connor, R.S. (2023) 'Exploring clinicians' experiences of engaging in collaborative music therapy and speech and language therapy for children with an acquired brain injury', *Approaches: An Interdisciplinary Journal of Music Therapy* [Preprint]. DOI: https://doi.org/10.56883/aijmt.2024.37
Catroppa, C. and Anderson, V. (2004) 'Recovery and predictors of language skills two years following pediatric traumatic brain injury', *Brain and Language*, 88(1), 68-78. DOI: 10.1016/s0093-934x(03)00159-7
Chapman, S.B. (2006) 'Neurocognitive stall: A paradox in long term recovery from pediatric brain injury', *Brain Injury*, 3(4), 10-13.
Chowdhury, S.R., Sahu, P. and Bindra, A. (2024) 'Nutrition management in pediatric traumatic brain injury: An exploration of knowledge gaps and challenges', *Journal of Neuroanaesthesiology Critical Care*, 11(9), 155-166. https://doi.org/10.1055/s-0044-1795103.
Cornwell, P.L., Murdoch, B.E., Ward, E.C. and Morgan, A. (2003) 'Dysarthria and dysphagia as long-term sequelae in a child treated for posterior fossa tumour', *Pediatric Rehabilitation*, 6(2), 67-75. DOI: 10.1080/13638490310001392891 0.1080/1363849031000139289
Crumlish, L., Wallace, S.J., Copley, A. and Rose, T.A. . (2022) 'Exploring the measurement of pediatric cognitive-communication disorders in traumatic brain injury research: A scoping review', *Brain Injury*, 36(10-11), 1207-1227. DOI: 10.1080/02699052.2022.2111026
Dennis, M. (2010) 'Margaret Kennard (1899-1975): Not a "principle" of brain plasticity but a founding mother of developmental neuropsychology', *Cortex*, 46(8), 1043-1059. DOI:10.1016/j.cortex.2009.10.008
Diener, M.L., Kirby, A.V., Sumsion, F., Canary, H.E., and Green, M.M. (2022) 'Community reintegration

needs following paediatric brain injury: Perspectives of caregivers and service providers', *Disability and Rehabilitation*, 44(19), 5592–5602. DOI: 10.1080/09638288.2021.1946176

Dodd, B., Hua, Z., Crosbie, S., Holm, A. and Ozanne, A. (2006) *Diagnostic Evaluation of Articulation and Phonology (DEAP)*. Harlow: Pearson Clinical Assessment.

Douglas, J., O'Flaherty, C. and Snow, P (2010) *La Trobe Communication Questionnaire*. Hove: Psychology Press.

Dunn, D.M. (2011) *British Picture Vocabulary Scale (BPVS-III)*, 3rd edn. Harlow: Pearson Clinical Assessment.

Enderby, P. and Palmer, R. (2008) *Frenchay Dysarthria Assessment (FDA-2)*, 2nd edn. Singular Publishing Group.

Forsyth, R. and Kirkham, F. (2012); Predicting outcome after childhood brain injury', *Canadian Medical Association Journal*, 184(11), 1257–1264. DOI: 10.1503/cmaj.111045

German, D. (2013) *Test of Adolescent /Adult Word Finding (TAWF-2)*. 2nd edn. Ann Arbor, MI: Ann Arbor Publishers.

German, D. (2014) *Test of Word Finding (TWF-3.)*, 3rd edn. Austin, TX: Pro.Ed.

Giacino, J,. Bodien, Y. and Chatelle, C. (2020) *Coma Recovery Scale-Revised (CRS-R), updated*. Rehabilitation Outcomes Center at Spaulding (ROCS).

Gilardone, G., Viganò, M., Cassinelli, D., Fumagalli, F. M., Calvo, I., Gilardone, M., Sozzi, M. and Corbo, M. (2023) 'Post-stroke acquired childhood aphasia. A scoping review', *Child Neuropsychology*, 29(8), 1268–1293. DOI: 10.1080/09297049.2022.2156992

Gill-Thwaites, H., Elliott, K. and Munday, R. (2004) *Sensory Modality Assessment and Rehabilitation Technique (SMART)*. London: Royal Hospital for Neuro-disability.

Gurgel-Juarez, N., Perrier, M-F., Hoffmann, T., Lannin, N, Jolliffe, L., Lee, R., Brosseau, L.and Flowers, H. (2020) 'Guideline recommendations for oral care after acquired brain injury: protocol for a systematic review', *JMIR Research Protocols*, 9(7), e17249. DOI: 10.2196/17249

Hammill, D.D., Brown, V.L., Larsen, S.C. and Wiederholt, J.L. (2007) *Test of Adolescent and Adult Language (TOAL 4)*, 4th edn. Austin, TX: Pro.Ed.

Hotz, G., Helm-Estabrooks, N. and Nelson, N. (2010) *Paediatric Test of Brain Injury (PTBI)*. Baltimore, MD: Brookes Publishing Co.

Kakonge, L., Charron, V. P., Vedder, J., Wormald, K., and Turkstra, L. S. (2022) 'Neuropsychological rehabilitation A mapping review of adolescent identity after TBI: what clinicians need to know', *Neuropsychological Rehabilitation*, 32(8), 1868–1903. DOI: 10.1080/09602011.2022.2071299

Kaplan, E., Goodglass, H. and Weintraub, S. (2004) *Boston Naming Test (BNT)*. 2nd edn. Ann Arbor, MI: Ann Arbor Publishers.

Kay, J., Lesser, R. and Coltheart, M. (1992) *Psycholinguistic Assessment of Language in Aphasia (PALPA)*. Hove: Psychological Press.

Keetley, R., Bennett, E., Williams, J., Whitehouse, W.P., Pilling, P. and Manning, J.C. (2021) 'Outcomes for children with acquired brain injury (ABI) admitted to acute neurorehabilitation', *Developmental Medicine and Child Neurology*, 63(7), 824–830. DOI: 10.1111/dmcn.14846

Kehoe, M. (2001) *CLEAR Phonology Screening Assessment*. CLEAR Resources.

Kelly, G., Dunford, C., Forsyth, R. and Kavčič, A. (2019) 'Using child- and family-centred goal setting as an outcome measure in residential rehabilitation for children and youth with acquired brain injuries: The challenge of predicting expected levels of achievement', *Child: Care, Health and Development*, 45(2), 286–291. DOI: 10.1111/cch.12636

Laane, S.A. and Cook, L.G. (2020) 'Cognitive-communication interventions for youth with traumatic brain injury', *Seminars in Speech and Language*, 41(2), 183–194. DOI: 10.1055/s-0040-1701686

Lefton-Greif, M.A., Okelo, S.O., Wright, J.M., Collaco, J.M., McGrath-Morrow, S.A. and Eakin, M.N. (2014) 'Impact of children's feeding/swallowing problems: Validation of a new caregiver instrument', *Dysphagia*, 29(6), 671–677. DOI: 10.1007/s00455-014-9560-7

Linden, M.A., McKinlay, A., Hawley, C., Aaro-Jonsson, C., Kristiansen, I., . . . Meyer-Heim, A. (2024) 'Further recommendations of the International Paediatric Brain Injury Society (IPBIS) for the post-acute rehabilitation of children with acquired brain injury', *Brain Injury*, 38(3), 151–159. DOI: 10.1080/02699052.2024.2309252

Lo, D., Waite, M. and Rose, T.A. (2023) 'Experiences of childhood stroke and aphasia during adolescence: An analysis of YouTube videos', *International Journal of Speech-Language Pathology*, 25(3), 403–412. DOI: 10.1080/17549507.2023.2182743

MacDonald, S. and Johnson, C. (2005) *The Functional Assessment of Verbal Reasoning and Executive Strategies (FAVRES)*. CCD Publishing.

McCabe, P., Thomas, D.C. and Murray, E. (2020) 'Rapid syllable transition treatment: A treatment for childhood apraxia of speech and other pediatric motor speech disorders', *Perspectives of the ASHA Special Interest Groups*, 5, 821–830. DOI: 10.1016/j.jcomdis.2014.06.004

McCauley, S.R., Wilde, E.A., Anderson, V.A., Bedell, G., Beers, S.R., Campbell, T.F., . . . and Yeates, K.O. (2012) 'Recommendations for the use of common outcome measures in pediatric traumatic brain injury research', *Journal of Neurotrauma*, 29(4), 678–705. DOI: 10.1089/neu.2011.1838

Mei, C., Anderson, V., Waugh, M.C., Cahill, L., Morgan, A.T. and TBI Guideline Development Group (2018) 'Evidence- and consensus-based guidelines for the management of communication and swallowing disorders following pediatric traumatic brain injury', *Journal of Head Trauma Rehabilitation*, 33(5), 326–341. DOI: 10.1097/HTR.0000000000000366

Mendell, D.A. and Arvedson, J.C. (2016) 'Dysphagia in pediatric traumatic brain injury', *Current Physical Medicine and Rehabilitation Reports*, 4, 233–236.

Meteyard, L. and Bose, A. (2018) 'What does a cue do? Comparing phonological and semantic cues for picture naming in aphasia', *Journal of Speech, Language, and Hearing Research*, 61(3), 658–674. DOI: 10.1044/2017_JSLHR-L-17-0214

Moll, D., Edwards, L., Kelly, G. and Hamilton, C. (2022) 'Using therapy outcome measures to identify the speech and language therapy needs of children and young people with severe acquired brain injury', *International Journal of Therapy and Rehabilitation*, 29(12), 1–13. DOI: 10.12968/ijtr.2021.0113

Morgan, A. (2010) 'Dysphagia in childhood traumatic brain injury: A reflection on the evidence and its implications for practice', *Developmental Neurorehabilitation*, 13(3), 192–203. https://doi.org/10.3109/17518420903289535.

Morgan, A. (2011) 'Management of oromotor disorder for feeding in children with neurological impairment', in P.L. Roig-Quilis (ed.) *Oromotor Disorders in Childhood*. Barcelona, Spain: Viguera Editores, pp. 225–245.

Morgan, A. (2014) 'Dysarthria in children and adults with TBI', in S. McDonald, L. Togher and C. Code (eds) *Social and Communication Disorders Following Traumatic Brain Injury*. 2nd edn. Hove: Psychology Press, pp. 1–25.

Morgan, A., Ward, E,. and Murdoch, B. (2004) 'A case study of the resolution of paediatric dysphagia following brainstem injury: Clinical and instrumental assessment', *Journal of Clinical Neuroscience*, 11(2), 182–190.

Morgan, A., Ward, E., Murdoch, B., Kennedy, B., and Murison, R. (2003) 'Incidence, characteristics, and predictive factors for dysphagia after pediatric traumatic brain injury,' *Journal of Head Trauma Rehabilitation*, 18(3), 239–251. DOI: 10.1097/00001199-200305000-00002

NHS England (2013) *2013/14 NHS standard contract for paediatric neurosciences: neurorehabilitation*. Available at: https://www.england.nhs.uk/wp-content/uploads/2018/09/Paediatric-Neurorehabilitation.pdf (Accessed: 28 November 2024).

Nippold, M.A., Mansfield, T.C. and Billow, J.L. (2007) 'Peer conflict explanations in children, adolescents, and adults: Examining the development of complex syntax', *American Journal of Speech-Language Pathology*, 16 (May), 179–188. DOI: 10.1044/1058-0360(2007/022)

Novak, I., Morgan, C., Fahey, M., Finch-Edmondson, M., Galea, C., Hines, A., Langdon, K., . . ., and Badawi, N. (2020) 'State of the evidence traffic lights 2019: Systematic review of interventions for preventing and treating children with cerebral palsy'. *Current Neurology and Neuroscience Reports*, 20(2), 3. DOI: 10.1007/s11910-020-1022-z

O'Hare, A. (2016) 'Management of developmental speech and language disorders. Part 2: Acquired conditions'. *Archives of Disease in Childhood*, 101(3), 278–283. DOI: 10.1136/archdischild-2014-306153

Pennington, L., Roelant, E., Thompson, V., Robson, S., Steen, N. and Miller, N. (2013) 'Intensive dysarthria therapy for younger children with cerebral palsy', *Developmental Medicine and Child Neurology*, 55(5), 464–471. DOI: 10.1111/dmcn.12098

Perkins, A., Gracey, F., Kelly, G., and Jim, J. (2022) 'A new model to guide identity-focused multidisciplinary rehabilitation for children and young people following acquired brain injury: I-FoRM', *Neuropsychological Rehabilitation*, 32(8), 1928–1969. DOI: 10.1080/09602011.2022.2100794

RCSLT (2024) 'Royal College of Speech and Language Therapists Position Paper on Childhood Apraxia of Speech', pp. 1–46. Available at: RCSLT-Childhood-Apraxia-of-Speech-CAS-Position-Paper-2024.pdfRCSLT-Childhood-Apraxia-of-Speech-CAS-Position-Paper-2024.pdf (accessed 13 March 2025).

Renfrew, C. (2010) *Bus Story Test (Renfrew Language Scales):* Revised Edition. Milton Keynes: Speechmark.
Renfrew, C. (2019) *Renfrew Action Picture Test (RAPT)*. 5th edn. Milton Keynes: Speechmark.
Renfrew, C. (2023) *Renfrew Expressive Vocabulary Test (REV)*. 5th ed. Milton Keynes: Speechmark.
Rispoli, M.J., MacHalicek, W. and Lang, R. (2010) 'Communication interventions for individuals with acquired brain injury', *Developmental Neurorehabilitation*, 13(2), 141–151. DOI: 10.3109/1751842090346846
Rosenbaum, P. and Gorter, J.W. (2012) 'The "F-words" in childhood disability: I swear this is how we should think', *Child: Care, Health and Development*, 38(4), 457–463. DOI: 10.1111/j.1365-2214.2011.01338.x
Royal College of Physicians and British Society of Rehabilitation Medicine (2003) *Rehabilitation Following Acquired Brain Injury: National Clinical Guidelines*, L. Turner-Stokes (ed.). London: RCP, BSRM. Available at https://www.headway.org.uk/media/3320/bsrm-rehabilitation-following-acquired-brain-injury.pdf (accessed 13 March 2025).
Scolding, N., Owen, A.M. and Keown, J. (2021) 'Prolonged disorders of consciousness: A critical evaluation of the new UK guidelines', *Brain*, 144(6), 1655–1660. DOI: 10.1093/brain/awab063
Shiel, A., Wilson, B.A., McLellan, L. and Horn, S. (2000) *Wessex Head Injury Matrix (WHIM)*. Harlow: Pearson Clinical Assessment.
Simpson, F. (2006) *Mount Wilga Assessment High Level Language Test (20th Anniversary Revised Edition 1)*. Available at: https://www.scribd.com/document/218341634/Mount-Wilga-High-Level-Language-Test-revised-2006
Slomine, B.S., Suskauer, S.J., Nicholson, R. and Giacino, J.T. (2019) 'Preliminary validation of the coma recovery scale for pediatrics in typically developing young children', *Brain Injury*, August 28, 16. DOI: 10.1080/02699052.2019.1658221
Swinburn, K., Porter, G. and Howard, D. (2023) *Comprehensive Aphasia Test (CAT)*, 2nd edn. Abingdon: Routledge.
Teasdale, G. and Jennett, B. (1974) 'Assessment of coma and impaired consciousness: A practical scale', *Lancet*, 2, 81–84. DOI: 10.1016/S0140-6736(74)91639-0
Togher, L., McDonald, S. and Code, C. (2014) 'Social and communication disorders following traumatic brain injury', in S. McDonald, L. Togher, and C. Code (eds) *Social and Communication Disorders Following Traumatic Brain Injury*. 2nd edn. Hove: Psychology Press.
Turner-Stokes, L., Williams, H. and Johnson, J. (2009) 'Goal attainment scaling: Does it provide added value as a person-centred measure for evaluation of outcome in neurorehabilitation following acquired brain injury?', *Journal of Rehabilitation Medicine*, 41(7), 528–535. DOI: 10.2340/16501977-0383
UK Specialist Rehabilitation Outcomes Collaborative (2013). *UK ROC UK Rehabilitation Outcomes Collaborative*. London: UK Rehabilitation Outcomes Collaborative (UK ROC), Cicely Saunders Institute of Palliative Care, Policy and Rehabilitation | King's College London.
Vanmechelen, I., Danielsson, A., Lidbeck, C., Tedroff, K., Monbaliu, E., and Krumlinde-Sundholm, L. (2023) 'The Dyskinesia Impairment Scale, second edition: Development, construct validity, and reliability', *Developmental Medicine and Child Neurology*, 65(5), 683–690. https://doi.org/10.1111/dmcn.15444
Wiig, E. and Secord, W. (2014) *Clinical Evaluation of Language Fundamentals Metalinguistics (CELF Metalinguistics 5)*. 5th edn. Harlow: Pearson Clinical Assessments.
Wiig, E., Secord, W. and Semel, E. (2024) *Clinical Evaluation of Language Fundamentals Preschool UK (CELF Preschool 3 UK)*. 3rd edn. Harlow: Pearson Clinical Assessments.
Wiig, E., Semel, E. and Secord, W. (2017) *Clinical Evaluation of Language Fundamentals (CELF 5 UK)*. 5th edn. Harlow: Pearson Clinical Assessments.
Williams, P. and Stephens, H. (2004) *The Nuffield Centre Dyspraxia Programme*, 3rd edn. The Miracle Factory. Available at: www.ndp3.org (accessed 28 November 2024).
Zimmerman, I L., Pond, R.A. and Steiner, V.G. (2011) *Preschool Language Scales (PLS-5)*, 5th edn. Harlow: Pearson Clinical Assessments.

18 Childhood onset eating, drinking and swallowing difficulties

Diane Sellers, Ailish Harrison, Sally Morgan and Mari Viviers

What you'll learn in this chapter

- Definitions of paediatric oro-pharyngeal dysphagia and Paediatric Feeding Disorder
- Biopsychosocial factors that influence eating, drinking and swallowing
- Different presentations across ages and stages of development
- Prevalence and aetiology
- Assessment and management of eating, drinking and swallowing difficulties.

This chapter presents information about eating, drinking and swallowing difficulties that arise in childhood. Deliberately, the term 'eating, drinking and swallowing difficulties' is used as an overarching term to cover what other authors might call 'feeding problems', 'oro-pharyngeal dysphagia', 'dysphagia', 'paediatric feeding disorders' and 'Avoidant Restrictive Food Intake Disorder'. The chapter provides an overview of paediatric eating and drinking difficulties as a route map to guide practice and further study.

Speech and language therapists working with children, from neonates to adolescents, require a solid theoretical understanding of the developing neuro-anatomy and physiology of feeding, swallowing, eating and drinking. It is essential to have a broad understanding of embryology, and the development and function of neurological, respiratory and gastro-intestinal body systems. It is also crucial to understand the interplay between different bodily systems in order to provide evidence-based care.

This chapter serves as an introduction to paediatric eating, drinking and swallowing difficulties. To develop your practice further, you will need to understand other features such as:

- neuroplasticity
- oral anatomy
- cranial nerves
- the concept of the valved system that supports skilled and safe eating and drinking
- the central pattern generators and the role of the brainstem and cortex in swallowing
- reflexes
- lung development and the impact of chronic aspiration on the developing lung tissues
- the impact of respiratory support on the larynx which reduces sensation, stents open the airway and decreases responsiveness to airway invasion.

Resources are given in the Recommended resources at the end of this chapter for further learning opportunities.

Key information about eating, drinking and swallowing difficulties

The number of children who have eating and drinking difficulties is estimated to be 20-50% of typically developing children and 70-89% of children with developmental disabilities (Benjasuwantep, Chaithirayanon and Eiamudomkan, 2013).

Infants start to develop the necessary skills to take fluid into the body by suckling and swallowing whilst in utero. The skills of sucking, swallowing, biting, chewing, and controlling food and fluid in the mouth continue to develop from early infancy, through the weaning process as a toddler and are refined in early childhood. These skills are developed against a backdrop of a changing and maturing biopsychosocial system. The process is typically complete by the age of 3 years, although greater skill and strength in managing more demanding food textures will develop with age and experience.

Eating, drinking and swallowing develop and change across the life-course. It is important to be aware of significant transition points in childhood. For example: moving from hospital to home as a newborn; introduction of solids alongside fluids; moving from care at home to nursery and then school; decreasing dependency upon others; increasing independence and competency in teenage years; and increased self-awareness and self-management with transition into adulthood.

Eating, drinking and mealtimes are important in all cultures, with family traditions, community foods, milestone celebrations, and sporting, cultural and religious festivals. All work in this area needs to consider the cultural and social context for the child and family.

Eating, drinking and swallowing difficulties: oro-pharyngeal dysphagia

The process of eating, drinking and swallowing requires co-ordination between different body systems to protect the airway and direct food or fluid into the stomach. Body systems that are particularly important are the respiratory, digestive, cardio-vascular, skeletal, muscular, and neurological systems. Disturbances to one or more of these systems may affect an individual's ability to eat, drink or swallow safely, comfortably and efficiently. When a baby is born prematurely, these body systems may not be mature enough to support the skilled co-ordinated movements necessary to take fluid into the body; this is illustrated in Freddie's story, at the end of this chapter.

Speech and language therapists (SLTs) working with children with eating, drinking or swallowing difficulties typically focus on those with 'oro-pharyngeal dysphagia'; this is when there are obvious disruptions to the body systems required to support the process of holding and processing food/fluid in the mouth, and moving this across a closed protected airway into the oesophagus and on to the stomach. For example, a child with cerebral palsy may experience disturbances to the neurological, musculo-skeletal, digestive and respiratory systems as a result of damage to the developing infant brain:

- Skilled movements to bite, chew and swallow food are affected by unstable posture and extra involuntary movements of trunk, head and limbs, jaw, face and tongue.

- It may be challenging to hold food/fluid in the mouth to co-ordinate swallowing with breathing; breathing may be laboured and uncontrolled.
- Bits of food or fluid may spill over the back of the tongue into the throat before the swallow is triggered to protect the airway and push the food/fluid into the oesophagus.
- Unco-ordinated, repeated or absent swallowing movements may lead to 'aspiration' when particles of food, fluid or saliva enter the airway which may contribute to respiratory illness.
- Disturbances to the digestive system may lead to hidden sources of pain and discomfort from reflux, constipation and delayed stomach emptying.

Different health conditions will have predictable and evolving impacts upon different body systems and associated function. Consider whether the underlying health condition that affects someone's eating, drinking and swallowing is present from birth, for example, Down syndrome and other genetic conditions, cleft lip and palate and other congenital malformations of the body and brain, or metabolic conditions. A child may develop typical eating and drinking skills until function is disrupted by degenerative health conditions that become apparent later in childhood such as one of the muscular dystrophies. Typical development and function may be disrupted and altered by acquired conditions such as traumatic brain injury, tumours, physical injury or body systems damaged by toxins, infections or injury.

Eating, drinking and swallowing may be disrupted by iatrogenic causes, that is where medical treatment or interventions cause or exacerbate difficulties, for example, a child may require a tracheostomy and/or long-term ventilation to support respiration, which will have an impact on their experiences and development of eating, drinking and swallowing skills; an infant experiencing repeated invasive procedures such as passing naso-gastric tubes may present with heightened stress, gagging and aversion around different food textures.

Children may have more than one co-occurring potential cause of their eating, drinking and swallowing difficulty. SLTs need to develop their skills in taking a full history to understand potential causes of someone's eating, drinking and swallowing difficulties, including multiple interacting strands.

Eating, drinking and swallowing difficulties: paediatric feeding disorder

SLTs are adopting a broader biopsychosocial focus with the recent consensus-based diagnostic term Paediatric Feeding Disorder, which is defined as: 'impaired oral intake that is not age appropriate, and is associated with medical, nutritional, feeding skill and/or psychosocial dysfunction' (Goday et al., 2019). This diagnostic term moves beyond a body systems approach to consider the area of dysfunction and needs of the child rather than the cause, acknowledging that difficulties in one of the four Paediatric Feeding Disorder domains can lead to dysfunction in all domains. For example, a child who has significant life-threatening food allergies can lead to dysfunction in all domains: the child's diet is restricted due to life-threatening allergies and reflux (medical), which may lead to a reduced diet range and food refusal (nutritional inadequacy), reduced opportunities to try new foods (feeding skill developmental delay) and high anxiety from parent and child about food impacting on all aspects of mealtimes (psychosocial dysfunction). All children with oro-pharyngeal dysphagia would fit within the wider label of Paediatric Feeding Disorder. However, not all children with Paediatric Feeding Disorder will have dysphagia, although many may have some level of feeding skill difficulty, such as difficulties with chewing despite an intact swallowing ability. Some infants and children with feeding aversion or a restricted diet may fit the criteria for Paediatric Feeding Disorder, while others may fit the criteria for Avoidant Restrictive Food Intake Disorder (ARFID).

There is ongoing debate around the use of diagnostic labels for infants, children and young people with feeding aversion and restricted diets. ARFID was introduced in 2013 in the *Diagnostic and Statistical Manual of Mental Disorders*, Fifth Edition (DSM-5) (APA, 2013), under the umbrella category of 'feeding and eating disorders'. Aligning feeding aversion with eating disorders has been contentious in the feeding and eating disorder clinical communities; this resulted in the definition and delineation of Paediatric Feeding Disorder. Paediatric Feeding Disorder's broad framework of medical, nutritional, feeding skill and psychosocial domains has many areas of overlap with the ARFID diagnostic criteria; agreement has not yet been reached as to how the two diagnostic labels coexist, which can be confusing and difficult to navigate, both for professionals and parents.

Stages of eating, drinking and swallowing

Changes and challenges to sucking, eating, drinking and swallowing for the growing child take place against a backdrop of changing anatomy and physiology (see the American Speech-Language-Hearing Association (ASHA) Pediatric Feeding and Swallowing in Recommended resources for anatomical differences in structures involved in swallowing from infancy to childhood). Nutritional and hydrational needs increase as a child grows as do expectations of greater independence and self-management. These and other changes associated with children's development and maturation may increase or decrease eating, drinking and swallowing difficulties. The infant takes in fluid only in the first months of life, with introduction of food as part of a process of weaning.

Difficulties may occur at one or more of the different stages of eating, drinking and swallowing. We outline the process in four stages:

Anticipatory stage

This stage includes emotions, memories, thoughts, actions and intentions that someone brings prior to the stage when food or drink enters the mouth. Personal and environmental factors will influence this stage when external cues from the environment meet an individual's senses (Leopold and Kagel, 1997; Shune, Moon and Goodman, 2016). These include:

- cognitive factors such as awareness, alertness, anticipation and motivation;
- emotional and physical readiness to eat and drink;
- hearing and understanding sounds linked to food and drink to be ingested;
- seeing, accessing memory stores and understanding physical properties of food/drink;
- feeling texture, temperature, size of pieces of food;
- smelling external cues, such as food and drink;

- proprioceptive feedback from reaching and grasping food/drink to be ingested;
- timing of mouth opening with arrival of food/drink at the mouth;
- skills to communicate needs and preferences to care-giver.

Disturbances at the Anticipatory Stage can affect children's engagement and enjoyment of mealtimes, as well as safety and efficiency.

Oral stage

The oral stage includes the processes involved in the mouth to prepare food and drink ready for swallowing (Matsuo and Palmer, 2008). This stage is sometimes divided into two separate stages: the Oral Preparatory Stage and the Oral Propulsion Stage. The processes include:

- taking food/drink into the mouth by the use of the lips, tongue and jaw;
- retaining food/drink in the mouth until ready for swallowing;
- biting food into manageable size pieces;
- chewing food and mixing with saliva until optimal for swallowing;
- positioning and holding food/drink in the mouth ready for swallowing;
- propelling food/drink backwards in the mouth to initiate swallowing.

Children and infants may experience disturbances at the oral stage affecting their nutritional intake, as well as the efficiency and safety of eating/drinking. The muscles and structures of the face, jaw and tongue work together to perform these skilled movements, informed by sensory feedback from the mouth. Changing dentition, oral hygiene and sources of pain in the mouth may have an impact on a child's food texture and temperature preferences and perception of eating, drinking and swallowing difficulties (Chow et al., 2024).

Pharyngeal stage

While the oral stage is mostly volitional, the pharyngeal stage is a rapid sequential activity or patterned response taking less than a second to complete (Matsuo and Palmer, 2008; Malandraki, Johnson and Robbins, 2011). It involves:

- propulsion of food/fluid through the pharynx and into the oesophagus, past the upper oesophageal segment;
- protection of the airway by insulating the larynx and trachea from the pharynx during the passage of food and fluid to prevent it entering the airway;
- protection of the nasal airway by elevation of the soft palate as food/fluid passes by;
- coughing and gagging to clear particles of food or fluid from the airway or back of the throat.

The pharyngeal stage involves mechanisms to protect the airway when food or fluid is in the mouth, including the closure of the vocal folds; pulling the larynx and hyoid bone upwards and forwards to tuck the larynx under the base of the tongue; and backwards tilting of the epiglottis to seal the entrance to the larynx. Disturbances at this stage will increase likelihood of particles of food or fluid entering the airway (aspiration).

Oesophageal stage

The pharyngeal stage of swallowing triggers the active opening of the upper oesophageal sphincter, allowing the entry of food/fluid into the oesophagus. Waves of smooth muscle contraction carry the food/fluid down the oesophagus, through the lower oesophageal sphincter into the stomach (Matsuo and Palmer, 2008). Disturbances at the oesophageal phase may include choking, reflux, regurgitation of food, and pain after swallowing.

Areas of complexity, challenge and risk

Airway protection

Airway protection is critical to swallowing, with serious consequences if the usual safety mechanisms fail. If the activities of swallowing and breathing are not tightly co-ordinated, it is possible that particles of food/fluid will enter the lungs, known as aspiration (Matsuo and Palmer, 2008). Strong reflex coughing or throat clearing is the body's usual protective response to aspiration, although altered sensation or weak and unco-ordinated movements will reduce this protective response (Arvedson et al., 1994; Matsuo and Palmer, 2008; Weir et al., 2009). Aspiration of food, fluid, saliva or stomach contents may occur at any of the stages of eating, drinking and swallowing outlined.

It is not possible to directly observe events taking place inside the mouth, throat and larynx when someone eats and drinks. Instrumental measures such as dynamic X-ray (videofluoroscopic swallow studies, VFSS) and fibre-optic endoscopic evaluation of swallowing (FEES) are used to visualise some of these hidden events in a limited time frame. The term 'silent aspiration' is used when aspiration is visualised using instrumental measures but is not accompanied by coughing, the expected response when food/fluid enters the larynx (Arvedson et al., 1994; Weir et al., 2009).

Some children may find it challenging to bite and chew food using precise jaw pressure in response to sensory demands of food, and lip and tongue movement to transfer pieces of food to molars for further chewing. The rhythmical repetitive vertical movements of the jaw in combination with rotary movements of the tongue and the co-ordinated activity of the lips and cheeks may be difficult to perform (Remijn et al., 2013). Lateral tongue movement is required to move food around in the mouth, mix it with saliva and dislodge it from tooth surfaces (Matsuo and Palmer, 2008; Remijn et al., 2013). Children may bite their tongues, cheeks or lips because of limitations in co-ordinating these movements (Matsuo and Palmer, 2008). If the child is unable to alter the properties of the food and reduce it in size suitable for swallowing, there is a considerable risk of choking and asphyxiation. The safety mechanism of gagging in response to large pieces of food at the back of the mouth may prevent someone from choking. However, a hyper-reactive gag reflex will impact someone's eating and drinking. Modification of food textures and fluid consistencies may reduce risks associated with biting, chewing and swallowing.

The consequences of aspiration and choking are highly variable, ranging from no discernible effects, through to airway obstruction or severe aspiration pneumonia (Cass et al., 2005; Matsuo and Palmer, 2008). Chronic or recurrent respiratory symptoms can occur when food, fluid, saliva, or gastric refluxate enter the lungs (Boesch et al., 2006); this may also contribute to premature death (Glover and Ayub, 2010). However, the presence of aspiration is not always correlated with respiratory morbidity (Cass et al., 2005).

Nutrition and hydration needs

Children with eating, drinking and swallowing difficulties may struggle to take enough food and drink into their bodies to grow and stay healthy. Researchers have used population studies to look at the impact of poor nutrition and hydration on the health and growth in children with cerebral palsy, who are at high risk of having eating, drinking and swallowing difficulties (Sullivan et al., 2002; Stevenson et al., 2006). Wherever eating, drinking and swallowing difficulties occur, there are increased risks of inadequate nutritional and/or hydrational intake with serious consequences for health. This includes children who are very selective about the foods they will eat.

Picky eating in infants, toddlers and children is very common. It is important to distinguish between children with 'picky eating' behaviours and infants, toddlers and children with feeding aversion or selective eating. Signs of feeding aversion may be recognised when the child appears to have a lack of interest in food or a poor appetite or when they become dysregulated during feeding and mealtimes. Children with feeding aversion might insist on mealtimes taking place in a certain environment, with a certain person feeding them; they may refuse to eat food based on the taste, texture, temperature or other sensory features. Children with food aversion may appear slow to eat, they may gag or vomit in response to foods they cannot tolerate, and mealtimes can become long and stressful. The child with food aversion may eat less food than is expected or required at their age and this may impact a child's ability to gain weight and grow. Medical professionals may become concerned at children's faltering growth and place pressure on families to increase their children's food intake, which inadvertently increases mealtime stresses, making it more difficult for families to stay calm and positive at mealtimes.

A child's feeding aversion may persist for some time, such that the child accepts only a very limited number of foods, known as 'a restricted diet'. Children restrict their diet because of their strong feelings about food which may include disgust and extreme fear; children with feeding aversion do not restrict their diet because of concerns about body image or cultural practices that require the child to only eat a select group of foods. Children who can only accept extremely limited ranges of food may develop nutritional deficiencies over time with serious health consequences, such as scurvy (secondary to vitamin C deficiency) and eye disorders (secondary to vitamin A deficiency).

Infants, toddlers and children with feeding aversion may have other medical complexities which impact their feeding and they may have a concurrent oro-pharyngeal dysphagia. Feeding aversion is more common for children with medical issues which impact enjoyment and associations with eating and drinking. Medical interventions and the associated trauma for children and their families may contribute to the experience of heightened stress and anxiety around food which is managed through extreme avoidance. Maladaptive strategies are understandable if eating and/or drinking is challenging, uncomfortable, painful or frightening. For some children, the feeding aversion remains long after the initial medical issue has been managed.

Neurodivergent children are also more likely to find eating and mealtimes more challenging; this may be due to unseen cognitive and sensory differences, communication difficulties, and altered interoception and exteroception. Feeding challenges may be one of the first signs of neurodiversity, long before a diagnosis is considered. In older children, neurodivergent burnout and mental health crises can lead to restricted diets, impacting nutritional status and weight gain. Neurodivergent burnout can involve losing skills or abilities that were previously accessible, and this can include struggling to eat the range or volume of food that was previously eaten. Similarly, mental health crises can also impact appetite and sensory tolerances which can present as restricted diet.

Important points about SLT practice in eating, drinking and swallowing
Parental and child involvement: person-centred care

SLTs are important members of the multiprofessional team. They should advocate and support family-centred and infant- or child-centred care across the different care settings. It is important to support the quality of life of a child and family within a functional approach. See Figure 18.1 for an annotated eating, drinking and swallowing difficulties adaptation of the 'F' words, based on the WHO International Classification of Function.

In a neonatal context, this will entail *family-integrated* care, which is equally applicable across paediatric settings. There must always be an awareness of the context of the family.

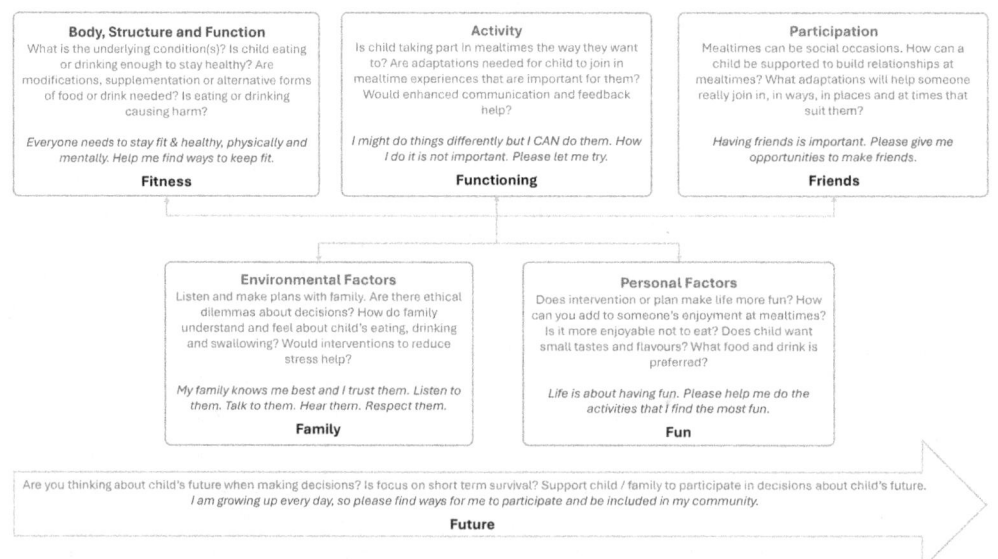

Figure 18.1 The ICF Framework and the F-words
Source: Rosenbaum and Gorter (2012), adapted from F-Words Knowledge Hub (www.canchild.ca/f-words) for person-centred care across the life course for those with eating, drinking and swallowing difficulties.

For example, there may be: long-term psychosocial harm arising from the separation of infants or children from their parents in Neonatal or Paediatric Intensive Care Units; or inadvertent tensions and disagreements created by ignoring family culture and practice, including food preferences.

The context of care

SLTs work across a range of settings with infants and children with feeding, eating, drinking and swallowing difficulties. This may range from child development centres, community clinics, health centres and school settings to hospital and rehabilitation settings and specialist children's hospitals. There are significant differences across the UK in how services for children with eating, drinking and swallowing difficulties are commissioned.

Acute hospital settings

SLTs support assessment and treatment of feeding, eating, drinking and swallowing difficulties ranging from birth in neonatal intensive care units (NICU), special care baby units (SCBU), to paediatric wards, paediatric high dependency units, paediatric intensive care units (PICU) and specialist outpatient clinics. Patient prioritisation will differ in the acute context, where establishing medical stability and supporting life-saving interventions are the priority. The SLT's role is to consider and support a safe route of nutrition/hydration to promote medical stability; in settings such as NICU and PICU, supporting a safe airway and respiratory support is prioritised appropriately over oral feeding, eating and drinking. A structured approach is required to ensure that the most urgent and complex cases receive timely intervention.

There are some key considerations for SLTs working in neonatal and paediatric acute settings:

- Assess the urgency and the severity: prioritise cases based on the medical stability of the infant or child. Those with severe feeding difficulties, high aspiration risk, no safe method or route of receiving nutrition/hydration or failure to thrive should be prioritised.
- Consider the level of complexity: cases with multifactorial problems such as neurological conditions, structural anomalies, and/or airway concerns may need immediate assessment and intervention.
- Use an evidence-based 'screening method' for ongoing caseload management: identify the severity of the feeding and swallowing difficulties. Categorize cases based on urgency and need for intervention. Re-evaluate cases to adjust priorities as medical condition and stability may change rapidly.
- Collaborate with the multidisciplinary team: work closely with paediatricians, nurses, dietitians, neonatologists, and allied health professionals to gather comprehensive information about the needs and medical history of each case.
- Develop clear referral protocols to ensure that cases needing speech and language therapy input are promptly identified and prioritised.

- Consider the concerns, preferences and culture of families. Families may provide insights into the urgency of feeding issues based on their direct experiences.
- Prioritise cases where families need immediate support and education to manage feeding/swallowing challenges.
- Work within resource constraints, such as available therapy time, equipment and staffing. Balance caseload priorities to ensure effective and safe service delivery.

Significant and distressing information may be shared with families for the first time in an acute setting, such as a diagnosis of paediatric feeding disorders or oro-pharyngeal dysphagia. The SLT may recommend the initiation of alternative routes of feeding, or support weaning from various types of feeding tubes.

SLTs work with pre-term infants to teenagers in hospital settings, and require a wide range of skills and knowledge to support diverse populations where ongoing growth, maturation and anatomical and physiological changes may rapidly occur. They may see more infants and children with medical complexity than colleagues in community settings; however, their involvement is likely to be of a shorter duration as infants and children will be discharged from hospital as soon as possible.

Community settings

SLTs may provide care for children with eating, drinking and swallowing difficulties from birth until adulthood. While children living in the community are medically stable, the need for interventions to support life may be ongoing. The focus of care will need to include all aspects of a child's life, represented in Figure 18.1. This may involve working closely with the family and others involved in caring for the child in pre-school and education services. Speech and language services are often arranged around education transition points such as entry to early years and school services, mainstream or specialist education settings.

In community settings, children with eating, drinking and swallowing difficulties are typically prioritised for assessment over children with communication needs alone. This is because of the associated risks to health outlined in previous sections. The central importance of working with the family is recognised, with a 'team around the child/family' approach, while co-working with a frequently large multidisciplinary team. SLTs in the community may liaise or work closely with colleagues in acute and tertiary services, as well as colleagues in mainstream and specialist health, education and social care services.

Following assessment and intervention provision, different services take various approaches to ongoing treatment and management, depending upon the complexity and ongoing needs of the child. In some services, children remain on the caseload until discharge to another service: during this time children's needs are regularly reviewed, targeted treatment is provided and liaison with relevant others is undertaken. An alternative service model is to discharge children after assessment and intervention provision with the request for re-referral when there is a change in the children's eating, drinking and swallowing needs. Changes may occur in health status, supportive seating requirements, or anatomical changes associated with growth throughout childhood that will be most marked during puberty.

Service provision in the UK for children with Paediatric Feeding Disorder is currently evolving, with some specialist services in hospital and community settings.

Understanding children's needs in eating, drinking and swallowing

The following section includes an outline of assessment tools, measures and processes used to diagnose eating, drinking and swallowing difficulties in infants and children.

Multidisciplinary team involvement

Speech and Language Therapy assessment and management of children's needs will be undertaken alongside other members of the multidisciplinary team. Team make-up will vary depending upon the setting, the child's need and the service factors:

- Medical assessment may include exploration of medical causes for the eating, drinking and swallowing difficulties, including underlying undiagnosed respiratory, cardiac, neurological and gastrointestinal conditions, and iatrogenic causes such as polypharmacy.
- Dietetic assessment will include exploration of nutritional adequacy of all nutrients (not just caloric intake) and adequate hydration across time, with the importance of constipation management essential. Measures of growth will also be considered over time.
- Psychologists may sometimes be available to explore the psychosocial factors that may have caused or appeared in response to children's difficulties.
- Occupational therapists may be involved to consider factors such as postural management, supportive seating, sensory issues or self-feeding.
- Physiotherapists may be involved to support understanding of a child's eating, drinking and swallowing difficulties in the context of the child's whole body, including their need for postural management, and potential sources of pain.

Multidisciplinary assessment of a 'typical mealtime' may not be helpful or possible because of the impact of being observed on the parent/carer and child and how this changes a 'typical mealtime'. It may be beneficial to supplement any observational assessment with other opportunities in different situations/times or consider other methods, for example, synchronous telehealth appointment or asynchronous observation of family mealtime videos. Services may also offer a multidisciplinary appointment with different professions meeting together with parent/carer and child to complete case history-taking, assessment and recommendations.

Clinical assessment

There are three key aspects to a clinical assessment of someone's eating, drinking and swallowing difficulties: case history, information gathering and direct assessment. Information can be gathered from the medical and clinical notes, and other involved professionals. This information can be clarified and expanded during case history-taking with a parent or carer. It is important to consider medical, nutritional, oro-sensori-motor and feeding skills, and psychosocial aspects alongside the child's developmental skills, including communication.

Parent/carers should be asked their key priorities and expectations of the assessment and intervention. Parents can be asked about signs of difficulties with the child's eating, drinking and swallowing during a mealtime, and associated consequences such as: prolonged or stressful mealtimes, chest infections, faltering growth, and impact of difficulties on activities at home and in the community.

The Royal College of Speech and Language Therapists (RCSLT) and ASHA have produced case history forms for professional use in assessing paediatric eating, drinking and swallowing difficulties, see the Recommended resources. There are other available measures including parent-reported assessments, for example, the Pediatric Eating Assessment Tool (PediEAT) (Thoyre et al., 2018) or the Feeding Impact Scales, both of which are available from https://feedingflockteam.org/ listed in Recommended resources.

An infant or child's readiness or willingness to participate in a direct assessment of their eating and drinking skills will depend on many factors, including their age, health, communication skills, physical, cognitive and emotional development. An assessment of cranial nerves and oral sensori-motor structures will require creativity and careful observation of oral movements and behaviours. Mealtime observations may be possible for children who are currently eating or drinking; information about mouth movements and sensitivities at other times such as brushing teeth can also be helpful.

It may be necessary to ask the parent/carer to bring familiar food, drink and utensils to the appointment which is at a time when the child may be ready to eat. Appropriately timed home visits may be the best setting for an assessment.

A clinical eating, drinking and swallowing evaluation needs to look at various different aspects, including:

- oral sensori-motor skills and function;
- mealtime interaction and behaviours of parent/carer and child;
- the range of signs and symptoms that could indicate difficulties with oral-sensorimotor skills, including swallowing ability, and potential signs of aspiration.

When assessing feeding skills, it is important to note the wider aspects of the mealtime, for example, the positions of the parent/carer and child, the food and drink offered, the equipment used, the environment, the timing and the pace. Each phase of eating, drinking and swallowing needs to be considered from oral-preparatory to oesophageal, with skills and abilities noted, for example, can the child take food from the spoon using the jaw and/or lip closure?; are rotatory chewing patterns observed?; is there lateral transfer of food from the centre of the mouth using the tongue?; is food, fluid or saliva lost? Note other mealtime behaviours, such as pacing, food or fluid refusal, selective eating and parent/carer responses to rejected food or fluid.

Overt aspiration events will be observable with strong coughing and voice changes. Silent aspiration events with weak or absent cough may be accompanied by subtle signs and symptoms, such as multiple swallows, change in respiratory rate, additional respiratory effort, wet breathing or voice sounds, throat clearing, stridor, wheezing, rattling chest, a snuffling nose, eyes filling with tears, skin tone colour change, gagging or vomiting (Benfer et al., 2015). The presence of aspiration can only be directly observed using instrumental means.

It is possible to enhance mealtime observations by listening to sounds of breathing and swallowing using a stethoscope placed on the child's neck, that is cervical auscultation (Frakking et al., 2016). The focus of listening is to ascertain whether wet breathing is heard before or after the swallow, as well as the quality of the swallow sounds. This approach can add an additional piece of information to an observational evaluation when used by ear-trained clinicians.

There are few validated measures of eating, drinking and swallowing. The Dysphagia Disorders Survey (Sheppard, Hochman and Baer, 2014) is widely used in North America, Australia and the Netherlands; the completion of an online registered course is necessary to develop the skills required to use the tool.

Instrumental measures and assessment

Clinical assessment of feeding and swallowing in the neonatal and paediatric population provides only partial information about risks to the airway from eating, drinking and swallowing. Instrumental assessment is used to visualise the swallow anatomy and function and to diagnose oro-pharyngeal dysphagia. Different instrumental assessments allow visualisation of different stages of the swallow and provide different types of images to the clinician and family.

Videofluoroscopic swallow study (VFSS)

VFSS is a diagnostic procedure that evaluates the swallowing function using real-time X-ray imaging. When performing the VFSS, the oral preparatory, oral, pharyngeal and oesophageal stages of swallowing are visualised. During the study, the infant or child is required to swallow various fluid and/or food consistencies mixed with a radiopaque contrast agent. Fluid and food consistencies should be identified according to its International Dysphagia Diet Standardisation Initiative (IDDSI) label to allow accurate shared understanding. VFSS enables the clinician to identify swallowing difficulties and risk of airway invasion (penetration/aspiration) and other related disorders, guiding treatment and management strategies.

The SLT performs the procedure alongside a radiographer and/or radiologist. The team of clinicians ensure the ALARA principles (i.e. 'as low as reasonably achievable') are followed during the study to limit radiation exposure but still obtain adequate information to develop appropriate interventions. Results of the study are typically shared with the referring medical professional and SLT as well as relevant members of the infant or child's wider multidisciplinary team.

Flexible endoscopic evaluation of swallowing (FEES)

FEES can also be used to assess the swallow function and anatomy. It involves the use of a flexible endoscope inserted through the nose to visualise the pharynx and larynx during swallowing. FEES allows clinicians to identify anatomical abnormalities, assess the safety and efficiency of the swallow and secretion management, and evaluate for airway invasion (penetration/aspiration) and other swallowing difficulties. FEES is particularly useful since it provides a real-time colour video of the swallowing process, enabling detailed observation of how saliva, fluid and food consistencies pass through the pharynx. The evaluation helps to guide treatment planning, including diet modification, therapy or surgical interventions that may be needed. It is often preferred for its lack of radiation exposure and it can be performed at the bedside on a neonatal unit, in paediatric intensive care, or in outpatient clinics or community settings. However, passing the scope through the nasal cavity is considered invasive and may not be tolerated by all infants and children. In comparison to VFSS, FEES does not allow visualisation of the oral stage and focuses on the pharyngeal stage with a period of whiteout observed during the actual moment of swallow onset. In the UK, the scope is typically passed by an ENT/medical doctor while the SLT reviews the images and guides the feeding, eating and drinking occurring during the study. In other countries, such as the USA and Australia, neonatal and paediatric SLTs are trained to perform scoping.

There are distinct risks and benefits associated with FEES and VFSS for neonatal and paediatric populations. The risks and benefits of any instrumental procedure should be discussed with parents/carers to obtain informed consent.

Benefits of FEES

- Direct real-time visualisation of the pharynx and the larynx during swallowing, providing detailed information on mucosal health and airway protection.
- No radiation exposure, making it safer for repeated assessments.
- Flexibility in positioning which may be beneficial for specific positioning needs.
- Useful to evaluate secretion management and airway protection, as no requirement for food or fluid with added radiopaque contrast.
- Assessment of swallow function during breastfeeding in real-time, supporting intervention plans, such as continuation of breastfeeding.

Risks of FEES

- An invasive procedure, as the endoscope is passed through the nasal passage; it may cause discomfort or distress.
- Limited view of the oral stage.
- Skilled clinician with appropriate competencies required for accurate interpretation and safe performance of FEES.

Benefits of VFSS

- Complete view of the oral, pharyngeal and oesophageal stages.
- Objective measurement of the swallow performance using quantifiable data such as timing, co-ordination and residue post-swallow to aid diagnosis and treatment.

Risks of VFSS

- Exposure to ionising radiation brings increased cancer risks to humans, especially when infants and children require multiple VFSS studies.
- Procedure and setting of VFSS can be stressful for families, infants and young children;

the fluoroscopy suite may be experienced as intimidating.
- VFSS can only be performed in medical settings with radiology departments or access to fluoroscopy suites.
- It cannot be used to assess swallow function and risk of airway invasion during breast-feeding; VFSS requires bottle feeding in neonates and infants.

The choice of instrumental assessment depends on the clinical context and the specific needs of the infant, child and the family. Risks and benefits should be discussed for each case, considering the medical history, the urgency of the evaluation and parental preferences.

Emerging instrumental assessment modalities

Pharyngeal manometry

- Specialised technique used to measure pressure and function in the pharyngeal region during swallowing.
- An invasive procedure, passing a catheter through the nasal passages to place in the pharynx.
- Growing use in infants and children to assess impact of pressure changes on swallow function. Objective data on the pressures generated during swallowing can aid identification of dysphagia and functional abnormalities.
- Evaluates timing and co-ordination of muscle contractions in pharynx, providing insights into the mechanics of swallowing for intervention and management. Useful diagnostic tool for tracheo-oesophageal fistula oesophageal atresia (TOF-OA), pharyngeal paralysis, muscular dystrophies, or other neuromuscular disorders affecting swallowing.
- Manometry is not widely available in clinical settings and may not be used routinely for assessment of swallow function.
- As research advances, pharyngeal manometry may become a more standard tool in paediatric dysphagia assessment.

Ultrasound

- An ultrasound scan, or sonogram, uses high-frequency sound waves to create a dynamic image of part of the inside of the body.
- A promising approach for assessing sucking, swallowing and laryngeal function in infants and children as it is less intrusive and invasive.
- Provides real-time imaging of tongue movement and the mechanics of sucking and swallowing and vocal fold movement for all, including breast- and bottle-fed infants.
- Current limitations are: the quality of the images depends upon the operator, limited visualisation of deep anatomical structures. and the lack of standardised assessment protocols.
- Ongoing research and development of standardised protocols may enhance its application and effectiveness in clinical practice across professional groups in a wide range of clinical settings.

Following clinical assessment, a classification of a child's eating and drinking ability will provide an agreed description of function that is meaningful for other professionals who may meet with the child and family in future. These systems are useful across different clinical and research contexts to ensure shared understanding of someone's eating, drinking and swallowing function. Suitable scales include the Eating and Drinking Ability Classification Scale (Sellers et al., 2014) and the Children's Eating and Drinking Activity Scale (Hanks et al., 2023).

Clinical assessment of neonates and infants

Early diagnosis of feeding and swallowing difficulties in neonates and infants is important to support appropriate feeding skill development and to prevent and minimise associated medical and developmental complications. The SLT observes and describes the nature of the feeding or swallowing difficulty and then proceeds to make the appropriate intervention to support health, nutrition, bonding and appropriate development. Feeding and swallowing difficulties in the neonatal period and during infancy are multi-dimensional, due to the complexity and variety of physiological systems involved in feeding and swallowing, and therefore require a multi-factorial approach to clinical assessment and treatment.

Most neonates or infants with feeding difficulties have at least one medical diagnosis as a contributing factor, and 50% of infants and children with dysphagia have multiple causative factors contributing to dysphagia. Pre-term infants experience other difficulties in addition to delayed oral feeding maturation. The prevalence of oro-pharyngeal dysphagia in pre-term and low birth weight infants is reported to be 25–35% (Zehetgruber et al., 2014).

A multidisciplinary team approach to assessment is required to comprehensively investigate dysphagia, and related diagnoses and pathophysiology. Physiological problems in neonates may result from the immaturity of the neonate's body systems; illness and/or dysphagia may limit the attainment of safe oral feeding. Observable signs and reported symptoms of feeding and swallowing difficulties may be different and even non-specific in neonates. Synactive Theory is a core theoretical underpinning for clinical assessment of neonatal and infant feeding; the five major subsystems of infant development are considered, to identify the infant's strengths, challenges and developmental accomplishments (Als, 1982). More recently, Thoyre and colleagues have developed the multidimensional view of feeding and swallowing difficulties, encouraging clinicians to use an asset-based focus to assess core components of physiological stability, oral-motor skills and suck-swallow-breathing coordination (Thoyre, Shaker and Pridham, 2005). Other models take a biopsychosocial perspective, highlighting the transactional relational nature of feeding, biomedical factors, interpersonal factors and behavioural and psychodynamic factors present within the feeding dyad (Berlin et al., 2009).

The core component of neonatal and infant feeding assessments is a comprehensive history of the prenatal, birth and subsequent time period from a parent/carer interview, the medical records, and discussions with members of the multi-professional team. It is important to understand the parental views of their role in feeding their infant and their choices of feeding method, the medical drivers of routes of feeding, and the observed feeding challenges. With clear targeted questions it may be possible to reveal subtle feeding and swallowing-related information.

The clinical assessment consists of observation of a full feed at an infant's feed time or when the parent/carer indicates that the infant is presenting with hunger cues, if they are demand-feeding. The SLT should support the parent/carer to prepare for the feed in as comfortable a position as possible. In a neonatal unit or hospital ward this may involve requesting the staff to sterilise bottle feeding equipment and provide the milk feed the parent is planning to use. If the mother is breastfeeding, a breastfeeding chair or comfortable seating with pillows to support comfort can be provided. The infant's pre-feeding state and physiological stability should be observed and then tracked during and for a few minutes after feeding. A comprehensive clinical assessment consists of observation and/or elicitation of:

- physiological parameters: heart rate, breathing rate, spo2
- state of the infant
- hunger cues
- oral-motor reflexes
- oral structure and function, including cranial nerve assessment
- observation of breastfeeding/bottle feeding: observe facial colour before/during/after feeding, especially the oral area, positioning, latch, seal, suck bursts, suck to swallow ratio, suck-swallow-breathe co-ordination, observable signs of possible aspiration (cervical auscultation can be used during quiet breathing and then during feeding to listen to breathing changes/swallowing sounds), feeding endurance
- for breastfeeding, explore how/if the parent experiences a let-down, nipple pain, swapping sides, and how the parent would describe the attachment to the breast
- stress cues during feeding
- parent-infant interaction

The first three of these useful validated tools are freely accessible on the Feeding Flock website – see Recommended resources:

- Early Feeding Assessment (Thoyre, Shaker and Pridham, 2005)
- Neonatal Eating Assessment Tool for breast, bottle or mixed feeding (Pados, Thoyre and Galer, 2019)
- Pediatric Eating Assessment Tool for breast, bottle or mixed feeding (Thoyre et al., 2018)
- Neonatal Feeding Assessment Scale (Viviers, Kritzinger and Graham, 2019).

Clinical assessment of children with restricted diets and/or food aversion

As with all clinical assessments, it is essential to take a thorough case history. The focus is to consider potential medical issues that may impact ease and enjoyment of early feeding; red flags include prematurity as well as disrupted neurological, respiratory, cardiac or gastrointestinal systems, food allergies or surgical interventions. Interruptions to the typical stages of feeding development may have an impact, including disruption to the feeding journey during sensitive periods for acceptance of taste and texture. The case history may reveal issues with the child tolerating transitions from milk feeding to complementary food and difficulties tolerating certain types of complementary foods, such as lumpy or textured food. It is important to establish the age at which feeding became more challenging for the child and the family. This may be around the neophobic stage when there is a natural increase in the child's independence and autonomy concerning food choices; it may be part of a wider developmental regression; or follow from a traumatic event such as a vomiting bug or choking event.

Broad sensory questions can provide initial information about any wider sensory sensitivities and a short dysphagia screen is important to rule out oro-pharyngeal dysphagia driving the restricted diet or food aversion. Information about the child's recognition of their appetite from infancy to present day is also important.

Gather information about the child's current intake, including: range of food accepted; volume of food and drink consumed; and how long the diet been restricted. Food diaries are useful when working with dieticians, including information about any multivitamins or supplements that are accepted. For all children with eating, drinking and swallowing difficulties, measures of height and weight are useful. However, for all clinical populations, this information is most meaningful when considered in the context of other height and weight measures plotted on growth charts over the life span. Children with restricted diets and/or oro-pharyngeal dysphagia can drift down through the centiles over time. It is important to gather information about the psychosocial impact of the restricted diet on the child and for the family.

Useful validated assessment tools include:

- Behavioral Pediatrics Feeding Assessment Scale (BPFAS): 35-item questionnaire assessing eating and mealtime behaviours, and skill-based feeding issues (Allen et al., 2015);
- Nine Item ARFID Screen (NIAS): screening tool using three main ARFID domains of selective eating/sensory avoidance, poor appetite/limited interest in eating and fear of negative consequences (Zickgraf et al., 2023);
- About Your Child's Eating scale (AYCE): set of parent-reported scales using three dimensions: Child Resistance to Eating; Positive Mealtime Environment; Parent/Caregiver Mealtime Aversion (Davies et al., 2007);
- Pica, ARFID, and Rumination Disorder Interview (PARDI): a comprehensive semi-structured clinical interview (Bryant-Waugh et al., 2019).

Supporting children's needs in eating, drinking and swallowing

Children's eating, drinking and swallowing needs will be supported in different ways, depending upon diagnosis, the severity of the impact, the prognosis, the context of care and the family circumstances. A holistic evidence-based approach (Sackett et al., 1996) is beneficial, taking account of the different domains represented in Figure 18.1. In the absence of a clear research evidence base, it is important to draw upon clinical expertise, multidisciplinary shared decision-making, practice-based evidence, and clinical consensus. SLTs have an important contribution to the management of risks to health and wellbeing from aspiration or choking, poor nutrition and hydration, limited/restricted diet and limited communication or self-management skills. Working in partnership with the infant, child and family is essential.

Therapy may be aimed at providing habilitation, helping the individual to attain, keep or improve skills and functioning for eating, drinking and swallowing, such as learning to bite and chew new food textures. Rehabilitation may be required for children to support them to regain previous eating, drinking or swallowing skills, lost or limited as a result of injury, illness or acquiring a disability. Some interventions will introduce or restore function to the individual while others will compensate for limited function, making aspects easier to manage. Other strategies will introduce and maintain adaptations to the environment to support better function.

The SLT may be well placed to work closely with the child to support their understanding of their eating, drinking and swallowing needs. These conversations will need to happen at different points over time as the child's communication and cognitive skills change. A child's priorities may change over time with improved understanding and may be different from their parents' or carers' ones. An assessment of mental capacity may be necessary to support a young person's decision to eat and drink at acknowledged risk.

The following strategies may support the infant and child to stay fit, remain actively engaged in mealtimes, participate in social occasions, be part of the family and find enjoyment and fun around mealtimes over the life course.

Frequently used intervention strategies

Balance safety, nutritional and hydrational needs, mealtime duration and enjoyment – all are important. Aims include habilitation, rehabilitation, compensation and adaptive strategies. Here are some frequently used intervention strategies (see also the FEEDS toolkit in Recommended resources) (Taylor et al., 2022):

- Modify the environment by changing the mealtime physical or social setting to suit the child.
- Provide supportive and/or appropriate seating or positioning at mealtimes, for example, the child sitting upright with head support.
- Limit food and fluid intake to avoid harm, with reliance on alternative means of nutrition and hydration such as gastrostomy or supplementation. Consider tastes or flavours of food for enjoyment and participation.
- Modify food and fluid consistency to reduce aspiration or choking risks or meet sensory and emotional needs of the child (see IDDSI levels in Recommended resources).
- Modify other aspects of food, such as taste, temperature, amount or presentation on plate.
- Modify placement of food or fluid in mouth to help with chewing or swallowing.
- Introduce new and/or more challenging food and fluid textures in carefully controlled ways to support the infant or child to learn new skills.
- Modify equipment used at mealtimes to support increasing mealtime independence and/or participation.
- Provide graded exposure to new foods, textures and fluid challenges, meeting the infant's or child's sensori-motor skills with appropriate 'just right' challenges.

- Enhance communication at mealtimes with agreed communication strategies for the child to indicate readiness to feed/eat or drink, food and fluid choices, such as 'more', 'enough', 'not ready', 'finished', etc.
- Respond to the infant's or child's cues and help others to recognise readiness to feed or eat through noticing breathing patterns, repeated swallowing, etc.
- Reduce mealtime demands on the infant or child with enhanced communication and feedback strategies, making adjustments to timing, pacing and expectations about food and fluid volumes.
- Create a sensory and emotional environment that is supportive of calm, engaged feeding, eating and drinking. This may include sensori-motor routines to address the child's or infant's altered sensory needs and adverse reactions.
- Provide physical support to the child to improve oral movements needed to bite, chew and swallow.
- Practise oral movements with non-food items to increase awareness and oral control at mealtimes.
- Use visual supports such as Social Stories to support the child's understanding of what happens during a mealtime.
- Timing of feeds or meals may need to be changed to maximise participation. Consider the impact of child factors, such as emotional regulation and modulation, tiredness, epilepsy, physical, cognitive and communication skills and adjust accordingly.
- Change behaviour at mealtimes, such as encouraging the child to stay seated for a meal.
- Model the desired behaviours by giving the child the opportunity to learn from other children or adults at mealtimes.
- Support independence and skills in self-feeding, including hand under hand support.

It is important to share strategies designed to support children's eating, drinking and swallowing with others. Changes to mealtimes will need to be agreed with parents/carers and children. Key messages need to be communicated clearly and consistently to all. SLTs may use a consistent format of mealtime guidance or a mealtime mat to do this, covering such things as: food and fluid textures, positioning, equipment, pacing, child's preferences, techniques, communication methods, risks and signs of aspiration or choking (Morgan et al., 2018).

Interventions with other members of the multidisciplinary team

SLTs may work with other members of the multidisciplinary team to support shared care and decision-making. A child may require interventions by others to support eating, drinking and swallowing. This may include medical interventions to manage disruptions to the different body systems and stabilise an individual's health. Surgical interventions may be necessary to repair or compensate for anatomical or structural differences, such as cleft lip and palate, cranio-facial conditions, tumours, heart conditions, tracheo-oesophageal fistula trachea oesophageal atresia (TOF-OA), or orthopaedic deformities with functional impact. Some individuals with neurological conditions may undergo surgical procedures to treat dystonia, such as deep brain stimulation, or high muscle tone using selective dorsal rhizotomy which impact the eating, drinking and swallowing function. The provision of alternative means of receiving nutrition and/or hydration or medication such as gastrostomy feeding will require the input of surgical, medical and allied health professional colleagues.

Treatment of an infant's or child's underlying issues with reflux, constipation, food allergies and intolerances may support improved participation in eating and drinking. Here are other interventions that may improve safety, participation and enjoyment at mealtimes:

- Work with others to eliminate sources of pain which may be linked to postural management, musculo-skeletal issues, gastro-intestinal system, neurological impairments, oral or personal hygiene.
- Change teeth cleaning routines to improve child's participation in essential oral care; reduced aspiration risk during teeth cleaning and better oral care will both contribute to reducing the consequences of aspiration.
- Address issues of anterior and posterior saliva loss which may reduce aspiration risks and increase mealtime safety, enjoyment and efficiency.
- Consider ongoing respiratory illness which may not always be linked to mealtimes; day or night-time positioning and/or tube feeding may increase risk of aspiration of stomach contents or saliva.
- Work with others to optimise medications to provide the child with a suitable basis for eating, drinking and swallowing. For example, a child with cerebral palsy may experience high and variable muscle tone throughout the body which interferes with trunk and head control; medication adjustments may facilitate greater ease of function at mealtimes.

In all cases, it is good practice to understand an individual's needs and preferences, providing neuro-affirming care.

In cases where children have a restricted diet or food aversion, the SLT should work with others to optimise nutritional and hydrational intake from the earliest emergence. Adults around the child need support to understand the drivers for the child's restricted diet; they may need to adjust their interaction style and the environment around food and mealtimes to create a positive eating experience for the child or young person.

Ethical decisions and dilemmas

Eating, drinking and swallowing are essential to maintain human life. Eating, drinking and swallowing can be extremely important in forming, maintaining and defining human relationships. Disruptions to an infant's or child's eating, drinking and swallowing can be profoundly challenging for families, including parents, siblings and the wider family. Recommendations that an infant or child be switched to non-oral feeding may be distressing and meet with much resistance or disbelief. The SLT may be a member of the multidisciplinary team that recommends non-oral or restricted oral feeding to the family. They may be involved in developing strategies with families to maximise activity and participation while maintaining a child's enjoyment and safety around meals. The ethical concerns and dilemmas associated with eating, drinking and swallowing difficulties are set out in a multidisciplinary position paper produced by the Royal College of Physicians in the Recommended resources.

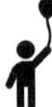

Freddie's story

Freddie was born 10 weeks prematurely, needing respiratory support and a feeding tube during his time on the neonatal unit. SLTs working on the neonatal unit supported his parents and staff to read Freddie's cues and signs that he was ready and medically stable enough to start oral feeding. When it was the right time for Freddie to start trying to feed by mouth, SLTs and lactation consultants supported Mum to breastfeed Freddie, alongside his feeding tube to make sure that it was as baby-led, safe and as enjoyable as possible for Freddie. Freddie was discharged home with his feeding tube still in place because he would get tired when breastfeeding and needed the tube to top up his nutritional intake.

SLTs in the community supported his parents at home, making sure that they were able to problem-solve and supported in Freddie's feeding journey, which included graduating from needing the feeding tube to introducing some complementary foods when it was time to wean at 6 months corrected age. Freddie was later than expected at meeting general developmental milestones and Freddie found managing textured foods and fast-flowing drinks challenging. The family received assessment and advice from SLTs to reduce the risk of possible choking and aspiration and to support his feeding skills development. Over the years, it became clear that Freddie had specific likes and dislikes when it came to his food and drink. He liked his meals to be presented the same way every time, including only eating certain brands of foods. If one of his preferred foods was not quite right, he would rather go hungry than eat it. His diet became limited to a small group of preferred foods. By the time he entered primary school, he was receiving support for his overall learning and development, and he was referred for assessment for autism.

Summary

Childhood eating, drinking and swallowing difficulties can arise from a variety of biopsychosocial factors, with wide-ranging consequences across the life-course. This chapter has outlined the different stages of eating and drinking including associated risks. The different presentations across childhood have been considered: the early difficulties and the challenges in infancy may persist in childhood with food aversion or selective eating; damage to the developing infant brain may result in emerging eating and drinking difficulties with increasing demands as the child matures.

Holistic child- and family-centred care involves comprehensive clinical assessment by SLTs working as members of different multi-professional teams. Assessment may include instrumental measures of function as well as investigations of someone's nutritional and hydrational intake, growth, cognitive skills, and sensory preferences.

SLTs working in the field of paediatric eating, drinking and swallowing difficulties require a thorough understanding of developing body systems, and the interplay between each to support this area of functioning. Eating, drinking and swallowing difficulties will have an impact upon someone's fitness, functioning, family, relationships, quality of life and future, including participation in their community. SLTs can develop the necessary skills to provide assessment, therapeutic understanding, sensitive management and life-enhancing care to infants, toddlers, children and young people with eating, drinking and swallowing difficulties, and their families.

Recommended resources

Key information about eating, drinking and swallowing difficulties

- A comprehensive professional reference on the topic of paediatric feeding, eating, drinking and swallowing disorders with contributions from all members of the multi-professional team: 'Pediatric Dysphagia: Etiologies, Diagnosis and Management' (Willging, Miller and Cohen, 2020),
- Online article including written descriptions and video material: 'Swallowing and feeding in infants and young children' (Arvedson, 2006): https://www.nature.com/gimo/contents/pt1/full/gimo17.html
- American Speech-Language-Hearing Association portal: Pediatric feeding and swallowing: https://www.asha.org/practice-portal/clinical-topics/pediatric-feeding-and-swallowing/#collapse_5
- Pediatric Feeding Disorder: Consensus Definition and Conceptual Framework. (Goday et al., 2019): https://pmc.ncbi.nlm.nih.gov/articles/PMC6314510/

Neonates

- Neurology for the Speech-Language Pathologist (Abou-Khalil and Webb, 2024)
- *Netter's Atlas of Human Embryology* (Cochard and Duenas, 2024)
- Feeding Skills in the Preterm Infant (Barlow Steven et al., 2010): https://leader.pubs.asha.org/doi/full/10.1044/leader.FTR3.15072010.22

Clinical assessment

- Feeding Flock presents online resources and measures for professionals and parents, including Pedi-EAT, Feeding Impact Scales, Family Management Measure of Feeding: https://feedingflockteam.org/
- See Chapter 13 by Anna Miles, 'Pediatric clinical feeding assessment in dysphagia assessment and treatment planning: a team approach' (Leonard and Kendall, 2017): https://www.ibmmyositis.com/Leonard2019.pdf
- See Chapter 29, 'Oral motor feeding assessment', by Miller et al. in *Paediatric Dysphagia: Etiologies, Diagnosis, and Management* (Willging, Miller and Cohen, 2020).
- Toward a synactive theory of development: promise for the assessment and support of infant individuality (Als, 1982): https://nidcap.org/wp-content/uploads/2013/12/Als-1982-Toward-Synactive-Theory.pdf
- Dysphagia Disorders Survey online training course: https://sites.google.com/view/dysphagiaorg/the-dysphagia-disorder-survey
- Eating and Drinking Ability Classification System: www.edacs.org

Intervention frameworks

- Sequential-Oral-Sensory Approach to feeding (SOS) – see comprehensive web resources and training programmes: https://sosapproachtofeeding.com/
- Early Intervention Sensory, Motor, Attention and Regulation, and Relationships Together (EiSMART); https://eismart.co.uk/
- Family Integrated Care (FIC): https://familyintegratedcare.com/
- Newborn Individualized Developmental Care and Assessment Program (NiDCAP): https://nidcap.org/
- International Dysphagia Diet Standardisation Initiative (IDDSI) web resources; https://iddsi.org/
- Developing the FEEDS toolkit of parent-delivered interventions for eating, drinking and swallowing difficulties in young children with neurodisability: findings from a Delphi survey and stakeholder consultation workshops (Taylor et al., 2022): https://pmc.ncbi.nlm.nih.gov/articles/PMC9058804/

Training frameworks

- RCSLT Dysphagia Learning: https://www.rcslt.org/members/clinical-guidance/dysphagia/dysphagia-learning/, which includes: Pre-registration eating, drinking and swallowing competencies and Dysphagia Competency Framework
- See RCSLT VFSS and FEES competencies
- Modified Barium Swallow Impairment – preview of training: https://www.youtube.com/playlist?list=PL3St3Pv3sqw3-bf35yjBmR8ctJZL_wFtZ
- Core Capabilities Framework for Supporting People with a Learning Disability: https://www.skillsforhealth.org.uk/resources/learning-disability-and-autism-frameworks-2019/

Ethics and risks

- RCSLT eating and drinking with acknowledged risks guidance
- Mental Capacity Act 2005: https://www.legislation.gov.uk/ukpga/2005/9/contents
- Royal College of Physicians. Supporting people who have eating and drinking difficulties. A guide to practical care and clinical assistance, particularly towards the end of life. Report of a working party (2021): https://www.rcp.ac.uk/media/fw5pmtvw/supporting-people-who-have-eating-and-drinking-difficulties_3_0.pdf

References

Abou-Khalil, R. and Webb, W. (2024) *Neurology for the Speech-Language Pathologist*. 7th edn. Oxford: Elsevier.

Allen, S. L., Smith, I. M., Duku, E., Vaillancourt, T., Szatmari, P., Bryson, S., Fombonne, E., Volden, J., Waddell, C., Zwaigenbaum, L., Roberts, W., Mirenda, P., Bennett, T., Elsabbagh, M. and Georgiades, S. (2015) 'Behavioral pediatrics feeding assessment scale in young children with autism spectrum disorder: Psychometrics and associations with child and parent variables', *Journal of Pediatric Psychology*, 40(6), 581–590.

Als, H. (1982) 'Toward a synactive theory of development: Promise for the assessment and support of infant individuality', *Infant Mental Health Journal*, 3(4), 229–243.

APA (American Psychiatric Association) (2013) *Diagnostic and statistical manual of mental disorders*, 5th edn. https://doi.org/10.1176/appi.books.9780890425596

Arvedson, J. (2006) 'PART 1 Oral cavity, pharynx and esophagus: Swallowing and feeding in infants and young children'. GI Motility Online: https://www.nature.com/gimo/contents/pt1/full/gimo17.html: www.Nature.com.

Arvedson, J., Rogers, B., Buck, G., Smart, P. and Msall, M. (1994) 'Silent aspiration prominent in children with dysphagia', *International Journal of Pediatric Otorhinolaryngology*, 28(2-3), 173-181.

Barlow Steven, M., Poore Meredith, A., Zimmerman Emily, A. and Finan Don, S. (2010) 'Feeding skills in the preterm infant', *The ASHA Leader Archive*, 15(7), 22-23.

Benfer, K.A., Weir, K.A., Bell, K.L., Ware, R.S., Davies, P.S. and Boyd, R N. (2015) 'Clinical signs suggestive of pharyngeal dysphagia in preschool children with cerebral palsy', *Research in Developmental Disabilities*, 38, 192-201.

Benjasuwantep, B., Chaithirayanon, S. and Eiamudomkan, M. (2013) 'Feeding problems in healthy young children: prevalence, related factors and feeding practices', *Pediatric Reports*, 5(2), 38-42.

Berlin, K.S., Davies, W.H., Lobato, D.J. and Silverman, A.H. (2009) 'A biopsychosocial model of normative and problematic pediatric feeding', *Children's Health Care*, 38(4), 263-282.

Boesch, R.P., Daines, C., Willging, J.P., Kaul, A., Cohen, A.P., Wood, R.E. and Amin, R.S. (2006) 'Advances in the diagnosis and management of chronic pulmonary aspiration in children', *European Respiratory Journal*, 28(4), 847-861.

Bryant-Waugh, R., Micali, N., Cooke, L., Lawson, E.A., Eddy, K.T. and Thomas, J.J. (2019) 'Development of the Pica, ARFID, and Rumination Disorder Interview: A multi-informant, semi-structured interview of feeding disorders across the lifespan: A pilot study for ages 10-22', *International Journal of Eating Disorders*, 52(4), 378-387.

Cass, H., Wallis, C., Ryan, M., Reilly, S. and McHugh, K. (2005) 'Assessing pulmonary consequences of dysphagia in children with neurological disabilities: when to intervene?', *Developmental Medicine & Child Neurology*, 47(5), 347-352.

Chow, C.Y., Bech, A.C., Olsen, A., Keast, R., Russell, C.G. and Bredie, W.L.P. (2024) 'Influence of changing dentition on food texture preferences and perception of eating difficulty in Australian children', *Journal of Texture Studies*, 55(4), e12856.

Cochard, L. and Duenas, A. (2024) *Netter's Atlas of Human Embryology*. 2nd edn. Oxford: Elsevier.

Davies, W.H., Ackerman, L.K., Davies, C.M., Vannatta, K. and Noll, R.B. (2007) 'About your child's eating: Factor structure and psychometric properties of a feeding relationship measure', *Eating Behaviors*, 8(4), 457-463.

Frakking, T.T., Chang, A.B., O'Grady, K.F., David, M., Walker-Smith, K. and Weir, K.A. (2016) 'The use of cervical auscultation to predict oropharyngeal aspiration in children: A randomized controlled trial', *Dysphagia*, 31(6), 738-748.

Glover, G. and Ayub, M. (2010) 'How people with learning disabilities die', *Improving Health and Lives Learning Disability Observatory*. London: Department of Health.

Goday, P.S., Huh, S.Y., Silverman, A., Lukens, C.T., Dodrill, P., Cohen, S. S., Delaney, A. L., Feuling, MB., Noel, R.J., Gisel, E., Kenzer, A., Kessler, D.B., Kraus de Camargo, O., Browne, J. and Phalen, J.A (2019) 'Pediatric feeding disorder: Consensus definition and conceptual framework', *Journal of Pediatric Gastroenterology and Nutrition*, 68(1), 124-129.

Hanks, E., Stewart, A., Au-Yeung, C.K., Johnson, E. and Smith, C.H. (2023) 'Consensus on level descriptors for a functional children's eating and drinking activity scale', *Developmental Medicine & Child Neurology*, 65(9), 1199-1205.

Leonard, R. and Kendall, K. (2017) *Dysphagia Assessment and Treatment Planning: A Team Approach*, 4th edn. San Diego: Plural Publishing Inc.

Leopold, N.A. and Kagel, M.C. (1997) 'Dysphagia – ingestion or deglutition?: A proposed paradigm', *Dysphagia*, 12(4), 202-206.

Malandraki, G.A., Johnson, S. and Robbins, J. (2011) 'Functional MRI of swallowing: From neurophysiology to neuroplasticity', *Head & Neck*, 33, Suppl. 1(0 1), S14-S20.

Matsuo, K. and Palmer, J.B. (2008) 'Anatomy and physiology of feeding and swallowing: Normal and abnormal', *Physical Medicine and Rehabilitation Clinics of North America*, 19(4), 691-707.

Morgan, S., Luxon, E., Soomro, A. and Harding, C. (2018) 'Use of mealtime advice mats in special schools for children with learning disabilities', *Learning Disability Practice*, 21(2), 20-26.

Pados, B.F., Thoyre, S.M. and Galer, K. (2019) 'Neonatal Eating Assessment Tool - Mixed Breastfeeding and Bottle-Feeding (NeoEAT - Mixed Feeding): Factor analysis and psychometric properties', *Maternal Health, Neonatology and Perinatology*, 5(1), 12.

Remijn, L., Speyer, R., Groen, B.E., Holtus, P.C., van Limbeek, J. and Nijhuis-van der Sanden, M.W. (2013) 'Assessment of mastication in healthy children and children with cerebral palsy: A validity and consistency study', *Journal of Oral Rehabilitation*, 40(5), 336-347.

Rosenbaum, P. and Gorter, J.W. (2012) 'The "F-words" in childhood disability: I swear this is how we should think!', *Child: Care, Health and Development*, 38(4), 457-463.

Sackett, D.L., Rosenberg, W.M., Gray, J.A., Haynes, R.B. and Richardson, W.S. (1996) 'Evidence based medicine: What it is and what it isn't', *BMJ*, 312(7023), 71-72.

Sellers, D., Mandy, A., Pennington, L., Hankins, M. and Morris, C. (2014) 'Development and reliability of a system to classify the eating and drinking ability of people with cerebral palsy', *Developmental Medicine & Child Neurology*, 56, 245-251.

Sheppard, J.J., Hochman, R. and Baer, C. (2014) 'The Dysphagia Disorder Survey: Validation of an assessment for swallowing and feeding function in developmental disability', *Research in Developmental Disabilities*, 35, 929-942.

Shune, S.E., Moon, J.B. and Goodman, S.S. (2016) 'The effects of age and preoral sensorimotor cues on anticipatory mouth movement during swallowing', *Journal of Speech, Language, and Hearing Research*, 59(2), 195-205.

Stevenson, R.D., Conaway, M., Chumlea, W.C., Rosenbaum, P., Fung, E.B., Henderson, R.C., Worley, G., Liptak, G., O'Donnell, M., Samson-Fang, L. and Stallings, V.A. (2006) 'Growth and health in children with moderate-to-severe cerebral palsy', *Pediatrics*, 118(3), 1010-1018.

Sullivan, P.B., Juszczak, E., Lambert, B.R., Rose, M., Ford-Adams, M.E. and Johnson, A. (2002) 'Impact of feeding problems on nutritional intake and growth: Oxford Feeding Study II', *Developmental Medicine and Child Neurology*, 44(7), 462-467.

Taylor, H., Pennington, L., Morris, C., Craig, D., McConachie, H., Cadwgan, J., Sellers, D., Andrew, M., Smith, J., Garland, D., McColl, E., Buswell, C., Thomas, J., Colver, A. and Parr, J. (2022) 'Developing the FEEDS toolkit of parent-delivered interventions for eating, drinking and swallowing difficulties in young children with neurodisability: Findings from a Delphi survey and stakeholder consultation workshops', *BMJ Paediatrics Open*, 6(1).

Thoyre, S.M., Pados, B.F., Park, J., Estrem, H., McComish, C. and Hodges, E.A. (2018) 'The Pediatric Eating Assessment Tool: Factor structure and psychometric properties', *Journal of Pediatric Gastroenterology and Nutrition*, 66(2), 299-305.

Thoyre, S.M., Shaker, C.S. and Pridham, K.F. (2005) 'The early feeding skills assessment for preterm infants', *Neonatal Network*, 24(3), 7-16.

Viviers, M., Kritzinger, A. and Graham, M. (2019) 'Reliability and validity of the neonatal feeding assessment scale (NFAS) for the early identification of dysphagia in moderate to late preterm neonates', *African Health Sciences*, 19(3), 2718-2727.

Weir, K., McMahon, S., Barry, L., Masters, I. B. and Chang, A.B. (2009) 'Clinical signs and symptoms of oropharyngeal aspiration and dysphagia in children', *European Respiratory Journal*, 33(3), 604-611.

Willging, J.P., Miller, C.K. and Cohen, A.P. (2020) *Pediatric Dysphagia: Etiologies, Diagnosis, and Management*, 1st edn. San Diego: Plural Publishing Inc.

Zehetgruber, N., Boedeker, R.-H., Kurth, R., Faas, D., Zimmer, K.-P. and Heckmann, M. (2014) 'Eating problems in very low birthweight children are highest during the first year and independent risk factors include duration of invasive ventilation', *Acta Paediatrica*, 103(10), e424-e438.

Zickgraf, H.F., Garwood, S.K., Lewis, C.B., Giedinghagen, A.M., Reed, J.L. and Linsenmeyer, W.R. (2023) 'Validation of the nine-item avoidant/restrictive food intake disorder screen among transgender and nonbinary youth and young adults', *Transgender Health*, 8(2), 159-167.

Index

AAC *see* Alternative and Augmentative Communication
ableist approach *see* neuro-normative perspective
Acquired Apraxia of Speech 269
acquired brain injury (ABI) 257; dysarthria in 261, 265, 268, 269; dysphagia in 266-7, 270; dyspraxia in 261, 269; factors affecting recovery 258; impact 257; key assessments 262-5; long-term consequences 258; measuring therapy outcomes 271; principles of assessment 261, 266; principles of communication intervention 268-9; setting therapy goals 270-1; SLT role in rehabilitation pathway 259-60; unique features of SLT practice 258-9
acquired language disorders 261
Additional Support Needs *see* support needs
aided communication 55
airway protection 282, 290
alexithymia 189
Alternative and Augmentative Communication (AAC): AAC-specific assessment tools 57-8; attributes of AAC system or device 56; comprehensive assessment 56-7; definition and terminology 54-5; identity 53; intervention and management 58-9; service structures 53-4
anti-discriminatory 12, 211
anxiety 211-12
aphasia *see* acquired language disorder
Articulation and Oromotor Assessment (DEAP) *see* Diagnostic Evaluation of Articulation and Phonology (DEAP)

Articulation Disorder 90, 91-3, 95, 96, 245
Attunement 153, 159, 160
auditory brainstem implants 227-8
Avoidant Restrictive Food Intake Disorder (ARFID) 218, 280, 294; *see also* restricted diets and food aversion
AWEsome approach 14-15

babble: babble intervention in cleft palate +/- lip 246
Balanced System 20-1; Balanced System Outcomes Framework 22-3; Five Strands outcome areas 19-20
barriers to learning 153, 154, 167
BBC Tiny Happy People *see* CBeebies Parenting
bioecological *see* biopsychosocial
biofeedback in cleft palate +/- lip 248-9: electropalatography (EPG) 248-9; ultrasound visual biofeedback (U-VBF) 249
biopsychosocial 9, 187, 209, 213, 279, 292; *see also* ICF:CY framework
bone conduction listening devices 228

Capability, Opportunity and Motivation - Behaviour (COM-B) 250-2
CBeebies Parenting 131
cervical auscultation 289, 293
child development: core principles of 5-6
child: definition 5
Childhood Apraxia of Speech (CAS) 90, 96; *see also* Acquired Apraxia of Speech
Childhood Dysarthria 91, 94; *see also* oromotor assessment; *see also* Acquired Dysarthria

Children's Communication Checklist-2 141, 194, 215, 264
CIRCLE Framework 197
CIRCLE Inclusive Classroom Scale 195
cleft palate +/- lip: assessment of speech sound development 245-6; assessment of velopharyngeal function 244-5; co-occurring developmental concerns 241, 242-3; diagnosis 241-2; embryonic stages 241; intervention 246-7; language assessment 246; multi-disciplinary team and working with others 243-4; prevalence 241; phenotypes 241-2
cleft speech characteristics (CSC) 245
cochlear implants 227
Cognitive Behavioural Therapy (CBT) 180
Cognitive Communication Disorder (CCD) 261
COM-B see Capability, Opportunity and Motivation - Behaviour (COM-B)
Comic Strip Conversations 217
Communication and Cognitive Framework 154, 155, 160
Communication at the Heart of the School (CATHS) 153; assessment 157-9; communication-rich classrooms 161; components 154-7; partnership 159-161; principles 154; service delivery model 159
communication partners; communication needs and preferences of 65; empowering and upskilling 67-9; expectations of 65; goal setting with 66-7; involvement in understanding children's needs 64-5; possible challenges and how to overcome them 69-71; using Talking Mats with 70; what they can do 63; who 62-3; why they are important 63-4
communication passports 42, 49, 57, 198
communication profiling tools see communication passports
communication support tools 216-17
communication: barriers 11, 46, 214, 215; channels 36; cycle of disadvantage 40; definition 9; diversity 42; event 38; journey 38; models 10-11; situational factors 37; ways 36
communicative functions 155
congenital malformation of the larynx 103
Consistent Phonological Disorder 90-2, 95, 96
consultative model 144

core vocabulary therapy 95, 96
co-regulation 212
cultural inquisitiveness 12-13

deaf children: aetiology 226; frequency 225; levels of deafness 227; onset 226; speech and language therapy practice 228-236; terms 225; types 226
deficit see difference not deficit approach
Demands and Capacities Model 177
developmental age 154; see also severe and profound learning disabilities
developmental band 154, 155, 157
Developmental Language Disorder (DLD) 136; assessment 140-2; causes 138; co-occurring developmental concerns 138-9; definition of 136-7; diagnosis 139; differentiating conditions 138; early identification 139; intervention 139-40, 142-4; prevalence of 136; screening 139; terminology 137
difference not deficit approach 196
Diagnostic Evaluation of Articulation and Phonology (DEAP) 93, 94, 95, 96, 195, 264
dimensional approach see neurodevelopmental approach
dosage 64, 69, 95, 110, 144
Double Empathy Problem 196
Dynamic Temporal and Tactile Cueing (DTTC) 96
dysphasia see acquired language disorders
dysphonia see Voice Disorder

Ear, Nose and Throat (ENT) 102, 104, 105, 109, 228, 290
early communication intervention in cleft palate +/- lip 247
early language development: clusters of risks 121-2; early language surveillance 128-9; early preventative intervention 129; factors that influence 118-19; public health approach 124-8; trajectories 121-2
Early Language Identification Measure and Intervention (ELIM-I) 132
eating, drinking and swallowing difficulties 277-8; acute hospital settings 285-6; areas of complexity, challenge and risk 282-4; clinical assessment 287-9, 292-4; clinical

assessment of neonates 292-3; community settings 286-7; ethical decisions and dilemmas 297; frequently used intervention strategies 295-6; instrumental assessment 289-292; interventions with other members of the multi-disciplinary team 296-7; key information 278-9; multi-disciplinary team 287; person-centred care 284; stages of eating, drinking and swallowing 280-2
educators see communication partners
emotional development 208
Enhanced Milieu Teaching (EMT): Enhanced Milieu Teaching Plus Phonological Emphasis (EMT+PE) 247
EPIC approach 14, 15-16
equity 35, 42-3, 46, 119, 125, 130; see also anti-discriminatory; see also inequalities
evidence-based practice 13, 218
externalising 208-9

feeding difficulties see eating, drinking and swallowing difficulties
fidelity 30, 143, 144
Five Strands outcome areas
flexible endoscopic evaluation of swallowing (FEES) 282, 289-90, 300
Focused Stimulation 247, 249
Formulation 213
Future Plan 154, 158-9, 160, 161, 167, 168
F-Words 268, 284

Goal Attainment Scaling 270, 271

Hanen More Than Words 64, 68, 197, 201
hearing aids 227
High Dependency Unit (HDU) 259
hoarseness see Voice Disorder
human rights-based approach 7, 41, 67

iceberg analogy applied to stammering see overt and covert features of stammering
ICF-CY framework 9, 79, 104-5, 192-4, 197-8, 284
impact; how to measure 78-84
inclusive communication: definition 36-8; environments 38; for whom 38-9; implementation of good practice 42-9; importance 39-42

Inconsistent Phonological Disorder 90, 95, 96, 264
Inducible Laryngeal Obstruction (ILO) 103, 104
inequalities 12, 41-2, 120, 126, 130, 186
Informing and Profiling Augmentative and Alternative Communication (AAC) Knowledge and Skills (IPAACKS) 60
Integrated Phonological Awareness 95, 96
integrated working 19, 29
Intelligibility in Context Scale (ICS) 93
internalising 208-9
interoception 189, 284
intersectionality 186

Language for Behaviour and Emotions 218
language: definition 9
lateral progress 159
Lidcombe Program 180
life-course see lifespan approach
lifelong needs 159
lifespan approach 6, 120
low-demand, low-arousal strategies 212

masking: in neurodivergence 187
Maximum Phonation Time (MPT) 107
medical model 8, 28, 76, 159, 174, 190
medical needs 1, 104, 154, 167
mental health 208
microlaryngobronchoscopy 105
minimal pair therapy 95, 96, 69, 248
mode of communication 155
motor learning principles 110
multidimensional see ICF-CY framework
multifactorial see ICF-CY framework
Multilingual Children's Speech web resource 92, 97
multiple oppositions therapy 95, 96, 248
Multisensory Input Modelling (MSIM) 247

nasendoscopy 11, 245
neuro-affirming intervention; 10 key principles 200
neurodevelopmental approach: integrated neurodevelopmental services and pathways 191
neurodevelopmental differences 189

Neurodevelopmental Disorders: co-occurrence 188-9; definitions, diagnoses and prevalence 187-8; see also neurodivergence
neurodivergence 186-7; assessment to understand and plan to meet needs 191-5; neuro-affirming approach to communication support and intervention 195-200
Neurodiversity Movement 190
Neurodiversity Paradigm 190
neuro-normative perspective 195
neurotypical expectations see neuro-normative perspective
Newcastle Assessment of Phonological Awareness 93, 94
non-traumatic brain injury: definition 257
Nuffield Dyspraxia Programme: Assessment 94; Intervention 95, 96
Nuffield Early Language Intervention (NELI) 143
nutrition and hydration needs 283-4

oromotor assessment 93, 94
oro-pharyngeal dysphagia 278-9; see also eating, drinking and swallowing difficulties
outcomes-based framework see Balanced System Outcomes Framework
overt and covert features of stammering 169-72

paediatric feeding disorders 278-80; see also eating, drinking and swallowing difficulties
Paediatric Intensive Care Unit (PICU) 259, 271, 285, 290
Paradoxical Focal Fold Movement Disorder (PVFMD) see Inducible Laryngeal Obstruction (ILO)
Parent-Child Interaction Therapy PCI/ PCIT) 68, 179
parents see communication partners
Percentage Consonants Correct (PCC) 94, 96, 247
persistent stammering 172
personal amplification devices 227-8
Personal Communication Passports see communication passports
pharyngeal manometry 291
phonological awareness 92-6, 128
Phonological Delay 90-2, 95, 96
phonological therapy in cleft palate +/- lip 248
phonotrauma 103, 110

prevention: Mosaic of 124-6; Primary 126; Secondary (targeted selective) 126-7; Secondary (targeted indicated) 127; Tertiary 128
Profound and Multiple Learning Disabilities (PMLD) 153; see also severe and profound learning disabilities
Prolonged Disorder of Consciousness (PDOC) 259
psycholinguistic model 92, 247, 263
public health framework: components 126-8; qualities 129-131

Rapid Syllable Transition Treatment (ReST) 95, 96, 269
Recurrent Respiratory Papillomatosis (RRP) 103
remote listening devices 228
resonance disorders 94, 101, 109-10, 236, 242, 245
restricted diets and food aversion 280, 284, 293-4
rights of the child see human rights-based approach

S/Z ratio 107
SCERTS assessment process 194, 195, 196
SCERTS Observation Form 194, 195
self-advocacy 137, 143, 145, 199
self-regulation 212
SEMH see Social, Emotional and Mental Health
severe and profound learning disabilities: terminology 154; prevalence 153
Severe Learning Disabilities (SLD) 153; see also severe and profound learning disabilities
SLCN see speech, language and communication needs
social development 208
social model 8-9, 190
Social Stories 198, 217, 296
Social, Emotional and Mental Health (SEMH); evidence base for speech and language intervention 218; meaning of 208-9; needs in 209; social communication in 210, 213, 214, 218; speech and language therapy roles 215-18; speech, language and communication needs in 210; support 215; understanding needs 212-15
Special Care Baby Unit (SCBU) 285

Special Time 156, 178-9
Speech Disorder Classification System 91
speech motor delay 91-2
Speech Sound Disorder (SSD) 89; articulatory/motor interventions 95; assessment 92-4; classification 89-92; diagnostic protocol 93-4; differential diagnosis 89, 92; impairment-based intervention 92; phonological interventions 95; screening 92; specialist level 92
speech, language and communication needs (SLCN): what does it mean for a child to have 11-12
speech: definition 10
stammering 169; aetiology 172; awareness-raising 179; direct approaches 176, 180-1; environmental and indirect approaches 176-80; group therapy 181; incidence and prevalence 172; information-gathering 173-6; integrated approaches 181; terminology and context 173
stammering modification 180, 181
stammering-affirming practice 173, 176
Standards of Proficiency (Health and Care Professions Council): 1, 64, 69, 139
stimulability 93
Stoke Speaks Out 131
strengths-based approach 13, 70, 194
stuttering see stammering
Supervision 212
support needs: meaning of 6-8; see also speech, language and communication needs
Supporting and Understanding Speech Sound Disorder (SUSSD) website 96, 97

Talking Mats: to elicit child views 49, 57, 67, 194, 198, 214, 217, 219
Team Around the Child (TAC): 13, 64, 270, 286
telemedicine in cleft palate +/- lip 248
Therapy Outcome Measurement (TOMs) 80, 271
therapy partner: definition 63; role 63, 66, 69

tiered approach see Balanced System
traditional articulation therapy in cleft palate +/- lip 248, 249
transdiagnostic see neurodevelopmental approach
transient stammering 172
trauma: in SEMH context 209, 211-12
traumatic brain injury (TBI): definition 257

ultrasound 95, 96, 248-9, 291; see also biofeedback
unaided communication 54
United Nations Convention on the Rights of the Child (UNCRC): 7, 41, 67; see also human rights-based approach
Universal Neonatal Hearing Screening (UNHS) 229, 230
universal, targeted, specific and specialist see Balanced System

velopharyngeal incompetence (VPI) 242; importance of the palate for speech 242
videofluoroscopic swallow study (VFSS) 282, 289, 290-1, 300
videofluoroscopy 245
visually supported conversations see Comic Strip Conversations
Vocal Fold Nodules (VFN) 102, 103, 109, 111
Vocal Fold Paralysis 103, 105, 109
Voice Disorder: aerodynamic performance 107; assessment protocol 104-9; auditory-perceptual evaluation and acoustic analysis 106-7; classification 102-3; intervention 109-111; quality of life impact measures 106

What Well 158, 166
whole system approach: core delivery principles 27-31; how to build 21; rationale 18-19; what is involved 19-21

For Product Safety Concerns and Information please contact our EU representative GPSR@taylorandfrancis.com
Taylor & Francis Verlag GmbH, Kaufingerstraße 24, 80331 München, Germany

www.ingramcontent.com/pod-product-compliance
Lightning Source LLC
Chambersburg PA
CBHW080923300426
44115CB00018B/2926